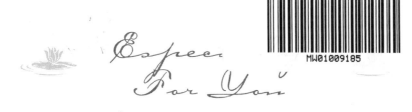

Especiali
For You

MW01009185

To: _____

From: _____

Special Message:

Copyright © 2007 Studer Group

ISBN-13: 978-0-9749986-4-0
ISBN-10: 0-9749986-4-8

Library of Congress Control Number: 2007929097

Published by:
Fire Starter Publishing
913 Gulf Breeze Parkway, Suite 6
Gulf Breeze, FL 32561

Cover and Interior Book Design and Production: Andra Keller, DeHart & Company Public Relations

Photo Research: Renee Annis, DeHart & Company Public Relations

A word about the graphics in this book. With a few exceptions, the images in *What's Right in Health Care* were selected only to add visual interest to the stories. They are *not* intended to represent the actual writers of the stories or the real people described therein.

All rights reserved. Printed in the United States. No part of this book may be used or reproduced in any form or by any means, or stored in a database or retrieval system without the prior written permission of the publisher, except in the case of brief quotations embodied in critical articles or reviews. Making copies of any part of this book for any purpose other than your own personal use is a violation of United States copyright laws. Entering any of the contents into a computer for mailing list or database purposes is strictly prohibited unless written authorization is obtained from the publisher.

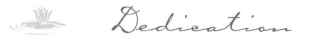

Dedication

To all those professionals who have accepted
the calling to make a difference
in the lives of patients, families,
and health care as a whole.

What's Right in Health Care

365 Stories of Purpose, Worthwhile Work, and Making a Difference

Compiled by Studer Group

Acknowledgments

To work on a book like this one is truly humbling. It makes us realize, in a profound and undeniable way, how many extraordinary minds, hearts, and hands work together to make America's health care industry the best in the world.

First and foremost, thank you to all the health care professionals from organizations across the nation who submitted the stories that appear in the following pages. Without your willingness to search your soul and share with readers the moments that most deeply touched and inspired you, this book could not exist.

Thank you to the Studer Group partners who work so hard every day to make the great health care they provide even greater. We are grateful for all we've learned from you.

And to everyone who works in the healing professions: You are making an impact in the world. You make people's lives better. You answered a calling and we are all better for it. You are what's right in health care. Thank you.

Studer Group

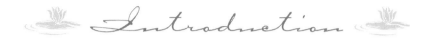

Introduction

"The task of medicine: Cure sometimes, Relieve often, Care always."

—Ambroise Paré
(1517-1590)

Since the earliest of days, people have used stories to convey a feeling, describe an experience, and reinforce learning. I know firsthand that while different people hear and absorb different parts of a talk, virtually everyone remembers the stories. That's why we believe a book filled with true, heartfelt, personal stories is one of the most powerful books that can be published.

I am an optimist about health care. Why? I am out in the trenches each week just like you. I have the great fortune to see the difference you make in the lives of others. We are surrounded by miracles, and everyone who works in the healing professions helps create them. What a responsibility we have—and what a privilege! That's what these stories convey.

In my book *Hardwiring Excellence: Purpose, Worthwhile Work, Making a Difference*, I shared many stories about you and your colleagues. The response to *Hardwiring Excellence* and the need to stay focused on the positives made a book about the difference people make in health care a natural.

The book you are holding is a collaborative effort. *What's Right in Health Care: 365 Stories of Purpose, Worthwhile Work, and Making a Difference* is about you. Leaf through it, and you may see your own stories and those of friends and colleagues. They chronicle this journey we're all on—the journey to make health care better.

This book provides a story a day to help health care professionals stay grounded. It is a daily reminder about why we answered this calling and why we stay with it—to serve a purpose, to do worthwhile work, and to make a difference.

Never underestimate the difference you can make!

Quint Studer

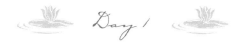

True Beauty

lternating her gaze from the clock on the wall to the mirror on her bedside stand, Mrs. Fischer found no peace in either. Her daughter would be here at 11 a.m. She promised she would be on time and take her home. The clock reminded her she was on her way. Looking back at the mirror, her eyes kept tracing the outline of the incision that now, to her, commanded center stage on a face she had looked at all her life. She had monitored the changes in this face, reflected through the years in the mirror, as the taut skin and soft cheeks of youth left her and the lines and wrinkles of her 78 years of life settled in. She accepted it with grace and dignity, affirmed by the voice of her beloved husband, who told her often, "You're beautiful." Maybe that's part of why she could not accept this brutal change. His voice and his message were silent now.

"I look horrible," she told Heather, her nursing assistant, that morning. "My grandchildren won't want to look at me." Heather continued gathering her belongings to prepare her for going home. "It will heal—you're going to be all right. Your doctor feels they got it all and that's the most important thing," she assured her. "Everyone who loves you will always find you beautiful." Those words, kind as they were, still didn't seem to help. The clock kept moving her closer to her daughter's arrival and that awful ride down the corridors, through the lobby and to the car. Staring at the mirror, she dreaded the spectacle she felt

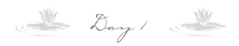

she had now become. Maybe if she had a scarf, she could wrap it around her face and no one would know. Did she bring a scarf with her? Perhaps when Heather returned from her break, she could look through her belongings.

The clock moved closer. The moment was nearing. Looking again in the mirror, as if something might miraculously change, it did.

Quietly, Heather stepped into the room. In her hands was a bag from the hospital gift shop. It rustled as she opened it, and she pulled out a wide-brimmed and lovely picture hat. "I thought you'd look nice in this," she said, and gently placed it on Mrs. Fischer, softly arranging her hair as she did. Stepping back a little, Heather said, "You're beautiful!" Those words seemed to echo a voice from a long time ago, resonating in the tears now trickling down her cheeks. "Do you want to see the mirror again?" Heather asked. "No…I believe you," replied Mrs. Fischer.

A lingering hug between youth and age marked the moment, and Mrs. Fischer left Beaumont hospital, her head held high, her dignity restored. She would forever cherish more than the gift of a hat…for that morning, she caught a glimpse of herself in the eyes of a thoughtful young girl, and it was good.

—Submitted by Rik Cryderman, Beaumont Hospital, Troy, MI

"Never underestimate the difference you can make."

2

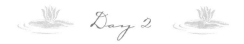

Guardian Angels

At one of my former hospitals, administrators often met with our staff about everyone's importance in delivering care to our patients. One year, after an outstanding JCAHO survey, we hosted an outdoor picnic for all of our employees to celebrate.

I sat down with a group of our housekeepers who seemed rather quiet and reserved despite the festivities around us. When I commented that the JCAHO surveyors had remarked how clean our hospital was, the housekeepers smiled and became more animated. They began to chat about the extra efforts they had made for the inspection.

I noticed one quiet housekeeper had multiple small angel pendants on the collar of her uniform. I asked about the pendants and she told me about their significance. "I call them my guardian angels," she said. "Well, they are very pretty," I said. "Oh, they're not for me," she explained. "When I clean a patient's room, I like to leave one on their bedside table when they're asleep. That way when they wake up, they see their guardian angel has come and has been watching over them. I hope it makes them feel better and know they're not alone."

Others around her laughed appreciatively. Another housekeeper spoke up about the time a patient came out of her room looking for "her guardian angel." When the patient found the housekeeper wearing the angel pendants, she rushed

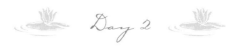

and hugged her tightly. "You'll never know how much that meant to me," the patient had said. "I was about to give up hope that I would ever recover and then I saw my little angel on the table. I just knew right then that everything was going to be all right."

The other housekeepers nodded approvingly and everyone stood to make their way back to the hospital. I didn't know what to say to them. I was just happy we had passed an inspection and wasn't prepared to be overwhelmed with such positive emotions for the people who had made it possible. I realized that these angels had left our table and would soon be back at work caring, in their own special way, for the needs of others.

—*Anonymous Contributor*

"Never underestimate the difference you can make."

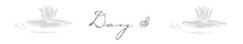

Mr. and Mrs. B

*T*he story of Mr. and Mrs. B touches my heart. These two dear patients were in their eighties and had been married for more than fifty years. Mrs. B's severe pulmonary disease required drastic measures and a very long stay in our Intensive Care Unit. Mr. B was as dedicated to his wife as he had always been and visited her each and every day. He would hold her hand as he talked to her and tried to make her feel comfortable.

As Mrs. B was being weaned off of the ventilator, Mr. B, who already had a history of cancer, was diagnosed with metastatic disease. He would require Hospice care and could no longer visit his wife. After the diagnosis, Mr. B had two requests. He wanted to tell his wife the news about his prognosis and he also asked that he be admitted to inpatient hospice so he could share a room with his wife.

There were countless reasons why this idea would never be approved. How would her dying husband's condition affect Mrs. B's recovery? How dangerous and error-prone would it be for two patients with the same last name to share a room? What would happen when one of them passed away? And the biggest concern, of course, was whether or not we would be able to convince the insurance company that inpatient Hospice was even warranted.

I am amazed by the dedication our nursing staff demonstrated in fulfilling this couple's wish. Their passion spread like wildfire as they advocated for Mr. and

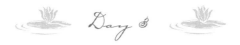

Mrs. B. The staff took it upon themselves to counsel with the respective physicians, family, Infection Control, Hospice, Nursing Leadership, Pharmacy, Lab, and Respiratory Care. They promised to micromanage the safety and infection control concerns.

After days of negotiations, everyone was finally convinced that this was the right thing to do. Mr. B was admitted to his wife's room where they lived together for three precious weeks, during which they were able to discuss their final wishes and say goodbye to each other. At the end of this time, Mrs. B was weaned off the ventilator and Mr. B was moved into home Hospice care. Though Mrs. B died several weeks after Mr. B's transfer, the nursing staff remained full of pride about this triumph of advocacy and autonomy.

—Submitted by Patricia Kurz, Good Samaritan Hospital Medical Center, West Islip, NY

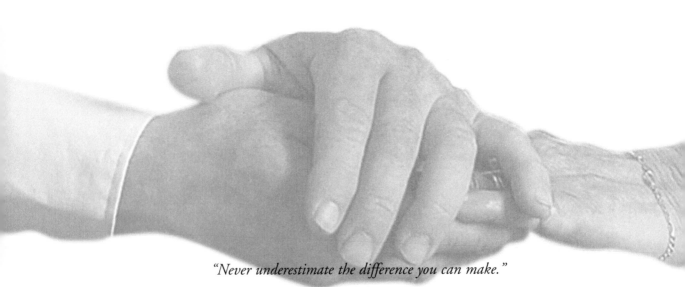

"Never underestimate the difference you can make."

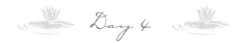

A Lasting Impact

Here is one story that I draw on to renew my faith as to why I love being a nurse. Eighteen years ago, I was a critical care nurse at Good Samaritan Hospital. We had cared for a young man in his high school years who was in our unit for several months due to complications from chemotherapy.

Several years ago, I was in line at our coffee shop buying lunch, when a young man in his 30s in a wheelchair stopped me and said, "Are you Linda?" I said yes.

He asked if several other nurses still worked at Good Samaritan and started to list some of the "old-timers" who were still there. He then identified himself as the young man several of us had cared for years earlier.

He said that as he grew up, he felt that it was the nurses who saved his life, even though he was wheelchair-bound. He went on to get a degree in physical therapy and now teaches new wheelchair patients how to adapt to their lives.

Day in and day out we are able to touch people in a way that can impact the rest of their lives.

—Submitted by Linda Hawes, Good Samaritan Hospital, Baltimore, MD

"Never underestimate the difference you can make."

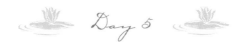

DENNY'S STORY

As a physical therapist at Carolinas Rehabilitation, I have had the pleasure of helping many people recover from life-altering strokes. In the fall of 2003, I was part of a rehabilitation team that worked with Denny H., a paramedic turned patient due to an unforeseen stroke that turned his life upside down.

The rehab team approached his recovery just as we would for any of our patients. We focused on the basics: eating, grooming, dressing, walking, and speaking. We wanted to prepare Denny and his family for life after the hospital, so we also began family training during most of his therapy sessions.

His recovery was slow, but gradually Denny improved to a point where he could get in and out of bed and propel himself around in a wheelchair.

Much of Denny's rehab mirrored that of other patients with a similar injury.

After he was discharged, the rehab team assumed that Denny would go on with outpatient therapy and hoped he would continue to improve.

Denny's wife, Linda, was kind enough to share her account of Denny's visit. The following is her story.

I'm no medical professional. My husband, Denny, was one for nearly thirty years. He was a paramedic, an instructor of PALS, BTLS, and ACLS courses for other health care professionals. He loved what he did.

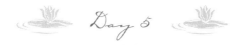

His career suddenly ended on September 2, 2003. Same-day surgery resulted in an embolism to his brain. He suffered a stroke, which left him in a coma. Luckily, he was at Carolinas Medical Center, a site which was participating in pre-FDA approved use of a new technology. A neurosurgeon was inside my husband's brain within 90 minutes, removing a fragmented blood clot. Denny survived. He came out of the coma three days later.

We spent well over a month at Carolinas Rehabilitation. Staff provided me with an air mattress and bed linens so I could stay with Denny. We began the long, slow process of physical, occupational, recreational, and speech therapies.

Denny struggled to perform even the simplest tasks. I followed him and his therapists as they worked, wiping his chin to keep saliva from soaking his shirt. More than once, vertigo made him vomit during therapy; more than once, his physical therapist had to clean himself up before we could go on.

The more we worked with his therapists, the more we learned about his condition, his deficits, and how our world would never be the same again.

Therapists at Carolinas Rehabilitation have a mission: to heal, to teach, to inspire. Staff quickly became family. They did not see my husband as "the massive stroke" or "the vestibular guy." They saw the person. Their realistic approach in training us to adapt to Denny's deficits were always coupled with deep affection, optimism, and empathy. We began to believe we could do the impossible.

When we were admitted to Carolinas Rehabilitation, Denny's condition was a one on their scale of one to seven. When we left, on October 21, he was a six. Our doctors were stunned.

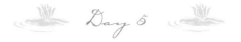

By December 5, before home therapy began, I very proudly returned his wheel chair. We had been able to get him mobile with a walker and a gait belt. We had six weeks of home therapy because riding in a car provoked vestibular vertigo and vomiting.

We have heard, time and again since then, that Denny (who now walks a little without a walker) "cannot possibly be doing the things he does." Our therapists have no trouble believing how far we have come. They are the ones who refused to put limits on what we could do if we were willing to work hard enough.

What's right in health care? An army of deeply committed physical, occupational, recreational, and speech therapists whose philosophy is this: "The difficult you can do right now. The impossible? It may take awhile, but you can do that, too."

—Submitted by Calvin Hung, Carolinas Healthcare System, Charlotte, NC

"Never underestimate the difference you can make."

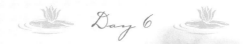

Pam and the Crying Woman

As I was exiting one of the buildings on our campus, I passed by a young woman who was crying. I considered stopping to see if she was okay, but I decided that I shouldn't intrude on her privacy. When I returned a few minutes later, I saw Pam, one of our dietary aids, talking quietly with the same woman.

I could see the compassion on Pam's face as the woman explained that she was new to our town and had experienced a miscarriage the day before. She had just picked up a prescription at our pharmacy and was overcome with grief and exhaustion. Her husband was at work and she didn't want to interrupt him at his new job.

Pam insisted that she drive the woman home and I volunteered to follow them so Pam could return with me. We also left our phone numbers just in case she should need anything. For several days afterward, Pam called the woman to check up on her and share in her grief for the lost infant. Weeks later we received thank you notes from the young mother—notes that revealed to us the difference Pam had made by deciding to "intrude" on someone who seemed to be in distress.

Pam was my mentor that day. I will never again let my fear of intruding allow me to pass by someone who may need my help. Over a year later, I can't meet Pam in the hallway without smiling at her, knowing that we shared a special experience. I am privileged to work alongside her as we serve the needs of our community. Pam is what is right in health care today.

—Submitted by D. Parker Haddix, Davis Health System, Elkins, WV

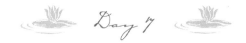

Delayed Travelers

Our hospital received this wonderful letter from the husband of a patient. It perfectly expresses what we believe is right in health care:

When I came into Raritan Bay Medical Center on Labor Day Weekend, I was "at my wits' end," as they say in Scotland. Our flight had been delayed on Saturday and we could not fly home until Sunday evening. The new airline security measures meant that my wife would not have been able to carry out her peritoneal dialysis for over two days by the time we would have arrived home on Monday. She was already showing signs of exhaustion while I was on the phone most of Saturday, liaising with Baxters to try and arrange a delivery of peritoneal dialysis bags to the hotel. But it was all in vain as the representative couldn't find anyone to deliver the supplies due to the holiday weekend.

When we arrived at the hotel, I called several of the local hospitals in an attempt to obtain some bags but this was also in vain as none of the receptionists could, or were willing to, help.

That is the reason why I ended up hailing a cab at 7:00 a.m. to go to your hospital. I just knew that if I could speak to someone who understood my predicament, all would be OK. Well, the response I received from your staff was tremendous!

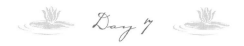

Angel, Sharon (emergency department RN staff), you were very sympathetic, friendly, compassionate, and humorous, too. Ann (nursing supervisor), I know at the end of the day, it didn't matter how kind the girls were. It was your decision to give me the medication and it was very much appreciated. You should have seen my wife's face when I went back to the hotel room with the bags!

I thank all of you from the bottom of my heart. In Scotland, we call our nurses "angels," and you three certainly fit the bill. I will never forget what you did for my wife and me.

We were home only five full days and just getting over our jet lag when we had a phone call from the transplant coordinator for Scotland. There was a kidney available in Edinburgh Royal Infirmary and it was a perfect match! We drove down through the night and she went through her operation on Sunday, a week to the day when I was in your hospital.

Margaret is home now and is doing great. If you had not supplied the much-needed peritoneal dialysis bags, she might not have been strong enough to go through the operation in the first place. And because of the complicated process in finding a match, it could have been many years before another opportunity, if any, arose. So again, we thank you! Your hospital has a lot to be proud of, and I sincerely hope that they know how fortunate they are to have such wonderful nurses on their staff.

—*Submitted by Deborah Jasovsky, Raritan Bay Medical Center, Perth Amboy, NJ*

"Never underestimate the difference you can make."

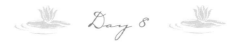

Pumpkin Pie

A few months ago, I received a request for a patient who was just admitted to inpatient Hospice. She was previously on a renal diet and all she wanted now that she had no dietary restrictions was a piece of pumpkin pie. So I scoured the refrigerators and freezers and much to my dismay, found that we had no pumpkin pie in our kitchen.

One of our cooks, Phyllis, heard that I was looking and was able to find just one can of pumpkin pie filling. She was ready to clock out and go home, but she stayed to make, bake, and serve this last wish to a dying patient. We delivered the warm pie, along with a huge bowl of whipped cream and lots of plates so that her family could spend quality time with her enjoying her pie. There must have been 10-12 family members in and outside the room. The patient was so thrilled at the gesture and she passed away a few days later. We were so happy to help fulfill her simple wish.

—Submitted by Sarah Hall, Shands AGH, Gainesville, FL

"Never underestimate the difference you can make."

14

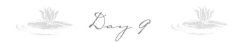
One Last Hug

At Genesis, we try to live our mission of providing quality and compassionate care to those who come to us in need as well as to their families. Sometimes the way the staff puts this mission into action makes us stop and catch our breaths in wonder and awe.

We recently had a patient named Walter who was nearing the end of his life. His family visited constantly and it was evident that this man was deeply loved by many. One evening Ursula, his wife of almost 70 years, was sitting at the bedside in her wheelchair crying quietly. Her nursing assistant approached her, gently touched her shoulder, and asked, "Are you all right?" With tears in her eyes, Ursula looked at the nursing assistant and said, "I'd just like to hug him one more time."

The nursing assistant went to talk with Walter's nurse. Together, they reentered the room and suggested a plan to Ursula. The two nurses carefully lifted Ursula out of her wheelchair and placed her on the bed right next to her husband. She turned to him and gave him a soft kiss and a caress on his cheek. Walter slowly opened his eyes, smiled back at her, and whispered in her ear. Then he placed his head against her shoulder and drifted back to sleep.

What Walter said to his wife remains a secret between the two of them. Their caresses and stillness took them on a journey of memories, all lived in a single touch and a shared smile. In moments like this, our mission to our patients and their families is exemplified in all its meaning, potential, and poignant beauty.

—Submitted by Lavonne Dwinal, Genesis Medical Center, DeWitt, IA

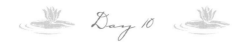

Forever United

I am a chaplain at St. Francis Hospital. The week before Memorial Day of 2004, I received a call asking if I would please perform a marriage ceremony for one of our patients. My first response was, "No," since weddings are not part of my job here at the hospital. But as I listened to the caller, who happened to be the patient's long-time girlfriend, I changed my mind. There seemed to be unusual circumstances where I needed to be more flexible.

The patient had been in and out of the hospital for some time and was not doing well at all. He had known his future wife all her life and now his time was running out. The couple wanted to be married outside on the hospital grounds so that the groom's elderly, much beloved dog could attend.

My husband, who is also a chaplain at the hospital, assisted with the ceremony, which took place on a warm Memorial Day in the shade of the trees outside the cafeteria. The groom came in his wheelchair with his nurse, and other wheelchair-bound family members were there as well. The dog wore flowers on his collar. Several doctors showed up, and people who were eating in the cafeteria came outside to watch. It was a wonderful occasion! There were smiles and tears.

After the ceremony, we went up to the patient's floor where family and staff had prepared a lovely reception. The groom was tired and did not stay too long. He had asked if he could go home for his "honeymoon," and he was discharged for the following weekend. However, his condition worsened, and he returned to the hospital where he died that week.

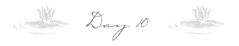

Two weeks to the day after his marriage, my husband and I conducted his funeral and burial. In the congregation were many who had been at the wedding. In our remarks, we emphasized the happiness of this couple, a special friendship that finally culminated in marriage. His wife told us that she felt her husband had hung on long enough for the wedding and that precious time together at home.

Being part of patients' lives is a privilege that we have as workers in health care. We may have an impact on them, but they can impact our lives in ways we can never imagine.

—*Submitted by Nancy O'Shea, Saint Francis Hospital, Memphis, TN*

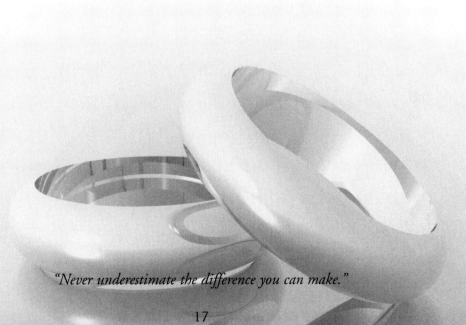

"Never underestimate the difference you can make."

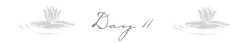

Kind Stranger

I was overseeing our main cafeteria and noticed an elderly man at the cash register who was holding up the line. I saw one of my employees, a food service worker, walk up to him and hand him money. It turned out the man was visiting a sick family member and had forgotten his wallet. When I asked my employee if she got his information to get her money back, she said, "Oh no, I did this out of the kindness of my heart. He has a very sick son. I don't expect the money back."

These are the kind of employees we have working here with us. They are kind and compassionate and truly care about people. They have a passion for what they do. I am proud to be on the same team with them.

—Submitted by Darlene Boggs-Pescuma, Lenoir Memorial Hospital, Kinston, NC

"Never underestimate the difference you can make."

18

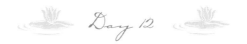
Loving Messengers

I am writing this story at a time that has been particularly difficult for my own family. My 22-year-old cousin, like many young men, is serving in Iraq. This is his second tour of duty. During his first tour, he was on a mission along with his best friend when a roadside bomb went off, killing his best friend. He was fortunate enough to escape without serious injury, but he was left with the pain of losing someone who was important to him.

He was scheduled to come home on Saturday, January 20, 2007. On the Monday prior to his scheduled return date, we were notified that while on his final mission, he had been shot in the face and was in very serious condition.

During the next few days, more information trickled in as his mother and many other family members prayed and hoped for the best. On the following Wednesday, Brenda, his mother, was informed that he would be shipped to a hospital in Landstuhl, Germany, where many military personnel are sent following injuries sustained during combat.

Upon hearing this news, I had shared this information with some of my employees at the hospital where I work in central Missouri. The lead CT technologist mentioned that her niece was a nurse at a hospital in Germany near where my cousin was to be taken. She and her sister-in-law, who is also employed here, took it upon themselves to contact the nurse in Germany asking if she could possibly get a message to him when he arrived. The nurse graciously agreed to do so.

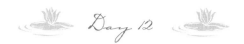

Later that evening I gathered messages from various members of our family to send to my cousin. I then compiled all of the emails and sent them to Jennifer, the nurse in Germany. The very next morning I received an email from her stating that she had received my messages and graciously forwarded them to a close friend of hers who worked at the hospital where my cousin was to be transported.

A few minutes later I received a second email from her stating that she had just gotten confirmation that he had arrived in Landstuhl, and her friend had personally given the email containing the messages to his nurse who would be reading those to him.

I cannot imagine how alone my young cousin must have felt without his family being able to be by his side, but because of special health care workers like Jennifer and her friend Shana, who went out of their way for complete strangers in another country, he was assured that he was in our thoughts and prayers.

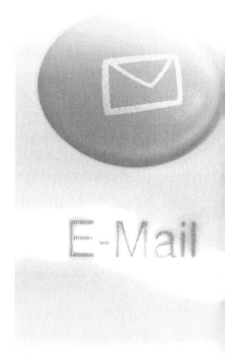

—Submitted by Gina Collier, Phelps County Regional Medical Center, Rolla, MO

"Never underestimate the difference you can make."

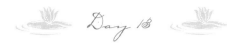

An Extraordinary Doctor

Dr. James Roach is a urologist who has practiced at St. Vincent's Medical Center in Bridgeport, Connecticut, for his entire career and everybody loves him. They love Jim for his empathy and response to others' needs and they love him for the legends, which have followed him during his entire career. You see, Jim does things that others would never consider. His practices stretch the standard of healer and Good Samaritan in a unique way and every time another story is revealed about Jim, it adds to his legend.

He has done many kind things, such as pro bono work or coming into the emergency department while his 25th wedding anniversary party was going on to catheterize a friend's son. He volunteers his time to clinics and community work and volunteers to care for the most at-risk populations.

What separates Jim from all of the other caring doctors of the world is the stretch of his kindness to others. Several years ago, Jim was contacted by the Catholic missions in Cambodia and asked if he would consider operating on a young boy who had a life-threatening tumor on his kidney. Without hesitation, Jim said he would be happy to do the procedure pro bono.

The missions called back to say that the patient needed to be sponsored to get into the United States. Naturally, Jim said he would sponsor the boy, but he was later told the sponsor had to be a relative of the boy. The boy had no relative in the U.S., so the next logical step for Jim was to offer to adopt him.

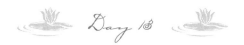

Thanks to Jim, the boy was able to come to St. Vincent's and have a successful surgery, which saved his life. He then joined the Roach family as their adopted child. In addition to rearing and educating his eight natural children, Jim Roach also put this young man through high school and college. Today the boy is a successful engineer with a family of his own.

Recently, Jim retired from his private practice and immediately began volunteering his time as a physician for Americares, an organization that serves the most vulnerable populations. He has also volunteered for more assignments at St. Vincent's clinics.

As a urologist, he treated a number of patients waiting for kidney transplants. Jim obviously helped many of these patients, but he wanted to do more. Incredibly, Jim made an appointment at the transplant center at Yale and told them he wished to donate a kidney. They asked him who the kidney was for, and he responded that it would be for whoever could use it.

Most people who hear this story, which has become popular despite Jim's best efforts to keep it quiet, are taken aback by this man's compassion for others. In many ways, Jim Roach's behavior challenges others to be better and to do more. While that may not be his intent, it is often the result. Some people say that being close to Jim Roach is like having your soul cleaned. I tend to agree with that statement. One thing is for certain: Jim Roach is a legendary caregiver.

—Submitted by Ronald Bianchi, St. Vincent's Medical Center, Bridgeport, CT

"Never underestimate the difference you can make."

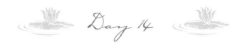

Blessing Quilts

As a new associate of Our Lady of Lourdes Medical Center, I was invited to do a short presentation at a Nursing Professional Governance meeting. The meeting proved to be anything but routine.

During the meeting, I was briefly distracted by the rumbling noise of a shopping bag. I glanced over to see the Vice President of Nursing, Barbara Holfelner, adjusting the overstuffed contents of a bag, which contained a large crocheted quilt. At first I thought that it must be a lost and found item, but I soon learned that this was no ordinary quilt.

We were all intrigued and we listened closely as Barbara began to tell us the story of the quilt. The quilt was made after a colleague learned of a hospital that improved end-of-life care by providing quilts for dying patients through a program called Blessing Quilts.

The Blessing Quilts are individually handmade and placed on the beds of dying patients. The quilts offer physical, emotional, and spiritual comfort to the patients themselves and provide a tangible sense of caring and support to their families.

Everyone at the meeting was moved and motivated by this compassionate project. We knew it was possible to create a similar program at Our Lady of Lourdes Medical Center and we immediately organized all of the different elements to consider in getting the program up and running.

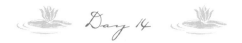

The first order of business was finding someone willing to make the quilts at an affordable price. This proved to be easier said than done. We checked with every local knitting, crocheting, and quilting service but came up with nothing. Barbara turned to an associate, Susan Woods, for assistance. Susan looked to the Internet for help and after a few weeks of inquiries, she tried eBay in a last-*stitch* effort.

Amazingly, Susan received a response from a woman over 3,000 miles away in Oregon. This stranger had heard about the Blessing Quilts and was eager to participate in the project. Much to our surprise and gratitude, she offered to make the quilts at a more than reasonable price. She explained to us that the reward of helping others through her quilts was much more enriching than any amount of money.

And so the Blessing Quilt project began. Financed by charitable contributions, the Blessing Quilts—each one beautifully different in pattern, size, and design—began to arrive in multiples, and soon the Vice President of Nursing's office began to resemble a craft fair.

Working with the Blessing Quilts program prompted me to think about my own life experiences and how items such as these had been so important during life's most momentous times: the knitted blue quilt my family had for many years, which gave my mother warmth in her final hours; the tiny knitted items given to me, a grieving new mother, by a delivery room nurse to help comfort me during a time of unimaginable loss; and the bright pink crocheted blanket that welcomed my new daughter. From these personal experiences, I know that sewn into each Blessing Quilt is a compassionate message that this patient was cared for until the moment of death—and that he or she was as complex and unique as the quilt itself.

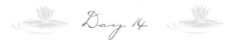

As nurses, we know the challenge of providing an environment for a peaceful death in a busy hospital setting. The Blessing Quilt program helps us find strength at these difficult times. We are able to offer the quilt as a gift to bond the grief-stricken with their loved ones forever. And we offer it with this very special message, "We cover our loved one with this quilt, this sign of our affection...that all the bonds of love that knit us together do not unravel with death."

—Submitted by Ann B. Townsend, Our Lady of Lourdes Medical Center, Camden, NJ

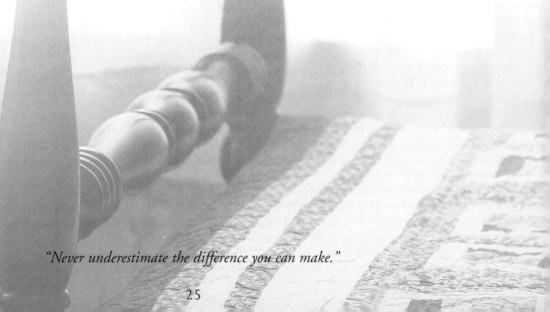

"Never underestimate the difference you can make."

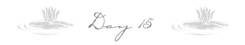

Hand Holders

One day last year I was called to a room in the emergency department. Lying on the gurney was an old woman. Her skin was wrinkled and freckled, her red lipstick almost as crooked as her bright red wig. She was leaning forward clenching the side rails, unable to speak and barely able to breathe.

In the corner of the same room was an old man, unable to take his eyes off the woman. He wore pants of brown polyester, secured by a white belt just below his armpits. His pale yellow shirt was tucked halfway into his pants and slightly wrinkled, resembling the lines in his forehead.

He inched forward in his tan, lace-up, patent leather shoes. As I approached the woman, I introduced myself as I put my hand slowly over hers. She looked up with her warm, brown eyes and managed a smile. I smiled and said I would help her breathe.

I wheeled my machine closer to the bed, smiling at the man in the corner. He told me that they had been married for 60 years and that she was the best woman in the world.

I walked over to the man, who was the cutest old man I had ever seen, took his hand and placed it in his wife's as I explained, "Hand holders are very important." That day, as I looked at the couple, I realized the most important thing in life is having someone special to hold your hand as you lie counting the dots on the ceiling…and I knew how fortunate I was to be the respiratory therapist in that very room.

—Submitted by Kimberly Havea, Mayo Regional Hospital, Dover-Foxcroft, ME

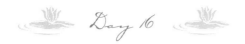

Care-full Nursing

I recently sent the following message to Michael Tarwater, our president and CEO, as a response to a presentation he made at our latest Leadership Development Institute. During the presentation, he stated that he would probably not make a good nurse because he would "tear up" when confronted with difficult situations. I have been a nurse for decades, and I thought that it was important to express to him how important a caring nature is when you are trying to be a great nurse.

Dear Mike,

I have been meaning to share something with you since the last LDI. Because it involved storytelling, I have a couple of my own to share. I truly appreciated hearing your story about the Christmas Eve flight and the response you felt when caring for the young child as you protected him from the weather. The feeling you get when you are able to help someone is, without a doubt, why most of us have chosen to work in the health care field.

I thought it was very interesting when you began to tear up and stated, "You can see why I could never be a nurse." I disagree with you. I think your compassionate feelings and caring nature are the characteristics that would make you an excellent nurse! Here is a story

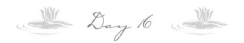

from my own experience that I hope will help you understand my point of view.

While in clinical as a student at Clemson University, I was caring for a nine-year-old child who had been badly burned. Before this day I had always thought I would love to be a pediatric nurse, but after caring for this child my thoughts changed and I almost left nursing forever. My job that day was to debride the burns on this young child, a task that involved taking off the old dressings, which stuck terribly to his wounds.

This was in the mid-1970s and we had not yet perfected our pain management techniques nor were we using a whirlpool to loosen these dressings. It hurt me then and hurts me now to think about how painful this procedure must have been for this child.

Unfortunately, despite the pain, it had to be done, so gowned and masked I went into the child's room to begin this tedious process. His burns covered his torso and most of the fronts of his legs. He begged me not to do the procedure. And he often cried out in pain and fear, asking me to stop over and over again.

The Demerol I had given him just wasn't enough to take away his fear and pain. It wasn't long before I was crying along with him as I futilely tried to convince him that what I was doing was necessary. Fortunately for me, my instructor, Ms. Brown, came in and, seeing my anguish, replaced me with another student who was able to finish what I had barely begun.

I felt ashamed and defeated. My instructor never gave me any constructive criticism other than telling me that I would need to learn to get my emotions in check. It was a devastating experience for me. I got in my little Pinto and began the drive home to my folks to confess to them

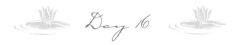

that I could never be a nurse. But I wasn't able to make that confession because I was also afraid of disappointing them. So I returned and continued my pursuit of a nursing career while hiding my emotions and fears.

Upon taking a job in the Intensive Care Unit at Charlotte Memorial Hospital in 1978, I learned a very valuable lesson that has helped me to be successful in educating new nurses. The incident took place during my first three months on the unit. Because I had seniority, I was in charge of a 21-bed unit. For these 21 patients, there were three RNs plus the Assistant Nurse Manager.

One weekend a 16-year-old boy came in who had been in a terrible automobile accident. On arrival he was near death and not expected to live. I elected to "break the rules" and let his family stay at his bedside while we cared for him moment to moment. It was not a popular move, and I knew I risked being reprimanded for my decision. As hard as we tried, we could not save this young boy and he died later that night. After my shift, I stayed on with his parents and stood by his bedside and cried with them.

About a week later the family came back to the unit. They were looking for me and reinforced to me that my decision to allow them to be with their child was the right thing to do. They said it made all the difference in the world to them that they were able to be there with him when he died. But most importantly they wanted to tell me how much it meant to them to see that I really cared about their son and them.

I was only 21 years old and didn't have children at the time so I couldn't have known how those parents were feeling. But somehow a

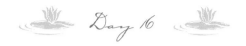

greater power gave me the strength to stand up and make the decision that night to break the rules and follow my heart.

That day was a huge milestone in my nursing career. From then on, I began to follow my heart and no longer felt like I had to squash my caring nature, which was the very part of me that would allow me to be successful in my job.

As I have had the privilege to work in many roles within CHS, I have been so thankful that I can share with new nurses the importance of holding on to the emotions that go along with our work.

Thanks for leading this organization in the wonderful way you do—with humility and a willingness to be vulnerable—but please remember those traits are excellent characteristics that would make you an excellent nurse!

Nursing is such a wonderful career choice and CHS is a wonderful place to practice. I have been blessed with a wonderful place to learn and grow in the nursing profession. This is my home.

Thank you,

Sara Masters, MSN, RN, Faculty, School of Nursing, Carolinas College of Health Sciences

—Submitted by Thomas Masters, Carolinas Healthcare System, Charlotte, NC

"Never underestimate the difference you can make."

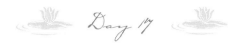

Bringing Them Together

A patient transporter, who just happens to be my daughter, Joy, moved an elderly man from his hospital room to another department for testing. A master at her job, Joy often talks to the patients to help keep their minds from worrying about the tests they are about to have. During their conversation, the patient told Joy that his wife was also a patient in the hospital. They continued talking and parted ways when Joy delivered the patient to the department for his test.

The next day Joy moved an elderly lady from her hospital room to another department for testing. Once again she talked to the patient to ease her stress. To Joy's surprise, the lady told her that her husband was also in the hospital. With tears in her eyes, the patient explained that they had never been apart in all the years of their marriage. Joy quickly realized that her patient from the day before must have been this patient's husband.

The next day Joy once again had to move the elderly male patient from a couple of days before. He was pleased to see her again and their conversation picked up where it left off as he talked about his family. The man talked about his wife and said he had been married over 50 years. With tears in his eyes, he told Joy—just as his wife had—that they had never been apart so long. Determined to bring this loving husband and wife back together, Joy told the patient she would wait for him to complete his test.

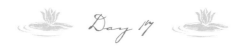

When the test was over, Joy told the patient they would be taking a detour on the way back to his hospital room. She pushed the patient onto the elevator and pressed the button. The patient noticed that she had pressed the wrong floor and pointed it out to her. She explained that this was all part of the detour. They soon reached the mystery floor and went down a hallway that was unfamiliar to the patient.

Joy went to another patient's room, knocked on the door, and asked if she could receive a visitor. The elderly female patient said, "Yes." Joy pushed the elderly male patient into the room, and he started crying when he saw his wife. Joy waited in the hall for a few minutes as they visited. On that day, though she wasn't a doctor, Joy was able to provide the best medicine possible for this elderly couple.

—Submitted by George Pelissier, Eastern Maine Healthcare Systems, Brewer, ME

"Never underestimate the difference you can make."

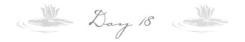

Fate Steps In

I am a 10-year survivor of breast cancer. I was fortunate enough to be working at the same hospital I work in now when I was diagnosed with the disease that eventually took one of my breasts but, thankfully, not my life or my spirit. But this story isn't about me.

As an administrative employee for over 17 years, my offices at this hospital have been away from the main campus. But a couple of years ago, I was relocated to an office in the same building that houses our Cancer Center.

A year and a half ago, I was walking down the hall when I saw a man and a woman, Jim and Jane, who appeared lost and confused. I stopped to ask them if they needed any help. Jane was wearing sunglasses and had been crying. They asked me questions about our Cancer Center.

She told me she had just moved here from Philadelphia and had recently been diagnosed with breast cancer. They had seen a television commercial about our hospital and wanted to check out our facilities in person. They explained that they were interested in talking to someone about receiving treatment at our center so they wouldn't have to commute back and forth to Philadelphia for treatment.

Jane was so distraught, scared, and tearful. Without giving it a thought, I told her I was a breast cancer survivor and briefly told her my story, offering encouragement with a sense of humor. I gave them directions to our Breast Center and the name of the director and then I walked them to their car. They

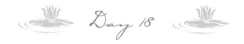

were so grateful to have run into someone to talk to and they thanked me over and over again. We all hugged and went our separate ways.

A few days later, Jim and Jane were at the Breast Center for an appointment and they came to see me to update me on Jane's condition. Again, I listened and offered support and encouragement. They were extremely happy and comfortable with our staff and doctors.

Our meetings became regular as Jane's treatment proceeded. Each time Jim and Jane came to the hospital, they would stop by to see me. The visits always ended with hugs and they never failed to show their appreciation for everyone they had met during Jane's treatment.

After these meetings, I always became tearful, not because the memories of my own experience with cancer were brought to the surface, but because of what Jane was having to experience. I knew her fears, felt her pain. I knew what it was like to wake up every day to a lump and not know what the final outcome of this journey would be. I knew what it was like to possibly be facing death. But I also felt that I might be making a difference for these folks…helping in a very small way. I often marveled at the fate that put us in that hallway at the exact same time.

After a couple of months without seeing them, I ran into Jim outside my building. He told me that Jane had her surgery and was being discharged from the hospital that day. I asked if it would be okay to visit and we walked over together. She had been through a lot, much more than I had, and it wasn't over. After a double mastectomy, she was now facing chemo. But she was positive and strong and sure that she, too, would survive. Again, Jane thanked me and referred to me as her guardian angel.

Over a year went by and I didn't see them. The time came for the annual Susan G. Komen Race for the Cure to benefit breast cancer research and awareness. I

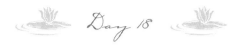
participate every year with my family, but this year my thoughts turned to Jane and I wondered how she was doing. After the race was over and we were getting ready to leave, I decided to go back by our hospital's booth one last time to say goodbye to everyone. I heard someone call my name, turned, and to my amazement, there were Jim and Jane. Fate had once again brought us together.

Although her hair was much shorter as it was growing back after her chemo, Jane looked radiant. I was so pleased to hear that she had finished the treatments and was doing great. I met her family and we chatted awhile. Again, she thanked me and insisted that running into me that first day made a world of difference. She said it was a true blessing. I was overwhelmed with emotion and was so happy for Jane and her family.

Whenever I reflect on the day I met Jane and Jim in that hallway, I wonder if it is one of the reasons I survived a disease that is still often fatal. If surviving breast cancer means I was able to help one person get through a devastating diagnosis, there is no longer a need to ask the question, "Why me?"

—*Anonymous Contributor*

"Never underestimate the difference you can make."

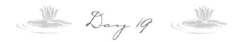

Miles from Home

Ursula Mansdorfer, or Ula as she is better known, is a nurse at Le Bonheur who really made an impression as we served a family who brought their child in all the way from Germany with a very serious brain tumor. The family had flown here with no family or friends nearby. The parents' English was good, but the little girl spoke no English. Imagine how comforting it was for the little girl to hear Ula speak to her in German.

Ula did far more than act as an interpreter. She went out of her way to help the family. She baked bread for them on her day off. She drove the father to his hotel. She rallied support from the local Jewish community so the family would get homemade kosher meals. Ula also arranged her schedule so she could drive the mother and the daughter to the doctor after the father had gone back to Germany.

One day, after the young girl's doctor's appointment, she took the girl and her mother to run errands and for a visit to the Children's Museum. During the young girl's care, the family repeatedly expressed their gratitude for Ula's incredible help and support.

—Submitted by Ruth-Ann Hale, Methodist Le Bonheur Germantown Hospital, Germantown, TN

"Never underestimate the difference you can make."

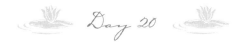

Whatever It Takes

I am the administrator of a critical access hospital in southeastern Washington. I'm honored to say that we have always been blessed with hospital staff who remember why they chose a career in health care and who have stayed true to those fundamental values.

Today's climate of "transparency" and "sentinel events" and growing scrutiny about the practices that take place in hospitals can jade the most optimistic and altruistic of any of us. And while we suffer our own version of disillusionment from time to time, I am proud every day to be associated with the employees, physicians, board members, and volunteers of our community hospital.

As you can see, I have chosen to not identify our name or city. The story I am about to tell could be interpreted by some as a reason for reporting improper activity. I assure you that we have expended efforts to review this case from many standpoints including an outside medical review. We are absolutely confident that this was neither a sentinel event nor that any inappropriate or unnecessary care was rendered. However, I feel compelled to protect individuals and the hospital from undue and undeserving criticism while I share this inspiring story.

On January 7, 2007, a four-year-old boy was brought into our emergency department by his parents. His dad had run over him with his truck. They had been out on the family farm doing chores just as they had

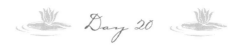

done many times before. Only this time, instead of going behind the truck to feed the cattle, the boy went in front of the truck. His dad simply didn't see him. When the boy and his father arrived at the hospital, the boy was alert and telling the hospital staff that his stomach hurt.

They began to quickly assess the extent of his injuries. Surgeons were called, and the OR call team was notified. They mobilized quickly. But before these teams could arrive, the boy went into cardiac arrest. Resuscitation efforts were started immediately. The staff soon determined that there was significant internal bleeding and blood products were ordered to be available for surgery.

The boy was successfully resuscitated but was now unconscious. In surgery, a tremendous team of professionals had assembled, some out of duty (they were on call) and others out of caring and concern. In the tensest throes of the case there were two general surgeons, an orthopedic surgeon who had just finished another emergency when the boy arrived in the OR, three anesthesia providers, a pharmacist, nursing staff, imaging personnel, lab staff, a house supervisor, a volunteer chaplain, the chief clinical officer, and the parents.

Everyone had a purpose. The orthopedic surgeon was manually massaging the boy's heart, the surgeons were attempting to locate the source of the injuries, the volunteer chaplain was trying to comfort the family, the lab staff was trying to understand the blood needs, and the others were tending to their myriad duties. Early in the effort, confusion arose regarding the availability of enough blood to transfuse. Concerned about the survival of the child, the surgeons ordered blood from another

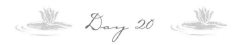

hospital. Fearing it would not arrive soon enough, one of the anesthesia providers said that he was an O negative blood type and offered to donate.

The surgeons decided to do the unorthodox and carried out a direct transfusion. The anesthesia provider lay on the floor of the OR and donated blood to this severely injured child. After an hour of trying every possible way to save his life, the child died. The injuries were too severe.

The emotional wrenching in the aftermath of this case has been extraordinary. Over a dozen staff people have sought out our organizational psychologist to try to cope with their feelings and questions. Did I do all I could? What more could I have done? What if I had done this instead? The second-guessing has been widespread. I observed a seasoned physician break down in tears when explaining the results of the autopsy. Yet, all reviews have indicated that no effort would have saved this boy. The autopsy revealed that his pulmonary artery had been detached from his heart when the tire rolled over his chest. His mortality was virtually 100 percent.

So, what do I hope to achieve by telling this story? I hope it serves as a reason for all of us to be grateful every day for people who are willing to put everything on the line for another person. We may have to answer as a hospital for "non-protocol" type of actions—a direct blood transfusion, confusion over availability of blood products, etc. But I will never apologize, nor suggest that any of our staff, physicians, or volunteers should not first do what is right without worrying about what is acceptable or politically expedient.

In our community hospital, people still see caring for people as their first priority and that is "What Is Right in Health Care." They still see that

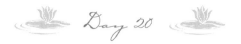
doing the right thing for that patient at that time is far more important than how it might look on the website or whether the protocol approves it, or whether they might get reviewed later. These dedicated professionals still know that ultimately they have to answer to themselves and be able to say that they did all they knew to do and then live with that. I am infinitely grateful to each of them. If it were my four-year-old child, I wouldn't have wanted it any other way.

—*Anonymous Contributor*

"Never underestimate the difference you can make."

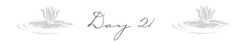

A Place to Stay

We recently had a homeless patient who had no identification and therefore was not able to be placed at any shelter or agency in our community. Over the next several days, Doug Jones, our amazing case manager, spent many hours calling around in attempts to get this man a place to stay where he could receive direction on treatment options. In the end, the patient was discharged to a homeless center in Indianapolis, which did not require him to have ID because they knew him.

The work that went into finding this man a place to stay was astonishing and it provides a great representation of what can happen when everyone works together to provide the best care possible for the patient. Take a look at what the staff had to do in order to find this man a place to stay:

- Doug Jones coordinated everything.
- Linda Zeese bought a bus ticket to Indianapolis.
- Pat Walker, JoAnn Stallter, Jackie Dotson, and Doug Jones pooled their money and gave the patient $35.
- Doug went "shopping" in the closet of extra clothes and put together a few outfits for him.
- The patient was given a cab pass to go to CVS Pharmacy to fill his prescriptions for free; the cab then took him to the bus station.

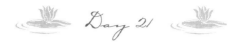

- Jackie found a cane and gave it to the patient.
- They packed the patient a bagged lunch along with his "new" belongings into a rolling cooler and sent him on his way.

I know that a lot of this is what our staff does every day, but the way in which this came together was just great! As a result of everyone's willingness to come together as a team, our patient received positive and beneficial care beyond his stay at our hospital.

—Submitted by Kathy Hawley, Saint Joseph Regional Medical Center, South Bend, IN

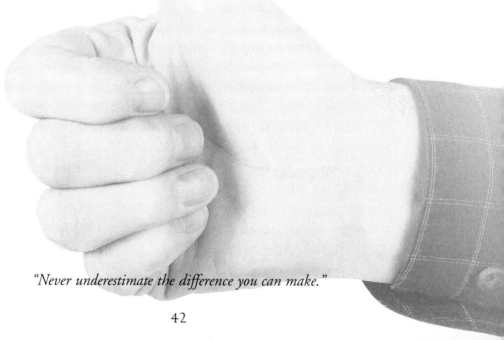

"Never underestimate the difference you can make."

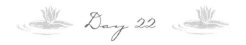

Welcoming Care

Several years ago I worked at a hospital in Bangor, Maine. As Bangor has the easternmost airport on the U.S. mainland, often times, if there was an inflight emergency, the plane would be directed to land in Bangor and the ill/injured person would be taken to our hospital for care.

One day, we received a call that an elderly gentleman had become gravely ill on a flight from Poland en route to the Midwest. The flight landed in Bangor and the gentleman, accompanied by his elderly wife, was transported to our hospital. One of our nurses, Helen, began the gentleman's care. She found a note pinned to the very worn and tattered suit jacket that the gentleman wore, which explained that he and his wife did not speak English and they were going to the Midwest to live with their nephew.

Despite all efforts to save this gentleman's life, he died. His wife was beyond distraught. Helen so very kindly said she would take care of the gentleman's wife. In typical Helen style, she took his wife home with her that evening. She helped make phone calls and arrangements for the gentleman's wife to accompany his body to the Midwest. And to top it all off, Helen also took the wife to buy a suit for the gentleman, which Helen paid for, so that he could be buried with dignity in his new country.

—Anonymous Contributor

"Never underestimate the difference you can make."

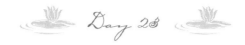

It Takes a Village

*T*he Friday afternoon before Hurricane Katrina made landfall, we sent our consultants on their way, noting the Weather Channel had changed the model. We stayed a few more hours to update our hurricane staffing plan for the Division of Quality/Case Management in the event that the hurricane came our way. We left voice mail instructions on our phones. We called staff and very methodically organized activities leading up to lockdown, landfall, and finally the All Clear.

On Saturday many in the department participated in the American Heart Association Heart walk in Gulfport. Of course, there was a lot of talk about what the storm might do, but at the same time, there were conversations about the beauty of the homes on Second Street. The weather was simply beautiful. Our focus at this point and up until lockdown was to discharge as many patients as possible. In actuality, only a few were discharged.

We went into lockdown Sunday at noon. The storm lasted all day Monday. And on Tuesday, despite the devastation that was around them, one by one our staff came back to work. They had to follow a path opened by emergency rescue vehicles. They dodged houses on the interstate, trees, refrigerators, dead animals, boats, and other debris. They drove over bridges that later were closed due to significant damage. They were stopped at checkpoints and often turned away. In uniform and with energy, they were all asking, "What can I do to help?"

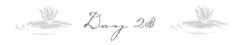
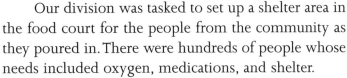

Our division was tasked to set up a shelter area in the food court for the people from the community as they poured in. There were hundreds of people whose needs included oxygen, medications, and shelter.

The food court was soon named, "The Village." These were people from our community and people we worked with who had been washed out of their homes or simply didn't have anywhere else to go. Their experiences were like something out of a nightmare. They were covered with mud and abrasions from having held onto trees while in the water. Some of them were still wet. The one thing they all had in common was the look in their eyes.

We set up a table outside the area to try to organize the chaos. At first all we had to offer was hot coffee. By Tuesday afternoon we had sandwiches. As the days went on and people came and went we were able to provide more and more. Several departments came together and established a makeshift pharmacy and filled prescriptions for a three-day supply. After three days we would refill them again. We did this for about eight or nine days until a local pharmacy finally opened. We also changed out oxygen canisters until we depleted our own stores. Finally a vendor from the community came forward and replenished our supplies and assisted the community.

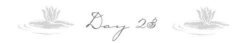

The hospital supplied formula, diapers, and personal care items. As patients were discharged from the hospital, many became a part of the growing group known as "The Village." The questions we heard from members of "The Village" were heartbreaking. *Where is my mother? My father? Where is the Red Cross? When will FEMA be here?* The anguish was overwhelming. It was such a lonely feeling. Everyone provided comfort to others. Not having the ability to control or to organize everything to make it flow better was agonizing.

After about sixty hours post-storm, we had the first sign of help from the outside. The military showed up and what a welcome sight it was. Sergeant Franklin showed up and took charge. He brought all of us order amongst the chaos. I knew then that we would be all right.

My staff came in and worked despite the fact that almost everyone in our division had lost their homes or sustained significant damage. Every morning they came back. We worked 16-hour days. We shared food and toiletries. Many people slept at the hospital because it was easier to stay there than go home; many stayed because they had no place to go home to.

Soon gas became a big issue. Some members of the staff were worried about being able to continue to come to work. The hospital arranged for a makeshift gas station to allow us to fill up our tanks. We did this after dark so as to not draw attention. On the third day, our division began transitioning from "The Village" to working case management and getting the appropriate patients transferred so we could decompress the hospital. Human Resources took over "The Village" at that time.

Still, trying to organize this chaos was the worst feeling. My staff rose to the occasion. They worked the phones and transferred hundreds of patients over a few days. We had several Chinook helicopters parked in the street. We had military

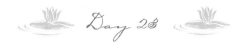

guards with machine guns outside the ED. It was surreal. The only sound outside was that of the helicopters.

The sight of my staff coming in on Tuesday morning at the regular time—or when they could get here—will forever be in my heart. The nurses, social workers, and secretaries came together and did what had to be done for each other and for our community. I know they would do it again because this is what we do.

During this very difficult time, the entire Mississippi Gulf Coast was devastated and communities were destroyed. Our hospital remained open and provided care to our community. We never stopped—not even as we faced a disaster.

—*Submitted by Karen Clarke and Melody Griffith, Memorial Hospital at Gulfport, Gulfport, MS*

"Never underestimate the difference you can make."

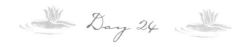

Letters of Thanks

In June 2006 we had a 20-year-old patient who presented with sepsis. She developed Acute Respiratory Distress Syndrome (ARDS) and ultimately suffered a cerebral bleed and died in our ICU. The following are two letters from her family. The first letter came just days after her death. To protect her privacy, the patient's name has been changed:

Sue's service is on this upcoming Monday, July 3rd, and our hearts are so full of gratefulness and appreciation to each and every one of you who so lovingly and graciously cared for "our beautiful rose" as she lay helplessly, fighting for her life. We watched each of you, with gentle skill and tenderness, make her as comfortable and beautiful as possible in her extreme illness and our hearts brim with so much respect, awe, and amazement at what you do every day, with every patient, without regard for color, race, or status in society. It was obvious that you "fell in love" with our Sue and we thank you. We continue to pray and hold each of you up before God for strength and wisdom as you continue every day to be the hands of love and skill for each person and family you care for. The care each of you gave could not have been matched by any other medical facility. Again, we say thank you. Words are inadequate at this time, so we hope the little expressions will shout what we cannot say. Each of you has our admiration, respect, and gratefulness.

This letter was accompanied by several small wooden boxes, each hand-carved, and hand-decorated with a rose on top for each staff member. We also received the following letter several months later:

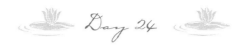

It has been five months since Sue's hasty exodus from our lives, leaving an empty place both in our hearts and in our home. As we reflect on these short months, we are so overwhelmed with gratitude and gratefulness for each of you who touched our lives in very personal ways. Again, we thank you for your kindness in our time of great need. Yes, the holidays are difficult, but we are comforted because you care.

To have touched a family in their darkest hours and to have them feel so moved by the care their daughter received that they needed to write letters, personally make gifts, and even stop by the ICU, validates for us why we stick it out in the hardest of times. A tragic event like this loss of a young life does not pass through without leaving its mark. And kind words like this carry the staff forward to the next.

—Submitted by Annette Cole, Merle West Medical Center, Klamath Falls, OR

"Never underestimate the difference you can make."

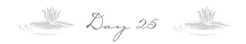

The Power of One

The laboratory department at Methodist Germantown went above and beyond the call of duty in giving volunteer Lori Siegal the opportunity to feel like she was valuable and needed. As a result of their work with Lori, members of the department were nominated by one of Lori's parents for a Miracles in Motion award, which is given to hospital staff members who have demonstrated exceptional customer service, going above and beyond their everyday roles to help patients.

Lori had Down syndrome and a severe congenital heart defect. Her hands and mouth were always blue as evidence of her failing heart. Most people would not have wanted to take the risk of allowing Lori to volunteer for them out of fear that her mental and physical limitations might get in the way of her work. However, this was not the case for the laboratory associates at Germantown.

Lori worked every Tuesday and Thursday for three hours and was friends with my daughter, Rebecca, who also has Down syndrome. Lori was always quick to tell Rebecca how important she was to the overall functioning of the laboratory at Germantown.

Lori was very high functioning and could do so much, but her heart severely limited her physically. Sadly, Lori died this year at the age of 25. At her funeral, her volunteer vest was proudly displayed with her pins signifying that she had volunteered for over 600 hours in the laboratory. Kelly Terry, director of the

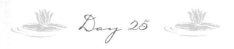

laboratory, spoke at Lori's funeral, sharing how valuable Lori was to each associate. Kelly was able to see past Lori's limitations and recognize her strengths.

It was obvious from the number of associates at Lori's funeral that she had touched every associate in the lab with her energy and excitement for life. And as a parent of a daughter with Down syndrome, I know how much the laboratory meant to Lori and her parents. The associates of the Germantown lab department looked past Lori's physical and mental limitations and gave her a chance to make a difference.

Lori Siegal represents the "Power of One." She proudly volunteered for Methodist Germantown even when her own heart was weak and failing. She valued her volunteer job and will be a continual inspiration to others with disabilities. My own daughter is following in her footsteps and is volunteering at Le Bonheur.

As a parent, I want the entire laboratory to know how thankful I am that they would accept, love, and make Lori feel that her short life made a difference. This is what the "Power of One" is all about—allowing each individual to use his or her gifts and talents to make a difference. The entire laboratory at Germantown has my gratitude and respect for giving Lori the chance to make a difference.

—Submitted by Ruth-Ann Hale,
Methodist Le Bonheur Germantown Hospital, Germantown, TN

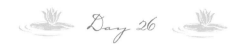

Blast from the Past

As the director of critical care for a Catholic hospital in Monroe, Louisiana, I have the duty of interviewing nurses to fill positions in critical care and telemetry. You never know what is going to happen in a fast-paced hospital environment, and I recently interviewed a nurse who took me way back to memories from the beginning of my nursing career.

When I began my nursing career, I was in a very busy critical care unit and had the opportunity to work with all kinds of patients from teenagers to the elderly. One patient in particular made a huge impact on me as a young nurse. My patient was in her early 30s and was dying from lung cancer. During the course of her treatment, I saw her gradually lose the ability to talk and respond to commands until she was totally unresponsive and finally drawing her last breath. It was an honor and a privilege for me to be able to care for this woman throughout her entire stay at our hospital.

During the course of her stay, I met her loving husband and two young daughters, one in the sixth grade and the other in the eighth grade. I became very close with them. We all cried together and shared stories, and even in her dying moments, she would thank us for caring for her. I told her it was my pleasure to be with her and her family during this time and reassured her that I was more

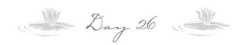

than happy to help in any way that I could. It wasn't long before she died and her suffering ended.

Many years later, I was interviewing a nurse I really liked. She was young, beautiful, and newly married. She asked a lot of the usual questions and then one question struck me as if a bolt of lightning had gone through my entire body. She said, "You don't remember me, do you?" I looked at her with a puzzled look and then she told me who she was. She said, "You took care of my mom."

I got tears in my eyes as I immediately realized who she was. She went on to tell me that I was the reason she went into nursing school. She said that I had been so compassionate with her mother and family that she wanted to be like me. I will never forget the words she shared with me during that interview.

Meeting this young nurse reminded me of all of the patients that I had helped over the years and made me wonder how many other lives I have been able to impact in such a positive way. In health care, you just never know how you impact the lives of others.

—Submitted by Donna Blackett, Saint Francis Medical Center, Cape Girardeau, MO

"Never underestimate the difference you can make."

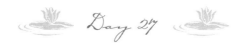

Day 27

A Beautiful Memory for Newlyweds

Like many couples about to get married, Ashley and Jeff put a lot of thought into every detail behind their wedding day. The one thing the couple hadn't planned for was a medical emergency. Just days before their big day in August, Ashley was rushed to Doctors Hospital in Columbus for near-kidney failure.

Although her condition steadily improved, Ashley's stay at Doctors Hospital meant she would have to miss her own wedding day. So Ashley's nurses devised an ambitious plan and asked us to help them create a memorable wedding day experience for the couple. The twist was that the ceremony and reception would take place inside the hospital in less than 24 hours, and ARAMARK Healthcare was going to cater it.

It was Friday afternoon by the time Niles Gebele, ARAMARK Healthcare's director of nutrition services at Doctors, got the news. No new food deliveries would arrive until after the weekend. The challenge was clear: create a delicious, upscale menu with no preparation or planning with only the ingredients they had on hand.

"We've always prided ourselves on providing the very best patient service," said Gebele, "and this situation was no different. It just meant we had to be more creative."

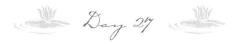

Overnight, Gebele and his team pulled together an impressive menu for the bride and groom and their 50 guests. At the reception they served beef Wellington, chicken saté, finger sandwiches, a fruit and cheese platter, and sparkling cider. They also decorated the reception area with centerpieces and flowers that were still beautiful and fresh from an earlier hospital event.

Our client, with whom we've had a seven-year relationship, was delighted with the outcome. In a thank you note to the ARAMARK Healthcare team following the reception, she wrote, "You created wonderful food, a wonderful atmosphere, but even more importantly, a beautiful memory for this couple."

—*Submitted by Stephanie Cziczo, ARAMARK Healthcare, Downers Grove, IL*

"Never underestimate the difference you can make."

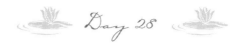

Out of the Mouths of Babes

When I chose to become a nurse, it was a decision by default (as I had originally planned to be a physical education teacher)—but one I have never regretted. I have had a fantastic career in nursing filled with memorable moments that attest to the impact we make on those we care for.

I loved working at Scottish Rite Pediatric Hospital in Atlanta, Georgia, as a float RN because it allowed me to care for all ages and illnesses. I have always had a passion for pediatrics because children give back so much more than they receive and because they are so versatile and resilient under the most devastating circumstances.

One morning I was going through my usual routine with an eight-year-old boy who had diabetes insipidus and a neurogenic bladder. The routine first consisted of a bath, during which I would have to firmly and repeatedly stop him from drinking his bath water. Individuals with this condition often have an unquenchable thirst and will drink any liquid available. I would then proceed to catheterize him, give him an injection, and literally blow about two ccs of a hormonal preparation through a tube up his nose.

Despite his situation, he was a very active boy and dressing him proved to be as difficult as trying to stop him from drinking his bath water and blowing medication into his nose. It took a bit of firm, but gentle coercing, and only after

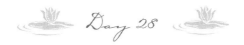

I had plucked him out of the air as he jumped around his bed—taunting me with cries of "you can't catch me"—was I usually able to dress him.

One day, when we had finished this harried routine and I was dressing him on his bed, he was standing at near-eye level with me when he put his arms around my neck, gave me a peck on the cheek, and said, "I really love you." I nearly died on the spot from overwhelming joy. Only a child could offer a reward of such value after being tormented with a catheter into his bladder, a needle in his leg, a tube up his nose, denial of sought-after water, and being plucked out of the air while pretending to be Superman. I knew at that moment I had made the right choice to become a nurse.

—Submitted by Durinda Durr, Rome Memorial Hospital, Rome, NY

"Never underestimate the difference you can make."

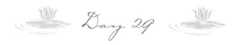

A Letter from a Mt. Airy Family Member

O ne of your staff from Environmental Services happened to be cleaning the room when my sister was experiencing a tearful period during my mom's final days. This loving woman offered her comfort in her beautifully accented English. When my sister asked her to say a little prayer for Mom, she responded sweetly, "Oh, I always pray for each patient and family, as I clean each day."

—Submitted by Bonnie Duncan, Mercy Hospital Mt. Airy, Cincinnati, OH

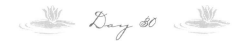

Getting Mrs. C
to the Wedding

My name is Kate Keohane and I am a registered nurse at New England Baptist Hospital on the medical-surgical unit. I have worked here for almost four years.

Over the course of my tenure here, I have treated a wide array of patients with issues ranging from cardiac to oncology to general medicine. Although I've only been a nurse for a short period of time—previously, I was a nursing assistant—I have had many experiences that have touched my heart. The story I share here is one that reminds me of all that is good with our chosen field.

Mrs. C was an oncology patient who frequently visited Four East due to an initial diagnosis of breast cancer in 1998, which had since spread to her lungs and brain. She needed to have part of her lung removed, which limited her lung capacity and caused breathing problems.

As she was only 44 years old, her hospitalization was not only emotional for her family but trying on our staff as well. Mrs. C was the mother of four children—all under the age of 19—and the loving wife of a caring and encouraging husband.

Around the beginning of January, Mrs. C was admitted to the intensive care unit for complications of her spreading cancer. She had been in and out of New England Baptist many times while trying to conquer her illness; however, this hospital stay would be an experience quite different from the others.

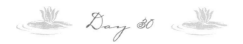

When she had stabilized, she was transferred from the ICU to my floor. When she arrived on our floor, we all took one glance at her and knew the prognosis was not promising.

Over the next couple of weeks, she had many critical instances where we thought she might not make it another day. She would then surprise all of us and show remarkable resilience and fight another day. As she stayed into the month of March, I was frequently assigned to work with her.

One day a discussion with Mr. C revealed that she had set a goal to attend her daughter's wedding in California, which was scheduled for the upcoming May. Although she knew she was terminally ill, she wanted more than anything to take part in this special occasion.

During one of the treatments, she received a severe setback and we were unsure as to whether or not she would make it through this experience. At this time, one of the physicians noticed her rapidly declining health status and pulled Mr. C aside to advise him to gather his family and contemplate the possibilities of moving the wedding to a closer location.

Considering that Mrs. C had become smaller and frailer, she would not be able to get out of bed, much less travel on a plane across the country. Taking the advice of the physician, Mr. C called his daughter and his wife's parents to fly in from California to be at Mrs. C's bedside.

In a couple of weeks, they were able to plan a small ceremony that Mrs. C could attend. As the wedding grew nearer, Mrs. C showed remarkable courage. With the assistance of the physical therapy team and her devoted husband, she was able to get out of bed daily.

Although hindered by her difficulty in breathing, she still displayed mental and physical strength to get up every day. There was no chance she was going to

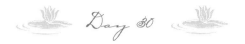

miss her daughter's wedding. As the date neared, many of the health care professionals at New England Baptist were busy planning her possible discharge so she could go from the hospital directly to the wedding ceremony and then home with Hospice.

Since I was most likely going to be the nurse the day of her departure, I knew that we would have to get Mrs. C ready for the wedding because her family would be busy with all the other intricacies of the day.

I requested that she be my only patient that day until she left for the ceremony. With the patience, compassion, and understanding of all the other nurses I work with, we all decided that my preparation time with Mrs. C was in her best interest.

I talked with Mr. C for a couple of hours and tried to the best of my ability to let him know what he may expect when they finally got home, how life with the Hospice team would be, and what to expect as Mrs. C began to pass on.

Heartachingly, he explained to me that he never thought this day would come and he always was hopeful that she would recover. This was overwhelming for him, and I wanted to help as best I could.

Knowing how hard she had fought to just stay alive until this day, I wanted to make Mrs. C look beautiful for her daughter's wedding. With the help of one of the nursing assistants, we got her showered, dressed, applied her makeup, and styled her hair. She looked more like a mother about to attend her daughter's wedding than a terminally ill cancer patient just out of her hospital bed.

When the ambulance driver came to pick up Mrs. C, everyone lined the hallways and remarked on how beautiful she looked. Her husband was so thankful to everyone. I think he hugged every single person on the floor. After they had thanked us all, tears began to stream down my cheeks as I watched

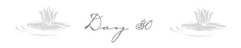

Mrs. C disappear into the distance as she was being wheeled down the hallway.

In the profession of nursing, there can be some very frustrating days and some truly remarkable ones. I have come to the realization that no matter how many bad days I may have, one day, like the day I made a difference with Mrs. C, makes all the hard ones worthwhile. This day was about much more than I even realized at the time. It was about life in general. One life that was, unfortunately, going to be taken from this world much too soon, another one just starting out as a newlywed, and the fact that my life intersected with both are the reasons I became a nurse…and love being one.

—Submitted by *April Hannon, New England Baptist Hospital, Boston, MA*

"Never underestimate the difference you can make."

Share Your Own Story

Throughout this book, you've read some stories that beautifully illustrate the life-changing power of a career in health care. Do you have a story you'd like to get down on paper—a story about an experience that connected you back to purpose, worthwhile work, and making a difference? Please feel free to write it on this page…and take a moment to appreciate the fact that you're a big part of what's right in health care.

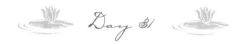

Going It Alone

I met Tony at a free clinic in town where I volunteer regularly as a nurse. When I met him, Tony was a very thin, frail 40-year-old, who had a very round, full abdomen, due to late stage liver disease. The physician and I worked with our hospital to get Tony's abdomen drained by the hospital radiologist. Startlingly, after only four days, Tony's abdomen was as large as ever, and it needed to be drained again. We attempted to get a shunt placed in him, but unfortunately, we were unable to do so.

Tony had never had his own place before and had just recently been able to get an apartment where he lived with his pet bird. He was working as a dishwasher at a local restaurant, which allowed him to pay his rent, but not much else. He was adamant about going to work each day even though it was difficult for him to ride his bike, his only mode of transportation, because of the discomfort he experienced when he hit a rough place in the road.

We continued to work with Tony, delaying the drawing off of the fluid as long as possible each time to avoid weakening him further. Tests confirmed he was suffering from terminal cirrhosis of the liver. In late October, I assisted the radiologist in drawing off more fluid. Tony was so relieved and thanked us profusely. He told us that it was his birthday and that he had just received the best present ever.

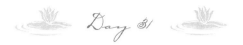

The physician at the free clinic asked me to assist him in talking with Tony about his prognosis, which was grim. Because I had worked with Tony often, the doctor wanted me to tell him that he was dying, that he had only several weeks or a few months to live, and that we needed to transition him to hospice care. First, I said a prayer for strength and then spoke with Tony. I asked him if he had any family. He said he was estranged from his family and had no contact with his mother. He said he would have to go through this experience alone.

On December 26th, Tony was admitted to our hospital for terminal care. The transition to hospice care went smoothly, and they were able to fast-track his disability payments, which allowed Tony to stop working. I went in to visit him and found that he was very concerned that his pet bird was not being fed and that his rent was not being paid. I referred his requests to the hospice nurse and knowing that these things were taken care of eased his mind. Providing him with even a little peace made me happy.

At this point, Tony looked so thin, probably weighing less than 100 pounds, but with a huge protruding abdomen. He was quite uncomfortable. He had one last consult with a specialist, who told him there was nothing else we could do. When Tony heard the last physician's report, he quietly went back to his room, where he died peacefully the next morning.

I truly learned a lot from Tony throughout the time I spent with him. He taught me to be thankful for family, to try as hard as you can for as along as you can, and to never give up!

—Submitted by Elaine Haynes, Carolinas Medical Center

"Never underestimate the difference you can make."

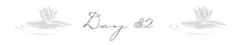

A Root Beer Float Is the Best Medicine

I am a radiation therapist. Recently, I started working with a new inpatient—a female with bone cancer in her shoulder and femur. She is 73 years old and a former lawyer. For most of her life, she had been fiercely independent. After being admitted to the hospital and losing much of that independence, she became very unhappy and she wasn't afraid to let everyone know how she felt.

One day, after her treatment, she mentioned under her breath that she would love to have a root beer float. The next day before her treatment, I brought in the makings for a root beer float and gave her one after her treatment. She was shocked to see that someone would do this for her, and you could see the walls that she had built around her fade away. After that day, she became a very pleasant lady.

My interactions with this patient have really taught me the importance of listening. Nine times out of ten simply listening to them is all they want you to do. And, through listening, we create great patient-caregiver relationships.

—Submitted by Scott Slous, Susan B. Allen Memorial Hospital, El Dorado, KS

"Never underestimate the difference you can make."

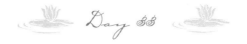

Kim's Caring

In our hospital's region, our facility paved the way in the area of magnetic resonance (MR) breast imaging. As we began seeing more and more women for MR breast imaging, Kim, one of our MR technologists, felt the need to become more than just the technologist who scanned them. Since the majority of the patients were near her age, they really hit a place in her heart and she wanted to give them more than just the run-of-the-mill care. She wanted to be there for them, to provide them with information about their newly diagnosed disease, and to let them know that she was always thinking about them.

Kim took it upon herself to make Breast Cancer Awareness bracelets for each MR breast patient. She purchased the beads and accessories necessary with her own money and made the bracelets on her own time. Kim gives each patient a bracelet after her scan. Accompanying the bracelet is a hand written card and a tag that reads, "Together We Stand Strong."

When these women reach our facility for the MR procedure, they are newly diagnosed with breast cancer. Some patients received this devastating diagnosis just days, or even hours, earlier. Naturally, they have lots of questions. Kim searched for information about breast cancer that could be put together and given to these patients. She met with our oncology service line and developed a packet that includes information about the cancer itself, support groups, inspirational stories, etc. Even if they choose not to read it in the very beginning,

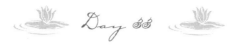

we've received a lot of positive feedback from women saying they are grateful the information is there for them when they are ready.

As radiologic technologists, we are not sufficiently trained on how to interact with patients, like these women, who are often distraught, angry, and confused when they come to us. Kim wanted to solve this problem. She felt it was important that all of the radiologic technologists knew how to give them the support they needed and to learn what to say to them when they opened up. To get answers, she organized an inservice training conducted by the oncology RN staff for the entire Diagnostic Center. The training helped give the technologists insight and guidance on how to care for these patients. Everyone learned the different stages of the emotional roller coaster these patients are on, gained a better understanding of this life-changing event, and learned more about the fear of recurrence that many of these patients have. The oncology staff provided the technologists with information on how to listen, and the importance of taking extra time with these patients if they finally open up and need to get their emotions out.

Naturally, we have received many letters and phone calls from patients whose lives Kim has touched by her actions. She has kept in contact and even formed friendships with some of her patients. Regardless of the patient, Kim always goes that extra mile to make sure they are well taken care of. For example, one patient mentioned to Kim how cold she always felt. Kim found a solution. Prior to this patient's appointment for a follow-up scan, Kim took the time to make her a blanket using Breast Cancer Awareness material. The patient sent her a card thanking her for the blanket and also for thinking of her.

Kim is an extraordinary technologist with a heart of gold. Her drive to let these women know that there are people out there that care about them has had

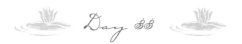
a tremendous impact on many of their lives. I have been in health care for over 20 years and have never met another technologist who has gone to the extent Kim has to make a difference in the lives of their patients. I truly believe that Kim is an exception, and I am very proud to have her on our team.

—*Submitted by DeAnn Utter, Midlands Hospital, Papillion, NE*

"Never underestimate the difference you can make."

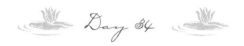

Tale of Two Hospitals

*I*n 1999, my grandson was born via C-section at Parma Community Hospital. During the procedure, he aspirated some amniotic fluid and, as a result, was having respiratory difficulty. He was subsequently sent via ambulance to Fairview Hospital.

I would like to comment on the kindness of the neonatologist, Dr. L. He came with the ambulance crew, checked out my grandson, and took two Polaroid pictures. At first I thought the pictures were probably for security purposes, but he laid both pictures on my daughter's chest as she was still lying down due to just having had a C-section. He took the pictures so that both she and my son-in-law could have one while their newborn baby was at a different hospital. The gesture was so touching that it brought tears to my eyes.

As my son-in-law and I walked with my grandson and the ambulance crew on the way out of the hospital to the ambulance, most of the hospital employees that we passed along our route told us "good luck." Their well-wishes were very important to us during such a difficult time.

The next day, when my son-in-law was allowed to hold his son for the first time, the Fairview Hospital staff videotaped the event and sent the video over for my daughter so that she could share in the moment. Although she couldn't be there herself, she still got to witness the wonderful experience. I will never forget

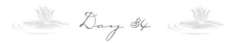
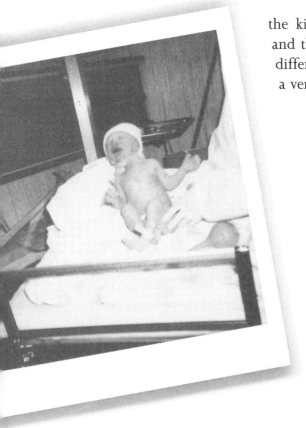

the kindness and thoughtfulness of that doctor and the staff at both hospitals. They made a big difference and provided a lot of comfort during a very difficult situation.

—Submitted by Mary Miller,
University Hospitals of Cleveland, Cleveland, OH

"Never underestimate the difference you can make."

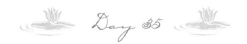

Correcting a Mistake

One day a very irate patient called our facility's Patient Financial Services Customer Service Department. It turned out that the woman had every right to be irate. Through a series of errors surely initiated by Murphy's Law, the patient's account had been placed with a collection agency and her wages had been garnished. The problem was—she actually owed nothing.

The patient was trying to purchase a house but was finding the process difficult with this unpaid debt hanging over her head. Suzanne Bowling was the customer service representative who took the very volatile call. Suzanne was so touched by the plight of the patient that she came to me, her boss at the time, and asked what we could do to make things right and to assist her in the purchase of her house. We got the agency to close the account, wrote a letter stating she owed nothing to the hospital, reversed the garnishment, and cut her a check to pay her back the money that had been taken out of her paycheck.

I then asked Suzanne to accompany me to the lady's work. On the way, we stopped and bought some flowers. We presented the patient with the money, the letter, the flowers, and a sincere apology. The patient was very touched by our efforts to correct the errors, and when Suzanne gave the patient a big hug, the patient broke down and cried tears of joy and appreciation. This was one of the most rewarding service recovery experiences in my 27 years of financial services experience.

—Submitted by Lee Evins

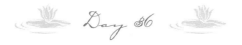
Act of Kindness

*M*r. N was a patient in our telemetry unit who had been admitted with chest pain and eventually experienced a heart attack. On the day of his discharge, we found out that Mr. N was homeless. He had no way to go back and forth to the doctor or to even get his medicine filled so that he could live a better life.

The staff of our unit took it among themselves to collect money for his bus passes. The physician even kicked in. Peggy, our assistant nurse manager, clocked out on her own time and went to the bus station to pick up enough bus passes for this patient to go back and forth for his doctor's visit.

I can't tell you how much this simple act of kindness meant to this patient. He could not thank us enough. It is just one of the many wonderful things the nurses on our telemetry unit do for our patients.

—Submitted by *Kathy Beaver, Frye Regional Medical Center, Hickory, NC*

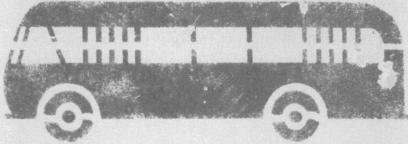

"Never underestimate the difference you can make."

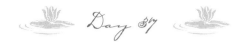

Lizzy, the Pet Volunteer

We had a volunteer that worked with our agency for five years. Her name was Lizzy and she was little different from our usual volunteers. You see Lizzy was a Shih Tzu, weighing only 8 lbs. but with enough personality to fill a room. She worked very hard at her job—going to the hospital, greeting people in the waiting rooms, cheering up very ill patients, and bringing a smile to everybody who saw her.

She was a certified pet therapist and everyone could tell she was very proud of her accomplishments. I remember the first visit to our hospital. We arrived on the Pediatric Care Unit (PCU) and announced and introduced ourselves. Dressed to impress, Lizzy was in her new vest and had her name badge on, looking very professional, and taking her job very seriously.

We asked for the patient list so that Lizzy could immediately begin her mission to cheer up as many patients as possible. We were told we could visit every room except for 201, which held a woman who had had a stroke and who would not know we were there. We visited all the other rooms and Lizzy was well received by all who saw her. She would get in bed with them while they would pet and cuddle her and talked about their own pets—past and present.

We stopped by room 201 on our way out to see if Lizzy could be of any comfort to this "nonresponsive" patient. Her eyes were open so we stepped in and I started talking to her—no response. I introduced Lizzy and told room 201

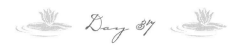

what and who Lizzy was, and then, I reached out and placed this patient's hand on Lizzy. We got a huge response—the lady moved her fingers in Lizzy's hair and made grunting noises that sounded like excitement. We stayed and visited for a while, and I think this was our best visit of the day. For the next five years, Lizzy and I continued to go to the hospital, nursing homes, and to visit homebound patients to help bring a smile or ray of sunshine to people who otherwise may not have had much to smile about.

Sadly, Lizzy became ill in May 2006 with an auto-immune disease. She passed away in August after a very brave and hard fight. I cannot begin to explain the impact this little bundle of joy had on this home care nurse and the other home care staff she hung out with not to mention the patients themselves. She had a special way of greeting all the staff as they entered the office and immediately brightened their day. Helping them to forget even for a little while about the difficult patients they had seen that day and helping to reduce the stress that we have as health care workers.

—*Anonymous Contributor, CMH Regional Health System Home Care Services*

"Never underestimate the difference you can make."

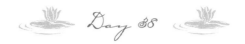
BREAKING POINT

aking an impact on someone's life is a powerful way to realize the effect your words and actions have on your patients. What we say, when we say it, and to whom can make a vital difference in the lives of our patients, and sometimes, we do not realize it until later.

I have been in health care management for the last 25 years and I've had the experience of being on the receiving end of health care. I have been a cancer survivor for more than 13 years and went through intense chemotherapy and radiation. During that time, many of my wonderful caregivers bestowed on me the blessing of quality care in every way possible. I have always been a very positive person and dealt with my treatments the way I dealt and continue to deal with life by keeping an upbeat, positive attitude.

My story starts very innocently. One day a patient presented at our outpatient registration area where I am the manager. If you've never had cancer, you may not know this, but there is a sort of kinship that forms between the people that have been through cancer treatments and those that are in the midst of cancer treatment. This patient in our outpatient area was having a bad day, not much was going right for her. She was very upset with the process, was having problems with her insurance, and was just generally feeling very down. After completing the process, she began to cry.

I recognized that she had reached her breaking point, and I was so glad I was there to help, because I had had several "breaking points" during the course of my treatment. I asked her to come into my office. I said, "Let's chat, sort it all out, and have a cup of coffee." During those 10 minutes, we became friends. She was able to vent to a completely uninvolved person who knew just how she felt. And the experience wasn't only helpful for her, I benefited too. It was a cathartic moment for me to stop and remember just how lucky I am as a survivor.

Over the next few months, during her multiple trips to the hospital, she would poke in her head to say, "Hello." We would exchange hugs, and one day she said, "You get me to come here for this—otherwise I would have stopped a while ago." She went on to tell me that the day we first met, she was deciding whether to proceed with her treatment, but seeing me—someone who had been there and "came out the better" for it—was enough to convince her that it was worth it.

I was stunned. I had no idea that I had impacted her life this much. I held in my emotions until I was able to return to my office and then I just let go and began to cry. One simple chat and a cup of coffee had impacted someone's life, and I had no idea.

Sadly, as time went on, I saw my friend start to fail. Ultimately, she was not able to beat it, but the fight she fought was so important. I am proud to have been, though it may have been in a simple way, a part of her fight. I miss seeing her face. Nothing else during the course of my career has had such a large impact on my life. I try to tell this story to everyone who works in health care. You may not always receive one-on-one recognition of it, but our impact as health care workers is so critical, important, and necessary.

—*Submitted by Stephen Hartman, Paoli Hospital, Paoli, PA*

"Never underestimate the difference you can make."

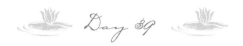

Acting Like Family

*I*n the neonatal intensive care unit (NICU) at Methodist North Hospital, there was a premature infant experiencing respiratory difficulties. The baby's family had no extended family to provide social support. Angela Warren, who works in the NICU at North, bonded with the baby's mother. She gave the mother her home telephone number and told her to call if she needed to talk.

Soon after, the baby was transferred to Le Bonheur for a tracheostomy because of its inability to be weaned off of the ventilator. The baby's mom, alone and frightened at Le Bonheur during her baby's surgery, called Angela at home to talk. In order to comfort the woman, Angela sent her own child to her mother-in-law's to stay and went to Le Bonheur to sit with the mother during the surgery even though it was her day off.

Since that time, Angela has maintained contact with the mother, and the baby has since gotten better and has been discharged from Le Bonheur.

—Submitted by Ruth-Ann Hale, Methodist Le Bonheur Germantown Hospital, Germantown, TN

"Never underestimate the difference you can make."

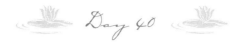

JOE

*I*n January 2004, during the "Janet Jackson" Super Bowl show, I received a telephone call from Kansas informing me that my father was ill and was being taken by ambulance to Westmoreland Hospital. I soon learned that Kansas was in the midst of one of the worst blizzards that had occurred in many years. My relatives were snowed in and they could not get to my father. As my father's condition deteriorated, I knew I had to get to Kansas. My husband tried to convince me that if my Kansas relatives couldn't get to my father, how was I going to get there? I didn't know the answer, but I knew I had to be by my father's side. Being a southern California girl, I had never driven or flown in snow, let alone a blizzard.

I got a flight arranged out of Los Angeles that would land in Kansas City. Then I called every rental car company I could find, because I would have to drive 200 miles to Westmoreland, Kansas. None of the rental car companies could or would tell me the weather conditions and whether I would be able to reach my father. My relatives also told me that I was nuts for trying.

Frustrated and crying, I called Westmoreland Hospital. My father's nurse referred me to "Joe" the ambulance driver. He told me how much ice was on the ground and the snow conditions. He informed me that it should be smooth sailing on the turnpike and that it might get slick on Route 99. Joe told me not

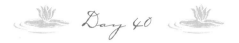

to worry, because he would come get me if I got stuck. Then he gave me his home number to call if I needed any help.

My father passed away, but I will never forget Joe. I wrote him a letter praising his compassion, and I sent it to the hospital's CEO. Joe felt that he was only doing his job, but in my opinion, he was doing much more than that. He was helping a daughter get to her dying father. Health care needs more Joes—a man with dedication, passion, and a true "fire-fighter!"

—Submitted by Joan Juarez, Little Company of Mary, Providence, RI

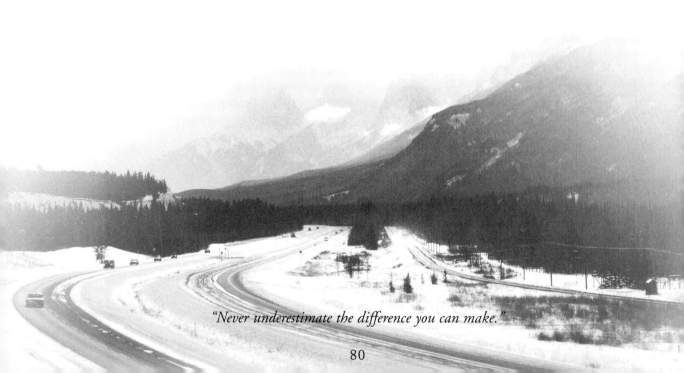

"Never underestimate the difference you can make."

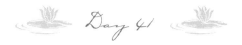
A Sacred Encounter

On a Sunday morning, junior volunteer Stephanie Jaw was dispatching for the Volunteer Messenger Service when she received an unusual call—a terminally ill ICU patient wanted some company so that he, as the nurse put it, "would not die alone." It is seldom that Volunteer Messenger Service receives calls to provide company for patients, but nonetheless Stephanie accepted the call and proceeded to the ICU—worrying the whole way there about what to say and how to act. Her time with the patient proved to be very special and beneficial for both. Several hours would pass by before she would return to the Volunteer Office, telling others with enthusiasm how friendly and kind the patient, Mr. M, had been.

Stephanie returned the next day, along with her friend, Jessica Wen, another junior volunteer and a fellow Junior Leadership member, to visit Mr. M again. This time, however, they brought him a homemade card, complete with a photograph of Stephanie and Mr. M. The two would spend the next few hours keeping Mr. M company while swapping stories and sharing laughter, all on their personal time.

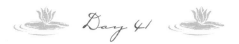

Stephanie and Jessica created a scrapbook and had planned on delivering it to Mr. M the following week. Sadly, Mr. M would pass on just two hours before the two arrived to deliver their gift of compassion. Stephanie and Jessica went above and beyond to help make Mr. M's last days less lonely. They are an example of what the volunteers of St. Joseph Hospital strive to be. Stephanie said that Mr. M "will forever be my inspirational hero." I think I speak for the volunteers when I say that these junior volunteers are both inspirational heroes to us all.

—Submitted by Micah Ting, St. Joseph Hospital, Orange, CA

"Never underestimate the difference you can make."

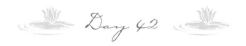

MAKING A DIFFERENCE

As Admission Coordinator for Central Intake and Referral of Covenant Hospice in Pensacola, FL, many people from the community call me looking for help.

One morning, I got a call from the bartender at the Moose Lodge here in Pensacola. They have a campground on the property where members of the Lodge can camp. The bartender called to tell me that there was a man camped there that was very sick. She explained that he had told them that he had a "bad liver" and was also estranged from his family. She said he was living in horrible conditions, and that the members were trying to help him, but that there was only so much that they could to. She told me that she thought he was dying.

I tried to get a doctor's order several times by calling the Veteran's Clinic where the man had gone before, but I couldn't get any one to answer my calls. I couldn't stand knowing that there was someone that needed our help and was possibly dying alone. So, I sent one of our nurses to the Lodge to see about the man even though I did not have a doctor's order. When the nurse got there she called me and said, "This man is dying, and he is living in filth. We have to get him out of here!"

I called our hospice doctor. She gave me an order to admit him to our services, and we transferred him to the Joyce Goldenberg Hospice Inpatient

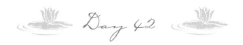

Facility. All of this took only two hours. They cleaned him, fed him, and medicated him. He died two days later, comfortable, clean, and safe.

Best of all, he was not alone. He had a peaceful death because a few strangers cared enough about another human being to step up and make a difference in his life.

A Heart of Hospice now hangs proudly in the Moose Lodge in Pensacola. Strangers truly can make a difference!

—Submitted by Debbie Magyarosi, Covenant Hospice, Pensacola, FL

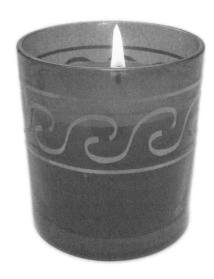

"Never underestimate the difference you can make."

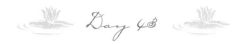

Personal Dignity Matters

A department supervisor was driving into work one morning when she received a call from a department lead. Although this type of "preemptive" call was a somewhat routine start to this supervisor's day, the situation I'm about to describe was not.

The lead said that a male patient had been brought to the facility's Emergency Department (ED) who appeared to be either homeless or indigent based on the state of his clothing. The caregivers had to peel and cut off the man's clothing to even begin diagnosis and treatment. Upon learning of the situation, the lead said she had commenced taking up a departmental collection to help buy the patient some clothes. When the supervisor heard this, she decided to help out, too.

Before arriving at work, she stopped at a local K-Mart and using personal funds, she purchased undergarments, pants, a shirt, socks, and shoes. She hoped a medium size would work, based on the minimal detail received about the patient's build. Immediately upon arriving at the facility, she went directly to the ED to bring the clothes to a somewhat surprised group of caregivers.

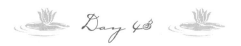

When asked to recount these actions later, the supervisor simply stated, "If in the end, he is well enough to leave the hospital, at least he can do so with some personal dignity." For both of these health care professionals, this way of thinking was not incidental. It represents how both of these women have consistently viewed their respective service support roles of direct patient care. They fully understand that "what's right" is always about that which is right for the patient.

—Submitted by Michael Rossi, Crittenton Hospital Medical Center, Rochester, MI

"Never underestimate the difference you can make."

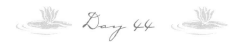

A Fire Starter in Action

*I*t's not always easy being a Fire Starter. I attended "What's Right in Health Care" approximately four years ago, came back to my organization, and attended the Studer Institute with nine other employees from my hospital. I have learned through experience that it only takes one person to "start the fire." This is my story.

I was on my way to a very important planning meeting and was running late. My vice president and several directors would be attending the meeting and the last thing I wanted was to walk in late. I am an educator with a background in counseling and social work and I pride myself on being a high performer with strong values and ethics around accountability.

On this particular day, I found myself in one of the large medical office buildings attached to the hospital. I was practically running down the hallway to make it to my meeting on time. I passed by an obese woman in her late fifties, walking with the aid of a walker. She was using oxygen and was clearly out of breath. I saw the panic on her face as she spoke with her adult son in the hallway. Her son was pushing a stroller with a very small infant and was obviously unable to assist his mother and care for the baby at the same time. I had seen that look many times before. It was a look that screamed, "I'm lost and I can't take one more step."

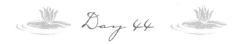

Even though I was late for a very important meeting, the Fire Starter in me stopped dead in my tracks. I knew it was the right thing to do, so I introduced myself, "Hi, my name is Marilyn and I work here at St. Rita's. I would be happy to give you some assistance. I have the time." Tears streamed down Mrs. R's face as she explained that she didn't know where her physician's office was located and she wasn't feeling well. The physician that she was seeking was located three medical office buildings away from where we were currently located. "I will take you there myself," I confidently replied.

I took Mrs. R's arm and quickly found her a place to sit as I retrieved a wheelchair. I needed a special wheelchair to accommodate her needs and I found one two floors away and returned to where I had left Mrs. R. I helped her into the wheelchair as her son left with the baby in the stroller to move their car to the correct medical office building parking lot.

The trip to Mrs. R's physician's office was a long one, or so it seemed at the time. The wheelchair escort was not an easy one. I'm 5'7" and 125 lbs. with not much upper body strength to move someone her size. Each office building is connected with an incline to the next building so it was uphill all the way. I pushed with all of my strength and wondered if I might need the oxygen myself. Thoughts began to race through my head and we pushed onward: *What if I keel over with a heart attack and Mrs. R rolls downhill? What if something happens to Mrs. R on the way to her physician's office? What if my own physical strength gives out? How am I going to call for help? I'm not a nurse!* Never once did I stop to think: "How am I going to explain missing my important meeting?" As a Fire Starter, I was doing the right thing and everything within me glowed with passion. I knew that my purpose that day was assisting Mrs. R, who was now no longer a stranger.

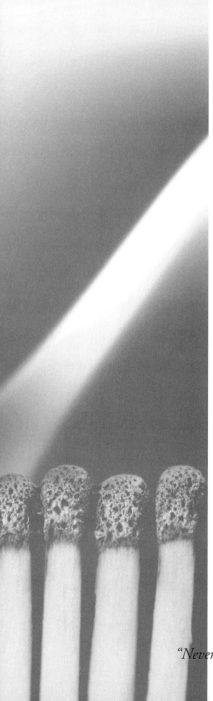

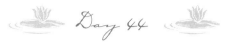

Helping the Mrs. Rs of the world is why I went into health care—not as a nurse, but as someone who cares about other people and about making a difference. Mrs. R and I arrived safely at her physician's office about twenty-five minutes later. When we arrived, her son and grandbaby were there to meet us. Mrs. R grabbed my hand and I knelt down beside her. "No one has ever had the kind of compassion for me that you have shown," she said. "I don't know what I would have done if you hadn't stopped to help me. Thank you so much."

I may never see Mrs. R again, but she is a friend for life. I will never forget her...and I know that I made a difference that day.

—Submitted by Marilyn Frueh, St. Rita's Medical Center, Lima, OH

"Never underestimate the difference you can make."

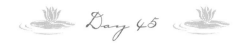

Changing My Perception of Nursing

M̲y nursing career started out very stressfully. I always considered myself a caring and compassionate person, which was one of the reasons I chose nursing as a profession. My workload just seemed so heavy at the time and that sometimes inhibited me from utilizing my basic human qualities that contributed to my being an excellent nurse.

Thankfully, one experience changed this for me. It was a typical night on my inpatient unit at a Louisville hospital. I came in to work for my 7 p.m. shift, in charge and assigned seven patients. Several had the diagnosis of chest pain, one was a DNR who was dying, and then there was the "VAD patient," as the staff referred to him.

This patient was critically ill but stable. He was a man in his late 30s who had acquired cardiomyopathy. I will refer to him by his first name, Chris. He had been sick only for a short time before he died at home and was resuscitated by an emergency response team. Chris was flown from his home in Kansas to a Louisville hospital, where he was implanted with a ventricular assist device (VAD). This device did the workload of his left ventricle while he awaited a heart transplant.

He was on a transplant list, awaiting a suitable donor. Prior to that night, I had never cared for Chris. I had only heard stories from other staff that he was grumpy and unpleasant. He was a large man with curly red hair and a beard to match. He looked as if he were straight off the pages of a biker magazine. Not

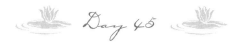

only did I consider him scary, he was connected to a VAD. One false move by me, and it was over.

Normally, I probably would have assessed him first being that he was my sickest patient and a full code. Instead, I checked his rhythm on the heart monitor and proceeded to my other patient rooms first. After completing my other assessments, I went to assess him. He was as grumpy as reported and had very little to say to me. I performed my work as required, gave him his medications, and hurried out of his room. I had to make several trips in there during the remainder of my shift, but I kept each visit as brief as possible because I did not want to upset the "scary biker man."

Avoiding any possibility of conflict, I gave him what he requested and probed no further. The night was uneventful with Chris. I was thrilled when my shift was over. After my initial night with Chris, I found myself assigned to his care more often.

With time, I learned a little more about his family dynamics from casual conversation. He had a wife and a teenaged son and daughter, all living at home in Kansas. They owned farmland where they bred and raised heifers. His wife had to continue working to pay bills while he was hospitalized. Once Chris had been stabilized on the VAD, she had returned to Kansas. She flew to Louisville only on weekends to visit. Frankly, I was timid about meeting her as well. Once I met Kareen, however, I started to see Chris for the person he really was. He was happy when his wife came to visit. When Kareen went home, he was grumpy just as before.

As they grew to know me better and respect me as a nurse, they shared more of their life story with me. Chris was required to stay on our unit in the hospital while awaiting a transplant for at least six months. In that time, more VAD patients

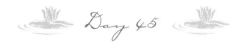

were placed on our unit and they all followed one another's situations closely. When one suffered a stroke, the others knew and worried.

In growing to know Chris as a person, not just a patient, I too felt his concerns. He was not grumpy, as we had all earlier believed. He was rightfully and understandably depressed. He had a great life. He worked hard and loved his family. That was all abruptly interrupted when he became ill. He knew he cheated death once and was scared he would not be so lucky the next time.

Once I opened my eyes to the entire picture and took the time to see what was so clearly in front of me, my life was changed forever. I no longer went in to see Chris last at night because I dreaded going into his room. I went in there last so I could spend more time with him. I would go in his room, sit down, talk about the day, my life, his life, joke, laugh, and change his television to the station where my boyfriend would be on as he hosted the nightly lottery drawings. He counseled me just as I did him. Something came alive in him during those months.

After befriending me and several other staff members, he no longer had that sadness in his eyes. He missed his family so much, as they did him, but the incredible thing was that we became their extended family. We celebrated with them and we cried with them. When we learned of their anniversary, I brought in takeout food on my day off, and we set up a candlelit dinner for them to share. The hospital set up field trips for him where he could go to lunch or shopping with one of the nurses for short periods of time for a change of scenery.

That is when Chris became healthy. Prior to his transplant, his new spirit prepared him for the surgery and recovery that awaited him. I will never forget the morning we got the call that they had a matching donor heart for Chris. I was just going off duty when the transplant team called with the news. Kareen had

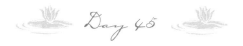

just flown back to Kansas the night before. Tears filled my eyes as I hung up the phone after speaking with the doctors. I got to tell Chris the moment he had been waiting for was finally here, after all of these months.

Several of us went into his room and shared the news. To this day I'm not sure if he really accepted it. He had been waiting for so long and had thought about giving up so many times, I think he truly wondered if there would ever be a day he would receive his new heart. Of course, the first thing we did was allow him to call his wife personally. We told her to get back on a plane as soon as possible. She was nervous the entire return trip, worrying if she would make it on time and if this long-awaited moment was really going to happen. It was one of the most memorable days of my life—and I'm sure theirs as well.

Chris received his new heart and recovered well with few complications. He remained in Louisville for several months following the surgery. With time, he finally returned home with his family. Thankfully, we have kept in touch ever since.

Initially they had to return to Louisville occasionally for more tests. When they did, they stayed with me at my home. In return, I traveled to Kansas to visit with them on a few occasions. Chris and Kareen remain two of my closest friends.

It amazes me when I think of my first feelings of trepidation with caring for Chris, and how that has evolved into my having an extended family that has impacted my life so greatly. Providing nursing care for Chris opened my eyes to how I needed to reach out to more patients in similar situations, so I obtained a position on a similar unit at another hospital where I have remained. If I ever find myself doubting what contributions I am making, or asking myself why on earth I subject myself to the stress that is health care, I think of Chris. A school textbook

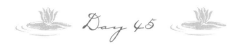

could not have prepared me any better for my experience with him. It was the actual experience itself that gave me valuable knowledge I could utilize with my patients in the future.

It opened my eyes to what is really important and valuable in the health care setting. As a nurse, I do have a purpose, my work is extremely worthwhile, and I really do make a difference in the lives of others every time I walk through the hospital doors. My career has since taken a different direction. I now work as the nurse manager of a Transitional Care Unit. Now I not only continue to make a difference in patients' lives, but am also afforded the opportunity to reinforce this with other health care workers. It is an honor and a privilege to be welcomed into others' lives and be afforded the opportunity to assist them during their time of need.

—Submitted by Mary Beth Polston, Baptist Hospital East, Louisville, KY

"Never underestimate the difference you can make."

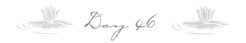

Mike

Mike was an RN in the neonatal intensive care unit (NICU) where I am currently the director. He grew up in Kentucky, loving the Kentucky Wildcats more than a normal person should. Before becoming an RN, he had served our country bravely in the army for fifteen years as an MP and a "dog handler."

Upon leaving the military, he decided that he wanted to become a nurse. His wife joked that he admitted it was because he liked seeing women in nurse's uniforms. Knowing Mike, there was a lot of truth to that statement. I came to learn, however, that it had more to do with his compassion and his desire to lessen the intense suffering felt by our tiny helpless patients and their families in the NICU.

Mike struggled through nursing school, having a wife and two young children at home. But his intense work ethic and perseverance kept him going. He graduated from nursing school and was very proud of his accomplishment.

Mike began his hospital career as a unit secretary on the post partum floor. He transferred into the NICU before he passed his nursing boards and worked with us as a unit secretary and nurse technician. He would do anything it took to get the job done. He never acted like he was above doing any task asked of him. Mike passed his nursing boards and began working with us as an RN in September 2001.

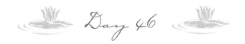

Mike was a favorite in our unit. He was a prankster, to say the least. He always knew when staff were feeling down or needed to feel silly. He would pop in with the craziest jokes, or say the corniest thing just to make you laugh. One of his trademarks was a set of "bubba teeth." The first time I saw him wearing them Mike came up behind me and smiled until I turned around to see who was there. It was both hilarious and frightening! He really enjoyed my reaction. Sometimes Mike would use the bubba teeth to cheer up the parents of his tiny patients.

In early 2004, Mike and his wife both developed sore throats. They both went to the doctor and began taking antibiotics. Mike's wife, Helene, got better. Mike did not. In addition to his throat pain, Mike began to suffer from severe neck pain and headaches. Several months later an MRI detected an abnormal growth that was the cause of his pain. The results were devastating—Mike was diagnosed with cancer of the neck and throat.

He began chemotherapy and soon became too sick to continue working. His wife had also had surgery recently and was still out of work. When Mike's paid leave ended, his insurance ended as well. His family was going to be devastated without his salary and benefits. My staff rallied together and donated a pool of vacation time and sick leave to him, so that his salary could continue and his insurance premiums would be paid. Mike underwent chemotherapy for the better part of two years. He was fighting for his life and refused to believe he would not win. The entire time, the staff of the NICU donated time to him, planned holiday dinners to take to his family, visited, sent cards, and worked to keep his spirits up.

During the 2005 holiday season, Mike was too sick to work. Our unit decided to take Christmas to him and his family. The only present Mike requested was a sponge bath from a nurse wearing a white uniform and fishnet stockings. We

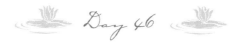

decided to surprise Mike by granting that wish. One of our male nurses dressed up in fishnet hose, heavy makeup, long nails, a wig, white uniform, and carried a sponge. Mike's children told us later that it was the first time they had seen their Dad laugh in weeks. As I was leaving the party I hugged Mike and asked him what I could do for him. His reply stunned me. "I want to come back to work," he said. His cancer made it very difficult to understand his speech so at first I thought that I had misunderstood him. I asked Mike to repeat himself and he calmly replied, "I said, I want to come back to work." I told him to come see me the next time he was at the hospital for his chemotherapy and we would talk.

Mike was in my office the next week. He was able to come back to work for the next seven months. Again, his work ethic was one you just don't see every day. He was receiving chemotherapy the entire time, and he still missed very few days. On a few occasions, I actually had to send him home from work because I could see that he did not feel up to being there. He still did not want to go home and I would feel bad for making him.

When Mike came into our hospital for the last time, the decision was made to move him into hospice care. The first person I called was the director of our chaplains, Skip Wisenbaker. I knew that I needed someone to tell me everything was going to be ok. Skip and his wonderful staff of chaplains, many of whom were volunteers, were always available to us and to Mike and his family. Mike was still denying that he was going to die. He was angry and he still had hopes of being cured. As health care professionals and chaplains we all knew he was dying but Mike refused to quit fighting. Instead, he wanted to go home and get ready for the next round of chemotherapy.

While he was in the hospice facility, he would try to communicate by speaking, but it became more and more difficult to understand him. We took him

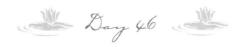

letter cards to use and we made sure he had a "write on board" so he could communicate with us. He would scribble notes to us that are so cherished today. A note to one of my nurses simply said, "I couldn't have done this without you."

Mike lost his battle with cancer on Nov. 11, 2006, which was Veterans' Day. He was buried in a beautiful new military cemetery in North Georgia on a hill overlooking Kentucky. Four doves were released at the funeral service to honor Mike. Three of the doves were dyed blue for Kentucky Wildcats. The fourth dove was white to signify Mike's spirit. The three blue doves immediately flew out of their cages and into the beautiful, clear blue sky. The white dove, however, did not want to leave its cage. Mike's wife, Helene, had to nudge the dove to get it to fly. When it finally flew out of the cage, the white dove flew a straight path to the female bugle corps personnel standing at attention on the hill. It was very comical seeing them so straight and serious, and then quickly having to dodge the dove! I am sure Mike was orchestrating the entire scene from somewhere in bubba-heaven.

As difficult as these months were for my staff, this painted a clear picture to me of what is right in health care. Mike went to nursing school to help heal the sick and comfort the grieving. It is when the healer is in need of healing themselves, and when the one who comforts the grieving is the one who needs the comforting, that the world changes. The uncertainty and unfairness of why things happen becomes real and strikes without warning. What is right is that Mike's co-workers and friends came together to support him and his family during their darkest hour. The compassion we learned in caring for others in the hospital setting was so beautifully displayed in the daily interactions and assistance provided for Mike and his family. I am proud of my staff. I am proud that Mike was able to return to work in a limited capacity for a few months before

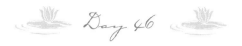

his death. I am proud of my facility for allowing me to make the decisions about whether he could work and how to schedule him.

I am in awe of Mike's positive outlook and the perseverance he showed for the two years he suffered through a devastating illness. I will never forget the love I saw showered on Mike and his family. Many days I saw posted notes reminding staff of Mike's need for more donated vacation time. These needs were always met. I learned secondhand of food drives underway for the holiday meals, of morale boosting notes and cards, and of funny things people would do for him. They didn't need me to plan or orchestrate these and many times, I was the last to know. When I visited Mike at the hospice facility, there were always numerous members of my staff with him. They were cracking jokes with him, rubbing his back, bathing him, or just holding his hand while he rested. Hours were spent with his wife and children, listening to them as they grieved for something for which they were simply not prepared.

One of his final expressions of love to my staff was a note he scribbled that simply said, "I love you all. Love, Mike". This was quickly framed for his funeral, and will be professionally framed for our unit along with Mike's picture. If anyone ever questions if health care workers are in this business for the right reasons, I hope they will hear the story of Mike and the unit who managed to reach out and extend the compassion they had learned as nurses to one of our own in need. I know I will never forget. This is what is right in health care.

—Submitted by Deborrah Furse, Southern Regional Medical Center, Riverdale, GA

"Never underestimate the difference you can make."

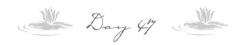

Selflessly Serving

Amy Craven, a radiology technician, works PRN in our system and occasionally works at the Methodist Diagnostic Center in Radiology. Recently, Amy performed a diagnostic test on an elderly gentleman, and noticed he was in dire need of hygiene care. She approached him and asked if she could clean him up a little, and he said he would be grateful.

Amy prepared a wash basin and bathed the elderly man and found a clean undergarment for him, since he arrived without one. She also took the time to wash and clean his electric wheelchair from top to bottom, including the spokes on the wheels, and she disinfected the cushions.

It was very touching to hear the man's expression of extreme gratitude and to see the tears in his eyes because someone—a stranger to him—cared enough to do what Amy did. She is a very caring person and treats all of her patients with the same compassion.

—Submitted by Ruth-Ann Hale, Methodist Le Bonheur Germantown Hospital, Germantown, TN

"Never underestimate the difference you can make."

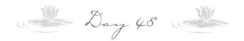

A Ray of Hope

G.R. is a 97-year-old woman who was referred to Home Care for an extensive cancerous lesion that had severely affected her left breast. According to her caregivers, the patient had had this open wound for more than five years, but now the drainage and odor had become problematic. G.R. lives in an assisted living facility and the other residents, unaware of her diagnosis, thought she was having episodes of incontinence.

Due to G.R.'s advanced disease and age she was not considered a surgical candidate and this was a terminal process. During her home care, she had several treatment goals, which included containing the odor and drainage. Once these problems were manageable, she would be transitioned to trained caregivers, since continued care for a chronic wound is not considered "skilled" under the Medicare guidelines. It was unlikely this wound would heal.

G.R.'s primary nurse immediately asked for an evaluation by a wound specialist. Upon examination, they found that the lesion was extremely friable—bleeding with the slightest provocation—but unlike 99 percent of patients with these kinds of sores, G.R. had absolutely no pain with dressing changes. On Dec. 27, 2006, the lesion measured 10.0 x 9.0 x 1.0 cm and exuded an odor and so much drainage that it soaked through her clothing. From our advanced wound

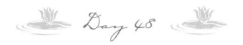

care product formulary, we created a system that we thought would be successful in treating G.R.'s condition.

On Jan. 10, 2007, her primary RN raced into the office and breathlessly reported that the wound was healing! It had begun to decrease in size and the patient was seeing improved results. Five days later she again reported that it had further decreased to 3.5 x 3 x 0.2 cm. The odor was gone and the drainage had decreased dramatically. This week, the RN reports the wound continues to close and the accompanying systems are improving drastically.

Although G.R. suffers from breast cancer, she no longer has to suffer with the open wound that plagued her for five long years. This wound may not close entirely but her quality of life and social dignity has been restored. This accomplishment was made possible through the expertise of home care services.

—Submitted by Susan Flow, Centura Health at Home

"Never underestimate the difference you can make."

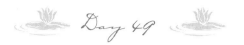

Bob

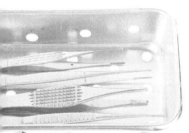

After a winter storm moved through Central Texas during the week of January 15, many employees were unable to drive to work at St. David's Medical Center in Austin. Despite rough road conditions, Bob Marrs, Director of Sterile Processing, was able to make the drive to the hospital.

Once he arrived, Bob did not leave. He wanted to be certain Sterile Processing ran smoothly so that it could provide the hospital with an adequate supply of sterilized instruments. He stayed from Monday through Thursday.

Bob has a true passion for Sterile Processing and is always making sure we have everything ready for our patients. He leads by example. If we are short of staff, he jumps right in to help clean and sterilize the instruments.

This particular week had the potential to be a really bad one for Sterile Processing and the entire hospital, but Bob helped make a difference by doing whatever he could to help everyone out. He would pass a cart around the whole Surgical Services area in the mornings with breakfast tacos from the cafeteria. He also gave vouchers for a free lunch to his employees that were there each day. Bob is a real inspiration and we truly appreciate his kindness and passion.

—Submitted by Tami Cass, St. David's Medical Center, Austin, TX

"Never underestimate the difference you can make."

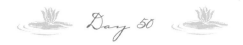

A Musical Gift

Two years ago, I played my guitar and sang Christmas songs for our hospital staff in the cafeteria. A gentleman, who was not a member of the hospital staff, sat listening intently.

As I finished and began putting away my guitar, he approached me. He said his mother was in our Clinical Decisions Unit (CDU) and was very sick. He asked me if I would come and play a couple of songs for her.

I had a meeting to attend and it really was not the best time for me, but I decided that I could "just be late" for the meeting and agreed to visit his mother. I entered her room and saw her son standing there by her bed holding her hand.

I played several Christmas songs. Then, she asked me if I knew any James Taylor songs. I played some of his songs for her and her eyes lit up. She was admitted several times after my first visit with her and with each admission she asked for me. I saw her each time.

When she passed away I was asked to come and play at her funeral. The church was packed and I was nervous. Her son told me he would never forget what the hospital did for his mom. At that time, I saw more clearly that he saw me as the hospital.

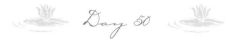
To this day, I keep in touch with her son and he stops by the hospital to thank me and CMC-Union for cheering up his mom and making her last days better. I know that I work at the hospital, but to know that our community sees no distinction between the person and the organization was a wake up call. Our community depends on us. I try to remember that every day.

—Submitted by John Danford, CMC-Union

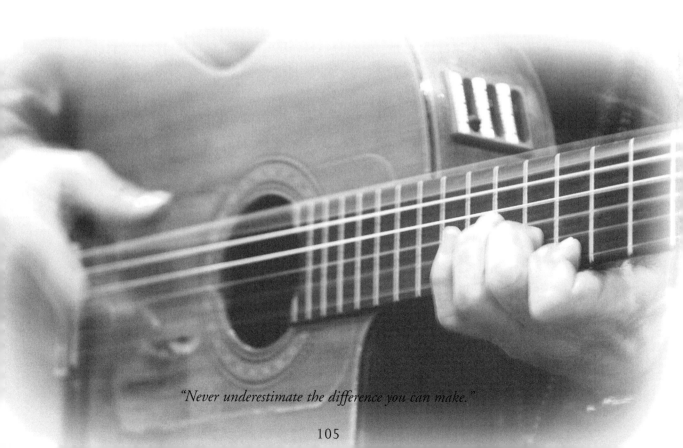

"Never underestimate the difference you can make."

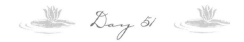

A Letter to My Lifesavers

The following is a letter I wrote to the colleagues who saved my life this past year:

This letter is overdue, but I believe I am just getting clear enough to write it now. I am asking that you share it in the right way with the right people in your organization. I am absolutely sure you will know what to do with this. I am an old nurse now—53 years young, but I am alive.

The events of early November 10th are crystal clear in my mind. I woke up early as usual and went to my office at home to study since I have been a lifelong student. It was about 4 a.m. and the routine that day was like an old familiar friend—coffee, CNN, and my computer. When I poured the coffee that day, I can still remember how good it smelled. I sat down at the computer and without any warning at all, the lights in my world went out. I woke up on the floor under my desk and was looking at the wall clock. I remember thinking that it was about 45 minutes later since it was almost 5 in the morning, just like it is now. I was on the floor and there was a steady drip of coffee from the desk above and all I could think of was a phrase that some of us had taken to using while we were in Louisiana doing disaster relief the month before: "That ain't right." I tried

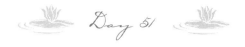

to stand up but sailed into the wall on the other side of the room and again thought; "That ain't right."

Since I have been an ER and flight nurse in years gone by, I knew that this was a major neurological event of some kind—a stroke, a bleed, definitely not good. Sitting on the floor, I looked at the phone on the far side of the room. I thought about calling 911, but for some reason, I decided that if I could just get to my family, everything was going to be okay. And so I began the crawl up two flights of stairs. About half way up the second flight, I succeeded in rousting Betsy. I just kept saying 911 and she got very calm in the way that she does and took care of business. The real symptoms began at that point—the intense pain in my head, the nausea, and the vomiting. Simply put, I was as frightened as I have ever been. The kids were scared too.

In what seemed like a heartbeat, the medics from the Allen Township Fire Department walked into our bedroom. By that time, I was on the floor and I remember their faces, but God forgive me because I do not know their names. I remember feeling very badly about being upstairs at that point because I knew they were going to have to carry me down again, and they did. They were sharp, they were professional, they were kind, and they patiently put up with me telling them what was wrong with me and what we needed to do about it. The medics very quickly took me to the ER at MHUC in Marysville, and I remember seeing Dr. Hoy who has often cared for my family in the years since we came to Marysville. He was outstanding, the nurses were as good as it gets, and the care was quick and professional.

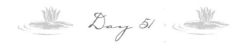

God, I was scared. My memory gets a little fuzzy at this point but I remember a CAT scan, and then I remember so clearly the face of an old friend—another nurse, Rita Johnson. I don't want to sound too corny here but I am telling you, when she walked into the room it was like an angel dropping in for a visit. I thought, *Okay, they decided to fly me. This is not good, but the good news is that Rita and MedFlight are here.* Then there was more very kind, very rapid professional care, cool air, and the old familiar sweet sound of rotor blades.

It was so ironic to be on that stretcher looking up at the place where I used to sit. Once again, God forgive me because I do not know who the medic and the pilot were that morning, only Rita and that smile. I heard there was a bleed and that we were going to Riverside. It really gets fuzzy here. I remember landing, cool air again, going through the back door of the ER at Riverside, seeing Rhonda and Dr. Yamarick. I remember thinking once again that I made it to my family and everything is going to be okay.

My next truly clear memory is somewhere around the first of the year 2006. There were so many heroes at Riverside in the weeks to come. I am really just hearing the stories about most of them who are in the ER, radiology, the neuro ICU, the rehab unit, 4 South, and so many other places. I wish I could name every single one of them and give them a hug but I just don't remember and probably never will. The last two months of 2005 are pretty much gone for good, I think. Then there is the unbelievably talented team in ER that just kept right on going without me and never missed a beat; for months. For those of you who may not know me, I have the good fortune to be the Director of Emergency Services at Riverside, and thanks to God and all of these wonderful heroes, I went

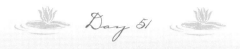

back to work today. It turns out that I had two cerebral aneurysms; one of them ruptured and caused a bleed. Dr. Pema, another hero, took care of that with incredible skill and a wad of platinum and here I sit with no deficits.

Trust me when I tell you that the health care system in this country and especially in Central Ohio is alive and well, just like me. The family of heroes I am referring to in this letter is a big one, like the ripples in a pond about a minute after the rock hits. At the center is my wife Betsy, my biggest hero, along with my kids, Bobby and Gabby. My brother Chip and his family are in there too. In this very true, very real life story, the rest of my family is in the ripples that go out from there. I cannot even begin to conceive of a way to say thank you to people that were so heroic in so many ways. How do you possibly thank someone for your very life?

You are all a tribute to your profession and I am so proud to be in your midst. Please do not ever make the mistake of thinking that your jobs are routine or meaningless because I am living proof that what you do is critical; it is God's work, and it matters so much to so many. You are honest to God heroes and He will be there for you some day, the way He, and you, were there for me on that day in November. Thank you all, from the bottom of my heart.

—Submitted by Bob Walsh, Ohio Health

"Never underestimate the difference you can make."

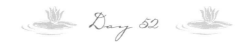

The Waiting Woman

It had been a long day at work. Nursing orientation was a little stressful, as a few of the presenters arrived late. I had to quickly come up with something interesting and engaging to fill the time. As it happened, I spoke about delivering patient-centered care which means keeping the patient as the focus of all that we do. It means fostering a "knowing relationship" with our patients and healthy relationships with our co-workers, while assuring that we don't neglect our own mind, body, and spirit.

I was already running late for an appointment when, exiting my office building, I saw a woman in a wheelchair waiting by the curb. I remembered seeing her in the same spot a few hours earlier. It was a little chilly, and I noticed that she was only wearing a thin sweater. Just as I asked her if she was waiting for a ride, one of the nurses who had attended the nursing orientation walked up. She was on her cell phone, trying to reach the patient shuttle service that had dropped the woman off for a 10:00 a.m. doctor's appointment. "I'm not having any luck," said the nurse. The woman told us that the shuttle bus was scheduled to return for her at noon, so she had asked staff from her doctor's office to take her outside to wait. "I've been waiting and waiting," she said, "I don't have a cell phone, and I'm too weak to roll myself back into the building, so I've just been waiting."

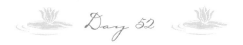

We looked around the parking lot to see only four cars, two of which belonged to the nurse and me. Just then, a patient walked out of the building. She had been in the same doctor's waiting room and had remembered seeing the woman in the wheelchair. "How long have you been waiting out here," she asked, "Don't you have a ride?" We quickly explained the situation to the patient. "I just had my eyes dilated and the doctor told me I shouldn't drive for a few hours," the woman said. "I was going to walk over to the restaurant across the street for dinner, then drive home. Why don't you join me, then I'll drive you home. Didn't you say you live in Illinois?" "Thank you, but no," the elder lady replied, "I'm so tired, I just want to get home and eat something there."

I looked at my watch, realizing it was 6:30 p.m. I was really running late and I knew that the other nurse had to get going as well. I called the nursing supervisor and she began to work on contacting the shuttle company on behalf of the woman. Then I called Security as we needed to have the woman picked up from the now-empty parking lot and taken to the hospital waiting room, while we worked on getting her home. The woman who offered a ride left after I assured her that I would not leave the elderly woman alone and that we'd get her home. She thanked me for caring. When security arrived we got the woman loaded in the truck, and off to the main hospital. The nurse waved goodbye, saying, "Isn't it ironic that we just discussed patient-centered care a few hours earlier, only to put it into action on the way home, with someone who's not technically our patient!"

I was still feeling uneasy as I got into my car. "Did I do all I could to help the woman?" I began to wonder, "What if she's in the waiting room all night? When was the last time she had something to eat?" After all, she was not a patient and did not have a registration number.

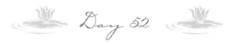
I called Pat Mohrman, our hospital president, and I brought her up to speed. "I'll just go meet her at the front door and get her something to eat. I'll take it from here," she said, "and thanks for letting me know." A tremendous weight was lifted off my shoulders, as I knew that Pat would absolutely ensure that the woman would get home.

The next day, I discovered that Pat had treated the woman to dinner, and that the shuttle company eventually arrived to take her home. I thought about how many people, like myself, must have passed by the woman in the wheelchair that day. It was as if she was on an island in the middle of a bay, with no way to move around, no phones with which to call for help. It felt good that a group of people cared and coordinated their efforts to get her home. She was truly at the center, and I think we're all the better for having put her there.

—Submitted by Yvonne Smith, Barnes-Jewish West County Hospital, St. Louis, MO

"Never underestimate the difference you can make."

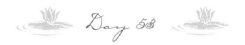

The Fuzzy Feline Christmas

I still remember it like it was yesterday. It was the holiday season in the Intensive Care Unit and I had drawn the short straw for the Christmas shift. I was scheduled for Christmas Eve and Christmas Day, working 12 hour shifts each day. I went in with a heavy heart but soon discovered that love can be shared no matter where one is.

I particularly remember the patient in Room 114. She had been in the Intensive Care Unit for so long that she seemed like a permanent fixture to us. The ICU staff had struggled through many an ailment with her and her prognosis was poor despite the finest medical interventions and nursing care we provided. As the holidays were drawing to a close, she made the difficult decision to stop the treatments that were sustaining her life.

At the time, dialysis was the only thing keeping her alive and she made an active decision to stop receiving it.

She knew that her treatment was coming to an end and she had just one wish before she died. Her husband informed me that her cat was her "baby" and she wanted to hold it one last time before she died. They had never had any children, he explained, and this cat meant the world to her.

At the time, bringing cats into the ICU was unheard of. However, I believe there are certain times when "rules are meant to be bent" and especially during the holidays! I formulated a plan with her husband. He was to get an egg box and

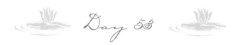

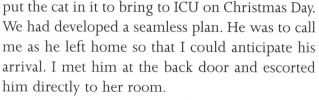

put the cat in it to bring to ICU on Christmas Day. We had developed a seamless plan. He was to call me as he left home so that I could anticipate his arrival. I met him at the back door and escorted him directly to her room.

We closed the door quickly and quietly. Her husband slowly opened the box to reveal the biggest, most beautiful Siamese cat that I had ever seen. At first she just lay in the box and skeptically glanced at the new surroundings. The patient was unable to talk so she gently clucked her tongue and gestured for the cat to come to her. Gingerly, the cat stepped from the box and onto her master's chest. In that tender moment the modern science surrounding us, all the beeps and whistles in the ICU faded away as the cat snuggled down to the familiar touch of its master. I have never felt such a sense of gratification as I did in that moment.

The time passed quickly. Soon, it was necessary for her beloved pet to go home. My patient actually smiled that day, something she had not done for weeks. I smiled, too, knowing that I had made someone else so very happy. She died just two days later but I know in my heart she died happy seeing her "baby" just one last time.

—*Submitted by Gina Flesher*

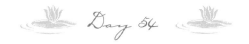

To Save a Tiny Life

Our Emergency Department, like so many others across the nation, was full, with patients waiting to be triaged, patients waiting to be seen, and patients waiting to go home. We were fully staffed with nurses and medical providers, and still, they kept coming through the front door. In a small community of only 30,000 and on this late Wednesday night, we were the sole source of medical treatment.

A young couple brought in their one-week-old infant stating that the baby was having trouble breathing. At first glance, the baby appeared healthy and responsive. Within minutes, his color changed and his breathing became erratic. His little toes and fingers were turning blue. We immediately knew that this baby was in trouble. The scenario that unfolded was classic emergency medicine. The Emergency Department physician saw the chest x-ray, diagnosed ductus arteriosus, and asked for help. The Emergency Department nurse rushed to the baby's bedside. We realized he needed to be intubated, stabilized, and transferred out of our Emergency Department for neonatal intensive care. Without this care, we knew that he would die. The parents were very young and they appeared so connected to each other and their baby. They immediately recognized the seriousness of their baby's illness and stood holding one another, tears quietly streaming down their cheeks.

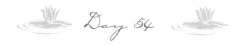

Within minutes, the bedside was crowded. Three experienced nurses shifted into full gear doing everything they could to speed up the baby's transfer. Two other nurses were trying to initiate an IV line, but as the infant's extremities became more mottled, peripheral access became more difficult. Attempts in intraosseus access were not successful. No medication could be given for the intubation that was necessary and time was running out.

The Emergency Department physician attempted to intubate, but the neonate airway was difficult to maneuver. We contacted the anesthesiologist at home to come and help. Although he was surprised at the request, he said he would be there, and he arrived within five minutes. As the charge nurse, I contacted the house supervisor to come and help us with this baby. We needed one more person to hold an extremity, to get medication, to access our resources. Even though it was the end of her shift, she came and immediately went to the bedside. The unit secretary was asked to start making arrangements for transfer to a tertiary facility over 100 miles away. After multiple phone calls, she learned that no helicopters could fly that night due to the weather. She started contacting the local ambulance providers to find transportation for the tiny patient. She did this in addition to her normal job duties, as there were still other patients in the department, and other providers writing orders. Despite a busy night for our local EMS, they said they would have a team there in 10 minutes.

The Emergency Department technician took over the care of the parents and grandparents. She made sure that they got to the bedside to see their baby, to talk to him, to hold his hand for what could have been the last time. The baby was intubated and the airway was secured as we worked to get the transfer underway. One of the Emergency Department nurses volunteered to accompany the baby to the new hospital. One of the respiratory therapists offered to go, even though he

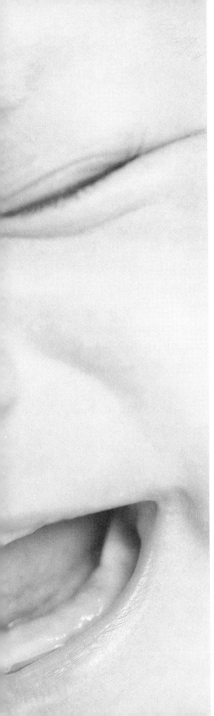

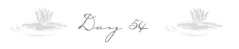
would have to double back in the morning. The Emergency Department call nurse was called in to help with the rest of the department and she arrived within 15 minutes. The remainder of the emergency staff were managing the department while keeping patients informed of the delays. The waiting patients seemed to know we were all working on a baby that night and not one person complained about the delay. The baby left and the Emergency Department team picked up where they left off with a full department and patients at triage.

This was when I called my director to come in and help me. I had enough nurses to handle the department, but I needed someone to help ease my burden. The stress of this baby, this crowded Emergency Department, and working my third 12-hour shift was enough to call for moral support. My director, a woman at least 10 years my junior, arrived in 20 minutes. With her presence, I didn't feel so overwhelmed any more. I broke down in tears when she arrived, but together, we kept it going.

This situation exemplifies our mission statement. The community of hospital workers pulled together to get this infant the care he needed. No one person could have accomplished this task on their own. In thinking back on it now, I can honestly say that we do this type of thing often, but it became clear to me that night. This was our job. This was our mission. This is Provena Health.

—Submitted by Mary O'Brien,
Provena United Samaritans Medical Center, Danville, IL

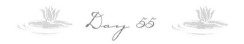
A Favorite Resident

As you all know, the Post Surgical Unit is a very busy place with patients coming and going all the time. Most people move on from the Post Surgical Unit fairly quickly, moving to other units to continue treatment and healing. However, there was one gentleman named Virgil that stayed with us from Nov. 24, 2006 to Dec. 26, 2006, waiting on his placement with a long term care facility that could meet his chemotherapy and radiation needs. With him, we shared several great moments.

Virgil's birthday fell on a weekend and all he wanted was to eat crab legs. His busy nurse took the time to call his physician and arrange a leave of absence. Then she called local restaurants until she found one that was serving crab legs for his birthday feast. Another nurse kept him supplied with his lottery tickets. He would let different personnel pick the numbers. He told them if he won he promised to take them on a cruise with him!

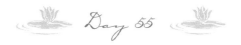

On another occasion, Dr. Ehrhard and his family came Christmas caroling. On Christmas Day, the staff placed a white tablecloth over the nurses' station desk and decorated it with the unit's Christmas decorations. The entire staff shared their Christmas dinner with Virgil. That night, a picture was taken of him and the staff and placed in a frame for him to remember us by. The next day he left for a local nursing home. The staff lined the hall and bid him farewell and well wishes as he entered the elevator. Tears were shared by all. The staff continues to visit him at the nursing home and sends cards. He is one resident that we will not soon forget.

—Submitted by Helen Massie, Memorial Hospital & Health Care Center

"Never underestimate the difference you can make."

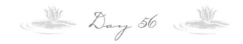

Changing a Life

My name is Jodi Langford and I am a patient educator at Saint Joseph's Hospital in Atlanta. I teach patients and their families about heart disease, diabetes, and how to make lifestyle changes in order to live a healthy lifestyle. Below is a letter from a patient of mine about the impact I made on her life. I have continued to keep in touch with this patient to follow her success. This is an example of a very determined person who is not letting any obstacles get in the way of achieving her goals. Here is her story…

Ending up in the Emergency Room last March with a heart rate of 265 BPM was the worst and the best thing to ever happen to me all at the same time. At the time, I had no idea that I was suffering from severe sleep apnea, diabetes, heart disease, and a thyroid disorder. In addition to suffering from severe depression, my heart was pounding away in my chest, I could hardly breathe, and I was exhausted 100 percent of the time. I had been living like that year after year, brushing it off as symptoms of menopause. Several times a day, I would become unable to catch my breath, and come close to passing out. The doctors implanted a pacemaker and performed an AV node ablation. After spending nine days in the ICU, I can now live without any of my prior symptoms.

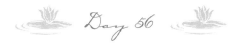

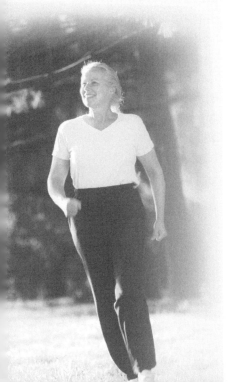

I never thought I would be capable of injecting myself with insulin. Now, with Jodi teaching me every step of the way, it has become the easiest thing I do in my daily health routine. As a severely overweight individual, I never enjoyed exercising. However with Jodi reinforcing the benefits of walking and managing my portion control, I have lost 50 pounds. I walk every morning in my neighborhood for an hour and I eat the correct foods. As a result of my life changes I have watched my strength and stamina slowly return. In the beginning, I could barely walk up a slight incline, let alone climb any stairs. Today, I do flights of stairs with no problem and even walk the hills in my neighborhood. Jodi always emphasized to me that losing just 10 percent of my body weight would help my diabetes so much. Breaking the changes down into those small increments is making it easier to continue my weight loss program. Now I exercise each and every morning because it is beneficial for my heart, my diabetes and my all around mental well-being. By doing something I don't want to do, it empowers me in all the other areas of my life.

Jodi took the time to help me when I was at the lowest point in my life. It reaffirmed to me that there are kind, considerate, and compassionate people in the health care arena. They are only there to help you. That is their sole purpose in being there for you everyday. This entire experience only makes me want to "pay it forward" to help someone else, exactly like I was helped by Jodi.

—Submitted by Jodi Langford, Saint Joseph's Hospital

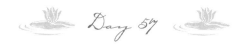

Setting the Example

Recently Dennis Duke, a physical therapy assistant at Methodist University Hospital, exhibited exemplary patient care and compassion by helping a young man from Mexico who had developed Guillain-Barré Syndrome. The young man was a musician, and his therapist put out a call for a loaner guitar. Dennis willingly brought in his own guitar, and let him take it to HealthSouth when he was transferred. While it was a challenge, playing the guitar was the perfect therapeutic task for him, providing great motivation and opportunity for exercise.

Dennis brought in a CD player, CDs, and checked on the young man regularly. He also volunteered to provide therapy on weekends, in addition to his other duties. When Dennis learned that the patient and his family were taking a cab to the airport to return home to Mexico, he volunteered to take them. He came up on his day off, helped them get prescriptions filled, and then drove them to the airport. The Rehab Department thanks Dennis for being such an inspirational example of the Power of One.

—Submitted by Ruth-Ann Hale,
Methodist Le Bonheur Germantown Hospital, Germantown, TN

"Never underestimate the difference you can make."

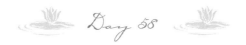

Giving the Gift of Life

I was working a 12-hour shift in the Emergency Department, assigned to the trauma room. I knew that this meant I should expect that anything could happen. I could be asked to care for simple things or I could be expected to care for a major trauma—but the likelihood of major trauma was low. We are a small community hospital with a designated trauma center located 15 miles away. Most cases that meet "trauma" criteria are usually directed to that center. This night was different.

We got a call from the Emergency Medical Services control center telling us to expect a patient who had been involved in a one-car motor vehicle accident. The vehicle had rolled over and the driver had been ejected onto the road. According to the Emergency Medical Technicians, the 30-year-old male was unresponsive and they were unable to secure an artificial airway. He was not breathing on his own and the EMTs were giving oxygen with a bag to breathe for the patient. When the patient arrived, his heart was still beating and the oxygen that the EMTs provided was sustaining him.

We immediately set about assessing the patient for injuries. We also started measures to establish an artificial airway and run the necessary tests to determine the extent of his injuries. When his family arrived, we described his injuries and potential diagnoses. Immediately, we determined that this man had no response to any stimuli we used, which was a very bad sign. He had no obvious injuries aside from a few superficial scrapes to his shoulder and his heart was functioning well enough to sustain a good blood pressure. At that point, we feared the worst—a devastating brain injury.

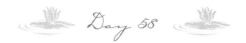

We prepared the family for this very distinct possibility. X-rays and CT scans confirmed that he was severely brain damaged. There was a large amount of blood on his brain and additional tests revealed no brain activity. After discussing with the family the probable outcomes and options, they made the difficult decision to donate his organs.

I contacted the Tissue and Organ Donor Network and began to prepare the patient for donation. I followed the patient and family through the process and asked to be allowed to follow the patient through the retrieval process. I stayed with the patient through the removal of his lungs, heart, liver, kidneys and pancreas for transplantation into various people. I felt a need to stay with him until the "end."

A few years later, I was attending a trauma conference in another city. I stopped at the Tissue and Organ Donor Network display, where I saw two people standing next to a display of my patient's picture. I inquired about the picture and verified that it was, in fact, my patient. A petite, middle aged lady asked me how I knew him. When I told her how I had cared for the patient and initiated the organ donation process, she immediately hugged me and began to cry. She was the recipient of this man's pancreas and kidney. She described to me how this transplant had saved her life and allowed her to have more time with her husband and small children.

In that moment, I truly knew that nurses, doctors, nurse aides, and many others in hospitals make a difference. When I was caring for this patient and going through the process with his family, I focused on comforting them and being there to get the process done. I never thought that just a few years later I would be hugged and thanked profusely by a person I did not know for what I considered to be "just doing my job."

—Submitted by Sandi Mahoney, Rome Memorial Hospital, Rome, NY

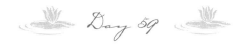

When Santa Claus Came to Town

Christmas 2006 was a memorable one for the participants of the Mary and Fran Ludington Adult Day Services Program of Sound Shore Medical Center in New Rochelle, New York, because Santa Claus dropped by to say, "Hello." Now, most people would not think that this is necessarily a big deal, but for one 94-year-old female, it was the dream of a lifetime.

Santa and his six "reindeer" (paramedics and EMTs from Emergency Medical Services and the New York City Fire Department) got out of their vehicle, adjusted antlers, beard and belly, and strolled into our street-level program. Some of our seniors wondered if this group had lost their way. Were they actually trying to find the pediatric clinic located above us? "No," we explained, "they are really here for us!"

Santa and his reindeer personally greeted and hugged all 35 seniors as well as our volunteers and staff. This was the first time in the 10-year history of the program that Santa had found his way to us. One of our ladies danced with him, one touched his curly beard, but it was Katie who brought everyone to tears. When Santa was about to leave, Katie called to him and said, "I need to tell you something." He walked over, bent down close to her and the room suddenly became silent. "I'm 94 years old," Katie said, "and my whole life I have always wanted to see you in person. Today my dream came true."

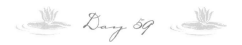
For a brief moment it was silent. Then the sobs could be heard and the tears began to fall. No one expected this—not even Santa, who cried silently. It was reinforcement for our staff of the special and unique gifts that we receive in return for our life's work. It showed us once again what we already knew—that we should never underestimate the power of a special gesture.

For us, this visit was as powerful as anything that could have happened that day and a perfect way to say farewell to 2006. We are forever grateful to our visitors who took time from their life-saving jobs to bring happiness to others. And, as they left that day, we noticed that Rudolph really did have a red nose!

—*Submitted by Pearl Hacker, Sound Shore Medical Center for Mary and Fran Ludington Adult Day Services, New Rochelle, NY*

"Never underestimate the difference you can make."

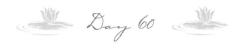

Reconnecting to Purpose

Brother Edward Francis and Sister Christine pause before entering the room of a gentleman newly diagnosed with cancer. They are a man and a woman of God yet they pause to find the "right words" and to consider what they will say to him. When they enter the room they are comforted by the one whom they came to comfort. "Like the bird that feels the light and sings when the dawn is still dark," so the patient restored their spirits.

Cis, a nursing leader for Studer Group, recalls a severely injured child that was declared brain dead. The child's family made the selfless decision for organ donation. Cis removed her badge as the head nurse that day and remained with the family through those long, dark hours. A month later she received a card in the mail, a card that transformed her life. The parents thanked her for her presence and for helping them to bear the unbearable. Cis carries that card with her to this day. Even though she cannot visualize their faces, those parents will never forget hers.

I reflect back to a nursing shift many years ago at St. Mary Medical Center in the Labor and Delivery Unit. The beds were full and overflowing. I was to care for a woman whose labor was being induced because her 18-week twins had died in-utero. The unit was very busy and our nurse chaplain was away at a conference. I felt angry for being given this assignment as I knew I would be mostly on my own to deal with it. I secretly hoped that the woman would deliver on the next

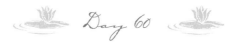
shift. However, her water broke and delivery was imminent so I called the obstetrician. In those quiet moments before birth I dimmed the lights and looked toward Heaven for some inspiration. I felt so ashamed of my earlier self-centered attitude. Although I had performed all the right nursing actions, I felt I could have done more to ease the family's suffering.

The first twin boy delivered and I held him in the palm of my hand. Then, the doctor arrived and delivered the twin brother. I realized that their delicate fingers were interlaced as together, they entered and left this world all at the same time. It was a sight of unimaginable beauty and awe I will never forget: birth, death, and eternal life all wrapped within those few moments. It was as if I could see through the eyes of our Creator and He in turn could feel my suffering. At the end of our days I am convinced we will receive much more than we ever gave. We allow God's love to flow through us and to us as we minister to and are ministered to by others…and there can be no greater purpose.

—Submitted by Pat Lucken, St. Mary Medical Center, St. Joseph Health System

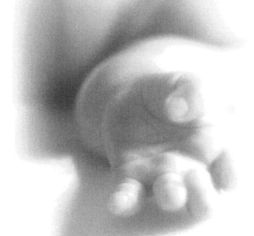

"Never underestimate the difference you can make."

Share Your Own Story

Please share an experience that connected you back to purpose, worthwhile work, and making a difference. You are a big part of what's right in health care!

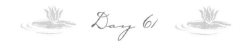

Going the Extra Mile

I am the nurse manager for General Pediatrics at my hospital. I work with a remarkable group of caring and compassionate people who make a difference every day in the lives of our children.

A while ago, we had an infant patient with serious cardiac disease. His parents were immigrants who spoke very little English, and they had no health insurance or outside resources to obtain the cardiac drugs essential for their child's health. The child was scheduled to be discharged on a Saturday—a time when many support services are limited. After many hours of searching for funding for the medication, it seemed clear that there would be no acceptable solution.

The nursing staff that day took matters into their own hands—they pooled their money hoping to help buy the medicine that the baby needed. After the work day was over, our Spanish-speaking nurse drove to three different pharmacies in the family's neighborhood to obtain the needed cardiac drugs. After intense searching, she was finally able to locate a pharmacy that had the needed medication. Upon hearing about the patient's dilemma, the pharmacist provided the medication at a drastic discount and took only the money the nurses had pooled. She drove back to the hospital with the medication and, in Spanish, instructed the parents how to give the proper dose to their baby. In the end, the child was able to be discharged safely, with the essential medication, proper teaching, and a plan for further obtaining the medication when needed.

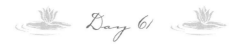
We sent a letter of thanks to the pharmacy that so graciously "did the right thing." Several weeks later, I received a note from the pharmacist citing the extraordinary care my nurses took in assuring this child's safety. We were all inspired by the extra effort made that day.

—Submitted by Diane Ohme, Hackensack University Medical Center, Hackensack, NJ

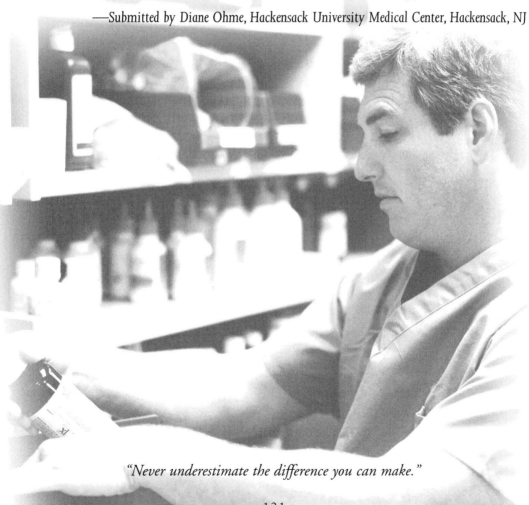

"Never underestimate the difference you can make."

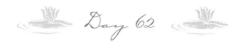

Saying Goodbye

"*D*on," the voice on the other end of the phone spoke, "I have a rather unusual request for you." Our CEO, I soon found, wondered if there was any way that we could accommodate the needs of a patient in our ICU. "His family called to inform us that his sister has died," continued our concerned CEO. "He is not well enough to travel to the funeral, and they wonder if there is anything we can do to help him say goodbye to her?"

Ready to help, that morning I called the funeral home. They were willing to arrange a private viewing for him if we could negotiate the space needed. I checked to see if our auditorium was available and luckily it was. I arranged for the viewing to take place later that morning. To make the experience as special as possible for our patient, we quickly redecorated the auditorium, trying to capture the ambience of a funeral viewing room. As we decorated, the ICU readied the patient and assigned a staff nurse to accompany him. We arranged for a local priest to do a blessing and to honor the religious needs of our patient.

Our patient was able to see his sister and say his goodbyes just as he would have done had he been well. I am certain that being able to have this final moment with his sister helped him fare better in the heart surgery he had soon after.

—*Submitted by Donald Shields, Markham Stouffville Hospital, Ontario, CA*

"Never underestimate the difference you can make."

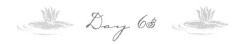

You Are My Sunshine

At Jackson-Madison County General Hospital, 9 West is dubbed the "cancer floor," and the nurses who work there are known for their compassion.

One afternoon, a patient named Libby received some disheartening news from her oncologist. Libby's nurse, Yvonne, sat with Libby as the young mother broke down and cried—and soon Yvonne found herself in tears along with her patient. The nurses on the floor realized Libby needed a break and so one of them secured Libby an afternoon pass, thinking some time outside of the facility with her husband, Brad, might cheer her a bit.

On their way out, Brad asked one of the nurses if Libby could be moved to a room with a view, as he thought that might help lift her spirits. All the nurses—Renee, Marie, Linda, Yvonne, Eloise, Judy, Julie, and Kim—devised a plan to put a smile on Libby's face.

Quickly, the nurses moved Libby's belongings to another room where sunshine streamed through the windows. But something was still lacking and the nurses decided the room needed further embellishment. Jessica, from Dietary, called one of her friends who was known for her flower garden, and she produced a colorful bouquet of fresh-cut flowers, which added a special touch to Libby's room. The caregivers all chipped in some money and bought Libby a new

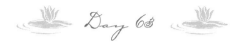

gown. And the nurses? Well, they had their reward, too. A wonderful smile lit up their patient's face once more. They felt the sunshine had truly returned.

When Brad and Libby returned from their afternoon out, the nurses were gathered in Libby's room, and sang "You Are My Sunshine" when she arrived. Both Brad and Libby were overwhelmed, greatly touched by the special caring these nurses had so freely shown.

—Submitted by Linda Pledge, Jackson-Madison County General Hospital, Jackson, TN

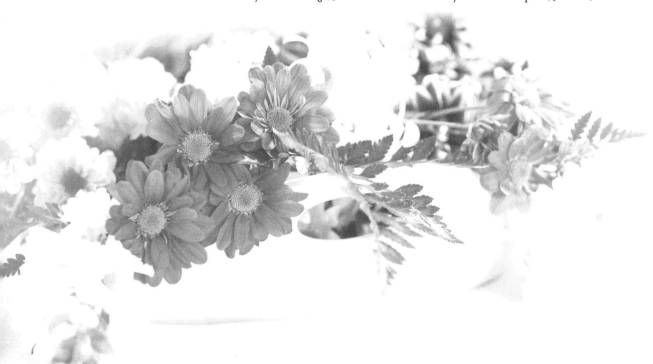

"Never underestimate the difference you can make."

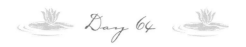

Nurses' Hearts Bleed Too

I came into work for a sixteen-hour shift one Wednesday afternoon in June. My assignment was to go to Angioplasty and receive a report on my next primary patient. She was a 20-year-old lady who was admitted to the hospital following multiple traumas with a grade IV liver laceration. She had already been through surgery but was still bleeding so she was sent to Angioplasty to uncover the source.

The adrenalin started to flow as I received the report that the angioplasty was completed. The results showed a small bleed in a branch of the hepatic artery. There was nothing more to be done to help "Angeline's" instability. Around 5:30 p.m., I brought Angeline back to the Intensive Care Unit but was struggling to stabilize her. The support that I received from the other staff members working with me was exceptional as I struggled to maintain Angeline's systolic blood pressure.

My biggest challenge still lay ahead. Approaching the family of the young lady, I did my best to support and educate them about her prognosis. As we spoke, I felt an immediate bond with them. I learned that Angeline was their only child and the absolute core of their lives. In addition, her boyfriend, Joe, was Angeline's first love.

After updating the family, I brought them into Angeline's room. As their eyes fell upon her, the overall "picture" was too much for her Mom, causing her to

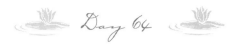

pass out in my arms. My heart was breaking for this family, but I forced myself to remain focused on continuing to provide the utmost care for Angeline.

The family had a bedside vigil and visiting hours were never discussed. I made myself work around this because I feared that Angeline did not have much time left. When I left in the morning, I told her parents that I would see them when I came back the next day for my next shift even though I felt in my heart that Angeline would most likely pass away before my return. When I returned to work the next day, I was greeted by Angeline's parents in the hall. They offered words of praise and a sense of relief that I was there. As I received the report at bedside, I learned that Angeline's condition had stabilized after going back to the operating room for exploration and packing. I remained optimistic and felt that Angeline's young and healthy heart might be enough to pull her through, even though she remained unresponsive and extremely critical. Then it happened!

As I was in the waiting room talking with her family, the staff that was covering for me summoned me. I ran to Angeline's bedside as resuscitative measures were initiated. Within what seemed like seconds, Angeline was in P.E.A. (Pulse less Electrical Activity) and was not regaining a pulse. We worked for over an hour to resuscitate her to no avail. I watched in disbelief as the physician ended the code, and Angeline was pronounced dead.

My heart was in my stomach, because I knew I had to go tell Angeline's parents that they had lost their only child. The screams and shrills that came from her mother pierced through me as I tried to console them. Angeline's father hugged me so tight that my own tears couldn't be restrained. Her mother's first words will live with me forever. "We waited all day for you, Mike," she said, "because if anyone was going to save our Angeline, it would be you." After hearing these words I felt as if I had failed them, even though I knew we had

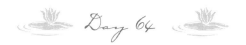

done everything we could to save their daughter's life. I went back to Angeline's bedside to prepare her body, then I brought them into see her. I stayed with them for a while then left them alone for their last hour with their daughter. I watched them looking from the picture of their beautiful little girl to the person in the bed and the emptiness in my stomach gave me the feeling of a failure.

As the family left, they hugged me and assured me that they knew I had done all that I could. It helped a little, but not enough. I felt the need for closure but did not know how to get it. Three days later, I went to Angeline's viewing. The moment her father's eyes caught mine he came over to me and hugged me as we both wept. I walked up to the coffin to kneel beside it and her family took pictures of me by Angeline's side. I wondered to myself if this was the closure that her family so desperately needed. As the cameras flashed, I felt my own sense of closure, because I knew now that they knew I did all I could to save the life of their beautiful daughter. Hopefully, Angeline knows this, too.

—*Submitted by Michael Beshel, Frankford Hospital*

"Never underestimate the difference you can make."

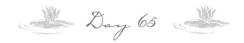

With Great Love

Robert Henderson, an occupational therapist at Le Bonheur Children's Medical Center, walked through the Rehabilitation Services door just two years ago, and since then, the Rehab department has never been quite the same. It's the small things that Robert does on a daily basis that make a big impact on the people who know him. He is loved and respected by patients and their families for his professional knowledge and personal involvement with them. Robert's connection and devotion to his patients extends beyond the 40-hour work week. It's not uncommon for Robert to clock out after a full day and remain in the hospital to visit patients on the floors, or to take the time to go eat lunch with one of his outpatients at school. His positive attitude is contagious.

The Rehabilitation Services department has gone through significant change, including shortages in staffing. One day, during a particularly difficult week, deli lunches just miraculously appeared in the department. Only after asking around and probing for information did we find out that the unknown benefactor was Robert. He wanted to cheer up the department and knew this would provide nourishment and save time for associates.

When times are difficult, Robert may be seen up on the therapy mat doing the Dog Pound Rock cheer (impossible to watch without smiling) or soliciting a group hug. His antics remind us that we are a team and we need to work as a team.

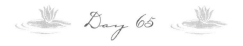

Robert represents the Methodist values even away from home. This past year, he served as a volunteer on international mission trips overseas, as well as stateside in the aftermath of Hurricane Katrina. Mother Teresa once said, "We can do no great things, only small things with great love." Robert does small things with great love and changes the lives of patients and coworkers in the most unexpected ways, and that is why he recently received the hospital's Miracle in Motion Award.

—*Submitted by Ruth-Ann Hale, Methodist Le Bonheur Germantown Hospital, Germantown, TN*

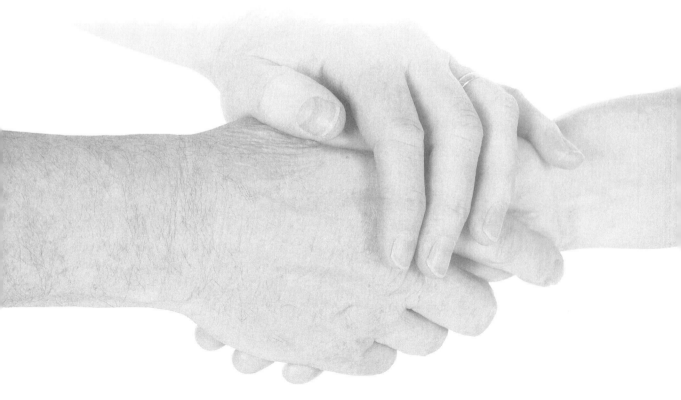

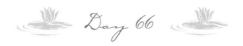

SAVING BABY CHRIS

*I*n 1987, my son Chris was born. Within 24 hours of delivery, he began to lose his peripheral pulses. The team at the hospital did a great job, and he was quickly diagnosed with Hypoplastic Left Heart Syndrome (HLHS). With HLHS, the left ventricle of the heart is not fully developed. While the diagnosis of HLHS was unfamiliar to me, my background in cardiac nursing had taught me the importance of the left ventricle and I couldn't imagine how anyone could live without it. The doctors shared with us that some of the larger medical facilities in the country were attempting to treat infants with this condition. If we chose, we could have our baby transferred to one of these facilities to see if anything could be done to save him. To save his life, we elected to transfer our baby.

When it came time to transport Chris, the NICU nurses packed him up in the Isolette and he was taken to the ambulance waiting outside for him. The plan was to take him to the airport where a plane would transport him to a major referral center. The transport team included a doctor, nurse, paramedic, respiratory therapist, and a pilot. Not even 24 hours after giving birth, I followed the ambulance carrying my baby because there was no room for me inside. At the airport, the Isolette was loaded onto the plane. I quickly counted the number of available seats to see if there might be room enough for me. My heart sank as I realized there was not a seat for me. Once Chris was loaded in, everyone took their places. I stood at the door of the plane to say what I thought could be the

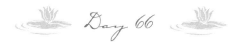

last goodbye to my baby. At that moment, the respiratory therapist jumped up from his seat. He suggested that there were enough clinical people on the plane that could cover in the event of an emergency and that I could have his seat. That respiratory therapist had a purpose, was doing worthwhile work, and made a difference in my life by simply offering up his seat.

Chris had his first open heart surgery when he was only four days old. While he was in the NICU recovering, I spent my nights sleeping in the waiting room. The nights were so long. Many nights, in an effort to pass the time, I wandered down to the cafeteria to get something to eat. One night, the cafeteria attendant who worked the night shift asked me how my "loved one" was doing. I shared with her that my baby had just had open heart surgery and that the doctors were giving him a 50/50 chance of surviving. She told me that she would be praying for him and asked if there was anything else that she could do. I mentioned to her that I really enjoyed the chicken salad sandwiches and pickles each night because they seemed so comforting to me. Every night after that, she over-stuffed my sandwich full of chicken salad and piled my plate with pickles. While it may not sound like much to some, it meant the world to this tired and discouraged mom. That cafeteria attendant showed me that someone cared about me...she had purpose, she was doing worthwhile work and she made a difference.

Chris was very slow to recover in the NICU. For a very long time, he required a feeding tube to eat and a ventilator to breathe. It was becoming discouraging for his father and me. We began to feel as though he was more the hospital's baby than ours. The nursing staff must have sensed our discouragement. Since the day of his birth, we had never been alone with him, never been able to hold him comfortably, and had never seen his beautiful little face without tubes and tape covering it.

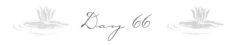

One night, while we were sleeping in the waiting room, we heard a knock at the door. We awoke wondering if Chris had taken a turn for the worse. We were confused because he had been progressing nicely and had even received orders to transfer to the floor the next morning. I couldn't imagine why they would awake us. I sleepily opened my eyes to see a nurse standing in the doorway with Chris in her arms! With a mischievous twinkle in her eye she said, "He pulled out his feeding tube and threw up all over me…he's your kid, you take care of him!" She handed him to us and walked out the door. It was one of the most precious gifts that anyone could have given us—time alone with our baby. I used that time to examine his beautiful little face and to recount his fingers and toes. His dad lay down beside him and they took the most relaxed nap that I had ever seen either one of them take. It was the nurse who made it happen. She had purpose, was doing worthwhile work, and made a difference in my life.

—Submitted by Lisa Binekey

"Never underestimate the difference you can make."

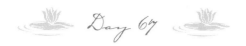

"Pasquale"

My 83-year-old father, Patrick, had suffered a serious fall that resulted in one trauma center visit and two hospital admissions. My mother had died a few months earlier, and his will to live seemed to be wavering. At one point, I had even heard him say, "The Lord can take me anytime." My father seemed disengaged in his health care process, but one afternoon this changed dramatically when Dennis Valera from Respiratory entered the room. He saw that my father's name was Italian, and calling him in the Italian version of his name he said, "Pasquale." He spoke another few words of Italian, causing my father's face to light up as he smiled. He immediately spoke in Italian as Dennis admitted that while he only knew a few words of the language he loved cannolis, lasagna, and manicotti. An immediate bond developed between the two.

Later the next day, I visited my Dad and inadvertently moved the inspirometer Dennis had given him off of his tray table. In a strong voice my father said, "Don't move that, it is very important. That guy Dennis told me that I have to use this several times a day. I have to do this, it is very important." A day later, Dennis arrived at the hospital with two small packages of mini cannolis. When I arrived to visit later that day, my Dad smiled and said that he had something for me. He gave me the box and told me that his "friend" Dennis brought them for the family. "Pasquale" began using his inspirometer regularly. Needless to say, I

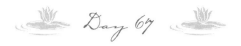

learned that day the difference a caring and engaged health care worker can have on one man's health.

My father was discharged from the hospital shortly after. Dennis appeared in a Santa suit on that day. The last picture I have of my Dad is with Dennis and me as Dad was leaving the hospital. On Christmas Eve, we received a telephone call from Dennis, asking if he and his daughter could visit "Pasquale" at home. They arrived with a violin in tow. His daughter played "Oh Holy Night," my father's favorite Christmas song, and indeed it was a holy night. My Dad died two weeks later, but he kept that inspirometer by his side. This was the difference one man was able to make in the life of another.

—Submitted by Patricia Tobin, Fawcett Memorial Hospital, Port Charlotte, FL

"Never underestimate the difference you can make."

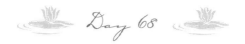

A Surrogate Family for Jason

Thirty-four-year-old Jason was admitted to Mary Immaculate Hospital on Oct. 30, 2006, seeking treatment for pneumonia. Within days of his admission, Jason experienced increased respiratory distress and required a transfer to the Intensive Care Unit where he was intubated and placed on the ventilator. During the following week, he became progressively worse, developing shock, renal failure, hemoptysis, and acute respiratory distress syndrome. The nursing staff and his family became very concerned for his welfare.

Jason's parents had lost their 29-year-old son only four months earlier and no one wanted to see them lose another child. Upon the family's request, the staff asked another physician to see the patient for a second opinion. Recommendations were made by the second pulmonologist, but they were not followed by Jason's initial doctor. As the patient's advocate, the staff encouraged the family to request the Critical Care Team, including the hospitalist and second opinion pulmonologist. After hours of making changes to the ventilator settings, the patient's respiratory status improved and the patient was much more comfortable.

During the entire ordeal of Jason's illness, the family became very close to the staff. On several occasions, the family showed their appreciation by making barbecue beef, pork ribs, and barbecue chicken for the staff to enjoy. On Dec. 1,

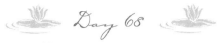
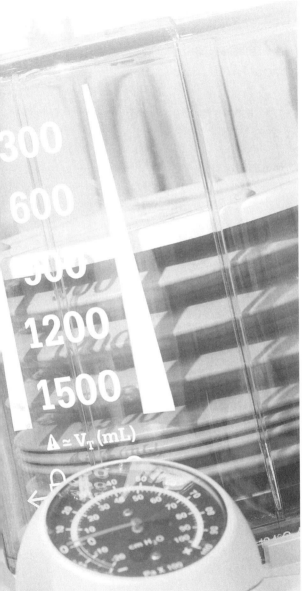

2006, Jason walked out of the hospital with his mother and father and there wasn't a dry eye in the entire department.

Today, Jason is living with his parents in Atlanta, and his physician reports that he is doing fine. The staff in the Intensive Care Unit at Mary Immaculate Hospital is the BEST! We live out the mission of this hospital and we care for all of our patients as though they were our own family. In this situation, we became a surrogate family for these people to keep them going when things didn't look promising, putting the patient first for the benefit of all.

—*Anonymous Contributor,*
Mary Immaculate Hospital-Bon Secours

"Never underestimate the difference you can make."

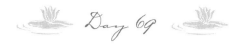

For the Love of "Sir Knight"

In January 2006, a patient at our hospital was identified as having no support person to be released to after his procedure. He was reluctant to follow through with the procedure because he did not want to leave his cat, "Sir Knight," unattended. It was discovered that both the patient and his cat lived in a makeshift shack along the Mojave River Bed, a sharp contrast to the affluent mansions that were just a stone's throw away. The shack was hidden away from view to prevent police or intruders from destroying his haven.

Our staff convinced him to follow through with the procedure he needed. One staff member even volunteered to take care of Sir Knight while the patient recovered. On the day of the procedure the staff took turns reassuring the patient that his cat would be cared for and that his shack would be safely waiting for his return. The following day the patient was discharged. A staff member and her husband visited him and brought him some chili to eat. They gave him a burner so he could cook warm food for his meals and most importantly they reunited him with his beloved Sir Knight.

Weeks later, the patient came to visit. Using his limited Social Security resources, he bought roses for the staff to let them know that they really made a difference. I believe that our staff had a sacred encounter with this patient, helping a homeless man and his only worldly possession, Sir Knight.

—Submitted by Joyce Rabor, St. Mary Medical Center, Apple Valley, CA

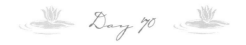

Selfless Giving

The volunteer knitters and sewers at Hackensack University Medical Center are amazing. Their talent, generosity, and anonymity make their efforts nothing short of philanthropic. These volunteers are never visible at the medical center; they make their items at home and then drop them off at the volunteer office. The employees and hospital volunteers have the joy of handing out these creations to patients. The donated items are often thematic, using colors for each holiday, such as red, white and blue for July 4th, green for St. Patrick's Day, and red for Valentine's Day.

Although there are many people who contribute these tenderly created items, two volunteers in particular, Stephanie Johnson and her late husband John, have consistently contributed 100 baby hats each week for nearly five years. The baby hats are made from 3" white stocking net donated by the HUMC Volunteer Services Department. Stephanie puts colored pom poms on each hat—blue for boys, pinks for girls, and matching colors for various holidays. The hats are particularly useful for premature babies because they can be made very small, are exceptionally soft, and stretch well.

Stephanie and John have also provided puppets for the children to help distract them from procedures as well as to keep their siblings entertained. This husband and wife team has created "angel gowns" for use when there is a loss of a baby. In addition, they make baby "pockets" which are used to wrap very small

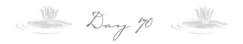

babies in after a loss, so the babies can be presented to parents who wish to hold them. The angel gowns and pockets have been lovingly constructed with lace trims and appliqués, and sometimes the parents want these items to be placed in a memory box that is provided by the medical center, and at other times, the baby is buried in the lovely items.

John Johnson recently passed away at the age of 93. For years, he helped Stephanie cut fabric, organize pieces and chauffered her to procure her sewing notions, as well as took her to the hospital to drop off her items. Despite losing her partner of so many years, Stephanie continues to make the baby hats, puppets, angel gowns, and pockets. She feels her work is her "saving grace," especially since losing John. However, the hospital family and volunteers who distribute her beautifully created items, feel she has blessed them—as well as the patients—with her selfless giving.

—Submitted by Catherine DiPasquale,
Hackensack University Medical Center, Hackensack, NJ

"Never underestimate the difference you can make."

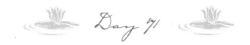

An American Hero

My nursing practice was changed not by a single patient but by an entire generation of patients. The following story illustrates what I mean:

W hen I came in to work one morning, it was reported to me that one of our patients had fallen at home and fractured his ankle. He went to the operating room and had an open reduction internal fixation. He was in his eighties and the analgesia and surgery can have severe side effects on a person his age. When he came out of anesthesia, he was having audio and visual hallucinations. During the day someone got him up and helped him onto a bedside commode. While he was on the commode, he got up on his own, fell, and fractured his hip. He went out of control—spitting, hitting, and carrying on like a wild man.

By the next morning, his mind had cleared. When I went into the room, I found a disheveled man in his bed. I introduced myself as his nurse and asked him if he remembered what had happened. He told me that there were only some parts he could recall. I explained to him that there was no way of knowing how a person will react to analgesia and told him that he had had quite a reaction. I started my assessment and realized that any movement he made was very painful, but he was able to

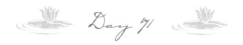

breathe deeply for me and didn't have any numbness or tingling in his affected extremity. He let me know how afraid he was to have his leg fixed because he was concerned that he may act violently again.

I sat down at his bedside. I explained to him that we now knew more information about how he is likely to respond to analgesia and that we could put a plan in place to keep it from happening again. Then, he asked me if his wife had called and I told him that she was on her way to come see him. "How long have you been married?" I asked. "We were married in 1946, which was one month after I returned from the war," he answered. He explained to me that he had served three years as a Marine in the South Pacific and that he still had nightmares from his time in the war. He began to cry and almost as soon as he started, I could see him fight it back. "You are an American hero," I told him, "and you deserve respect and compassion."

That's when it hit me—I was caring for the generation that changed the direction of the world. When the country called these men and women, they went without protest or complaint. They went to a war that was not on their shore. They went with the commitment that the whole nation was behind them. While I was having the time of my life, these men where facing horrors so terrible that 51 years later it still gives them nightmares. The only thing these men and women wanted when it was over was to raise a family. I am one of their children. These men and women are the people that made a home for us. Our mothers were in the home. Our fathers were building a nation. My safety was never in question. They are the men and women that paid the price with their lives and youth and now it is my turn to pay them back. It is my turn to help

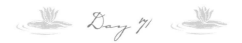

them through their twilight years. It is my turn to give them the respect and dignity that they deserve, and it is my duty to remind my coworkers who our clients are and why they deserve the best.

—Submitted by Kevin Williams, Saint Mary's Health Care

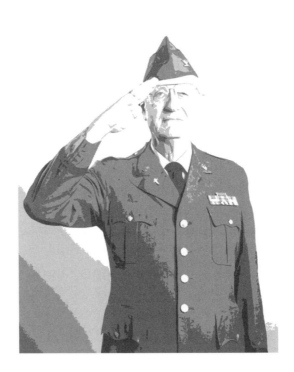

"Never underestimate the difference you can make."

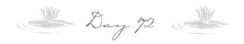

My Inspiration

When I was 16, I was diagnosed with cancer. I was given six months to live if I didn't have a radical hysterectomy. My physician recommended I go to a hospital in New York City. So off I went in the middle of January 1971. My mother stayed at a minister's home nearby so she could still see me, but I was very much alone in the hospital. And remember, this was before cell phones, so I couldn't just chat all evening with my friends. I was hundreds of miles from home.

It was a long painful surgery—emotionally and physically. Not only would I never be able to bear children, I was also afraid that I would die. Throughout the three weeks I was hospitalized there were two people who made a difference in my life. I don't know their names. I just know that they came and sat with me through many long evenings. One was a resident and one was a nurse. They weren't assigned to my case. They didn't have to be with me or spend time with me. Each sat at the bedside, talked, watched TV, and were just "there for me." That was when I knew I wanted to be a nurse. I knew then what it meant, even through the pain and loss—that through the gift of several minutes sent sitting by a patient's beside, some can make a difference. Thirty-five years later, it still makes a difference in the way my life has evolved.

—Submitted by Carolyn Laughlin, Wadsworth Rittman

"Never underestimate the difference you can make."

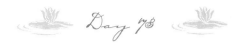

Going the Extra Mile

One of the most challenging aspects of being a health care professional is offering support to those who are suffering from a terminal illness. Part of this mission includes comforting family members who are often fearful and uncertain.

Christy, an RN at WellStar Kennestone Hospital, has a heart of gold and a gift for offering love and comfort, even to those she barely knows.

Mrs. C had been a patient on Christy's unit several times before. She was a strong soul who had suffered with cancer for many years.

During Mrs. C's last admission, Christy realized the gravity of her condition, as Mrs. C's immune system appeared to be losing the battle with cancer. Mr. C stayed at his wife's bedside as much as possible, even sleeping beside her with a mask on to prevent the spread of germs.

When his wife lost consciousness, the decision was made to transfer Mrs. C to hospice care. Despite Mrs. C no longer being on her unit, Christy checked on Mr. C to see if he needed anything to eat or if she could bring him anything, but Mr. C said, "No," and that he was doing okay. Again the next day, Christy called him to make sure he was doing all right in this trying time. He said he would welcome a visit if she could work that out. That night, after working a 12-hour shift, Christy drove in the opposite direction from her home to offer support to Mr. C as he sat by his wife's bedside.

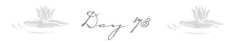

This has been Christy's nature—taking care of patients and their families as well. Such caring doesn't end with a patient's transfer, and Christy never hesitates to go the extra mile.

—*Submitted by Amy Little, WellStar Kennestone*

"Never underestimate the difference you can make."

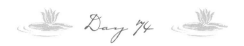

The Importance of a Smile

One of my coworkers, Alice, is able to comfort those around her without even saying a word. She projects a sense of calm and her positive spirit radiates a silent message to others.

When Alice was diagnosed with breast cancer, we all came together to pray for her as she underwent surgery, chemotherapy, and radiation treatment. Her endurance and recovery only emphasized the inner strength she possesses. Although we all knew she was fighting hard and enduring many trials, Alice managed to keep a smile.

When Alice returned to work, we knew her presence would once more influence patients in a positive way. One particular night, Alice was working with a patient who had been diagnosed with breast cancer. The patient had undergone a mastectomy but was having a difficult time recovering, both physically and emotionally. She had been depressed and the hospitalization was making her recovery even more difficult.

I noticed Alice had been in that patient's room for a long time before returning to the nurse's station. Later, when the patient's IV pump started beeping, I went in to investigate and reset the pump. While I was there, the patient stopped me and smiled. That was the first time I had seen her smile during her stay on our floor.

She started talking about Alice and what a special person she was. Of course, I wholeheartedly agreed with her. Giggling, the patient told me that she and Alice had compared their cancer battle wounds.

Because Alice had taken the time to communicate in a special way with this patient, she had relayed hope and helped this patient come to terms with her own fight with cancer. By projecting such a positive attitude about her own struggle, Alice had impacted this patient in a way no one else could. Alice had restored a sense of faith to a person who desperately needed it. Alice's friendly, caring demeanor, wrapped in her smile and positive attitude, had given this patient the gift of hope and put a smile on her face, as well.

—Submitted by *Amy Little, WellStar Kennestone*

"Never underestimate the difference you can make."

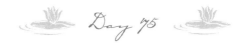

Providing a Helping Hand

Norton Healthcare in Louisville, Kentucky, was named after the Rev. John N. Norton, who was called "the Good Samaritan" by the people in the community he served. In his honor, the hospital instituted their Good Samaritan Award to recognize employees who perform extraordinary acts of service, outside the expectations of their job descriptions.

Travis Stowers, employed in the engineering department at Norton Southwest Medical Center, received the Good Samaritan Award because of his innovative method for helping a patient.

Travis was making routine maintenance rounds when a patient with limited hand mobility asked for help answering the phone. It occurred to Travis that this patient was going to continue having trouble answering the phone, so he contacted the physical therapy department to see if there was a device that could solve the problem. When Travis discovered there was nothing available, he proceeded to design one which enabled the patient to hold the receiver by sliding his hand between a bar and the handset.

After installing the device, Travis noticed that the patient also had problems holding eating utensils. Again, with no device available for that purpose, Travis created a second device so the patient could manage eating utensils.

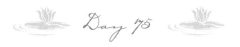

On subsequent hospital visits, the patient would contact Travis, who would install the devices in the hospital room, enabling the patient to perform these simple tasks with comfort and dignity.

The patient was delighted that his hospital visits were now more pleasant because Travis went out of his way to solve a problem and allow the patient more control over his environment.

Because of Travis Stowers' ingenuity and dedication, he received the Good Samaritan Award. More importantly, he made the hospital environment a more comfortable space for patients with limited hand mobility.

—Submitted by Janelle Picklesimer, Norton Healthcare

"Never underestimate the difference you can make."

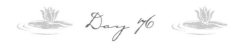

A Higher Purpose

A patient shared this heartfelt story with our organization:

It was on Monday, Dec. 20, 1999, just five days before Christmas—the day my life changed forever. I had worked as an electrician for almost 25 years, and on this day, I was inside a generator. We all thought the electricity was shut down. It wasn't. Suddenly, I was shocked with more than 12,000 volts of electricity—that's 60 times the power in your home.

The next thing I remember was waking up in the Burn Center two months later. I heard the soothing voice of my nurses and saw their faces for the first time. They told me I was the sickest person in their hospital. I had third-degree burns on more than 60 percent of my body and had to fight pneumonia, cardiac arrhythmias, and major infections. Every day was a new challenge, every week a new surgery—but day by day, week by week, I began to heal physically.

I am grateful to all my nurses, especially Mindy. Mindy is my angel. Besides caring for my physical needs, she cared for my soul. So many nights while she carefully cared for my raw skin, we'd talk and cry together. I could see my bandaged arms and my red, raw legs, and I was

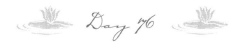

scared of how people would react to me. She was always there to listen to me.

Whenever I looked at my granddaughter's photo, I would just break down. I'd ask Mindy, "How do you explain to a 3-year-old that her Pop has been hurt—that he is deformed?" She would tell me, "Alexia will see beyond this and love you." And she does. In fact, Alexia has accepted the way I look better than I have. It takes special people like Mindy to care for people like me.

Outside every room in the Burn Center is a little plaque that says: "Those who care for burns will get their reward in heaven." I don't think they should have to wait that long. They should get the recognition now. It's been four years and 57 surgeries since my accident, and every day I think about Mindy and the people who saved my life. Sure, I have bad days…but I have good days, too. Mindy is always there for me and that makes the future bright.

I visit the unit often and I try to give something back. I share my story in the Burn Center to help other burn survivors put their lives together. During some of my toughest times, I would ask Mindy, "Why didn't I die?" And she'd tell me, "There's a higher purpose for you that someday you'll realize." Today I realize my purpose…it is to help others.

—*Submitted by Barbara Versage, Lehigh Valley Hospital Health Network*

"Never underestimate the difference you can make."

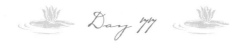

Day 747

I Do! I Do!

Imagine everyone's surprise at hearing "Here Comes the Bride" echoing through the halls of Emory Healthcare in Atlanta, Georgia. Over the past three years, the staff of Emory Healthcare's Bone Marrow Transplant Unit has planned a total of three weddings, giving a new meaning to the importance of teamwork and interdisciplinary planning.

The first wedding was that of a 25-year-old man diagnosed with leukemia. He had experienced several hospitalizations over several years with his girlfriend beside him as his main caregiver. She was with him through all his admissions and took care of his home care needs following each discharge.

After the young man completed yet another exhausting treatment, the couple shared with the staff their desire to get married. In an effort to grant that wish, Emory's team of nurses, aides, chaplain, social worker, and physician rushed to accomplish the feat with one week's notice.

The chaplain assigned to the transplant unit agreed to officiate and reserved the hospital chapel for the event. The rest of the staff took care of the arrangements, from securing a florist, to music selection, and premarital counseling. Various staff members agreed to donate hors d'oeuvres and booked a conference room for the reception. The hospital's food service provided a beautiful wedding cake.

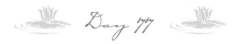

After the ceremony, staffers placed a "Just Married" sign on the groom's transport caddie, along with Styrofoam cups which streamed from the transport as he was wheeled from the chapel to the reception area.

News of this untraditional wedding quickly spread, capturing the attention of local media. Since that first wedding, two more have taken place on this unit and staff members report that patients occasionally ask to be admitted to a room on the "wedding planning" floor!

—*Submitted by Paula McGuire Saunders, Emory Healthcare, Atlanta, GA*

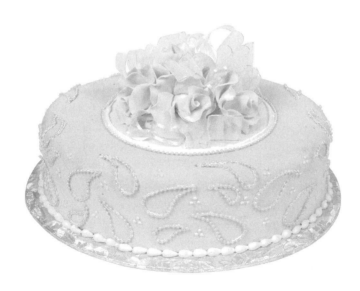

"Never underestimate the difference you can make."

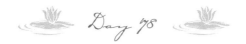

Touched by an Earth Angel

I believe in "earth angels." On July 4, 2005, my family and I were touched by one such angel at Norton Audubon Hospital. While picnics, parties, and fireworks were going on in the outside world, my family and I were in the waiting room of the Intensive Care Unit, after learning that my 44-year-old brother, David, had two malignant brain tumors.

That day was the worst day of my life to that point and I am sure that anyone observing my family could see our pain and dismay. And then, Peggy appeared.

Peggy was a kind, caring little cleaning lady, and she restored my faith and hope and my belief in angels on that July 4th day. She seemed to have appeared out of nowhere, but I believe she was sent to us. She was radiant, and I was immediately drawn to her. She spoke of the loss of her mother and of her pain and of the raw, empty, hopeless feelings that people experience at these trying times in their lives. She ministered to me, my husband, and my dad that July afternoon, telling us to "hold on."

When Peggy left the area with her cleaning cart, my husband and my dad both said, "There is something about her." We would find ourselves saying that again and again about Peggy in the coming days.

My brother was moved from the ICU and spent about 10 more days in the hospital. During that time, Peggy had searched for my brother and when she saw my parents one day, she asked about him. My parents took Peggy to visit David.

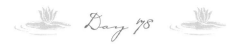

When they opened the door, about 15 other people were crowded in the room, but Peggy made her way through the many visitors to David's side.

Peggy talked to David and told him to "hold on" and pointed her finger up towards heaven. She told him his work was not yet done here. Then she sang "Amazing Grace." The room was silent and tears were flowing. When Peggy left, David said, "There is just something about her."

The next day, David had to make some hard decisions about his care plan. He was confused and scared and needed to make the decisions quickly. As the doctors were leaving his room, Peggy returned to visit. She walked in, handed David an envelope, and turned to leave. When she got to the door, she turned back to David and pointed upward with her index finger—a connection made without a single word spoken.

Within a moment of opening the envelope, David had made his decision. He called me and told me that Peggy had helped him make his decision. David explained that he had opened a card from Peggy and that a gold cross had fallen out of the card onto his chest. He said within that moment, he had been able to make a decision about his surgery. He added, "There is just something about her."

By the time David was finally discharged, he and Peggy had formed a special bond. David felt he had been touched by an angel. When David left the hospital, he faced a long, trying journey, but Peggy had infused him with faith, hope, determination, and a readiness to fight his aggressive form of melanoma.

During the months ahead, David endured brain surgeries, chemotherapy, radiation, lung surgery, and other tests too numerous to mention. Through it all, Peggy was there, visiting him on a regular basis, sending him music, bringing

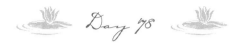

him flowers, and even giving him an angel figurine. In July 2006, David took a turn for the worse, with cancer taking over his brain. But Peggy continued to stay in touch and was a great source of comfort and strength to our family.

Near the end, Peggy came to visit David at home. She prayed with us and quoted scripture. The next time she would see David, he was an inpatient in the hospice unit.

David passed away on Sept. 7, 2006, at 8:15 p.m. I got out my cell phone to call Peggy and let her know, and there was a call from her I had missed—which came in at 8:15 p.m. It seems Peggy always knew when we needed her.

Peggy still calls us. She has been a dear friend to us all and truly, an angel. She touched our lives in a way no one ever has. To think a cleaning lady who works two full-time jobs and takes care of her own family would have time to be concerned about others is amazing.

As a tribute to this special "earth angel," David was buried with the gold cross Peggy gave him.

—Submitted by Janelle Picklesimer, Norton Healthcare

"Never underestimate the difference you can make."

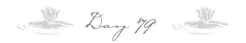

Making It Happen

Telemetry had a patient that needed a life vest, a vest that when worn by the patient is devised to "shock" the heart back into rhythm when needed. Because it was a weekend, the vest would not come in until late Saturday afternoon. The sales rep explained that he could not put the vest on the patient or teach them how to use it until Monday.

This meant our patient was going to have to stay an additional two days even though he had already expressed how much he wanted to go home. Amber, one of our nurses, truly stepped up to the plate. She drove down to the UPS store, picked up the life vest, paid the $5.00 postage, and brought it back to the hospital. And thankfully, the sales rep was able to get here late Saturday afternoon to teach the patient how to use the vest. The patient was able to go home to his family that day.

The patient and his family were very appreciative of Amber's kindness and willingness to do everything in her power to get him what he needed so that he could go home.

—Submitted by Kathy Beaver, Frye Regional Medical Center, Hickory, NC

"Never underestimate the difference you can make."

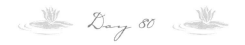

Making Connections

A little over two years ago, we opened the Lacks Cancer Center at Saint Mary's with the intent to focus on an exceptional patient experience. Through the Center, I had the opportunity to see first-hand the impact our team was making. I was on the way to the cafeteria for lunch when I ran into two new and very lost ambulance transporters. They had come to pick up one of our cancer patients to transport him to Hospice. They were in the main hospital building and needed to go to the inpatient unit in the Cancer Center so I offered to take them there. As we were walking, one of the individuals asked me if I knew of the patient and his cancer's prognosis. I could sense her uneasiness as she explained that she was new and had never taken a patient to Hospice before. I assured her that the staff was amazing and would give her the necessary info to help her feel more at ease.

When we arrived at the Center, I asked the unit secretary about the location of our patient. "He's in Room 4436 and I'm pretty sure his nurse, Maggie, is with him," she said with a pause, "I am so sorry to see him go." As we entered the room I introduced Maggie and our patient, Jim, to the transporters. Maggie was leaning over talking softly in Jim's ear and as she looked up at us I could see a tear in her eye. I went back to the desk and offered to guide the transporters back through the Cancer Center to the area where they entered when they were ready.

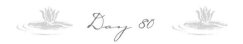

As the transporters left the room with Jim, I began to see a scene that I know will be in my heart forever. We were walking down a hall toward the elevator when one of our environmental service associates came toward Jim and whispered to him "It was an honor serving you," as she gently kissed him on the cheek. A few more feet down the hall, a PCA approached Jim and the transporters. She gave him an enormous hug and told him she would keep him in her prayers. Yet another nurse approached as we neared the elevator. She gently spoke in Jim's ear before departing with a tear. As we entered the elevator, Jim said to me, "You truly have angels here," and he broke down in a wave of silent tears. The transporters, too, had tears in their eyes as we got off the elevator and Jim departed.

I went back to my office for a moment and shed some tears myself. I knew that what I had just witnessed was something powerful and moving. I knew we were hitting our mark and truly making a difference in our patient's life. I went back up to the unit to share my experience with our nurse manager, Markaye and to tell our associates how very proud I was to be working with such amazing individuals. "You know, Amy," Markaye explained to me, "Jim doesn't have any real family or friends. He's had a pretty tough life and drove a truck for many years so he really hadn't made any real connections." Yes, I thought to myself, Jim did make some connections. And in turn *we* were the recipients of something very powerful.

—Submitted by *Amy Searls, Saint Mary's Healthcare*

"Never underestimate the difference you can make."

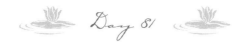

Providing Care from the Heart

Nurses not only provide care for our "precious gifts," but also provide the needed support and compassion for the immediate and extended families of their patients. This was demonstrated under extraordinary circumstances by the pediatric nurses at Inova Loudoun Hospital.

During the admission of an infant to the Pediatric Unit, the nurse noticed the mother seemed unusually worried and stressed. The mother mentioned that her family was new to the area and did not have any relatives or close friends nearby. To make matters worse, her husband was traveling on business and the family dog had been having seizures all day.

After the infant was made comfortable, the mother asked if it would be possible for her to briefly return home and check on the family pet. Although it is routine in the Pediatric Unit for a parent to stay with an infant, the nurse could sense the mother's concern and anxiety. The nurse was able to arrange for a staff member to stay with the infant so the mother could make a quick trip home.

While at home, the mother answered a phone call and learned her father had suffered a massive heart attack. Upon her return to the Pediatric Unit, the mother told the nurses about her father. Her distress was apparent and, without hesitation, the nurses and physicians provided emotional support for the mother as she cared for her infant and tried to deal with the possible loss of her father.

They listened compassionately as she discussed the possible scenarios that would enable her to travel halfway across the country to visit her father one last time.

Eventually, the phone call she was dreading came. She was advised that, if she wanted to stay goodbye to her father, she would have to leave immediately. Understanding that the infant was not ready for discharge, the pediatric nurses developed a plan for providing additional staff to care for the infant in the mother's absence. The nurses assured the mother that the infant would be well taken care of, if she needed to leave. Most importantly, the nurses told the mother it was okay to leave the infant and be with her father. Fortunately, the mother had a friend with a private plane who was available to transport her to and from the hospital where her father was a patient. The mother was assured the entire trip should not take more than 12 hours.

When the mother received the call that her friend was waiting at the airport, she tearfully said goodbye to her infant and left for the airport. The infant had an uneventful night in the Pediatric Unit, receiving extra TLC from the staff. Early the next morning, the mother arrived back at the hospital to find her infant being held, content, and continuing to recover.

As the nurses gathered to hear how her trip went, the mother became overwhelmed at the care and concern given to both her infant and herself. "It is hard to find words that describe the amount of compassion and caring everyone has shown my family," the mother stated. As the mother held her infant, the phone rang. Her father had passed away just hours after her visit.

Although the nurses were saddened to hear of the passing of the mother's father, they were also overcome with pride. This young mother had enough confidence in them to leave her infant overnight. This type of caring and compassion is truly what's right in health care today.

—*Submitted by Diane McFarland and Sheree O'Neil, Inova Loudoun Hospital, Leesburg, VA*

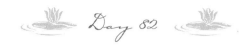

Letting Go

Mrs. B was a frequent admission to the ICU at Inova Loudoun Hospital. Her emphysema required that she be placed on a ventilator. During one particular admission, Mrs. B and her daughter, Alice, had decided it was time to "let go," with no use of extraordinary means to prolong her life.

As the shift began, Mrs. B's nurse, Dolores, was once again caring for the familiar patient. Although Dolores had cared for Mrs. B on many previous occasions, this time was different. In addition to providing care for her critically ill patient, she was helping Alice make preparations to take her mother home to spend her last hours with her family.

Throughout the day, as Mrs. B's condition worsened, it became apparent that time was of the essence. While Alice made home health care arrangements, it became necessary that she leave her mother's side. Recognizing the urgency and stress of the situation, Dolores promised to stay with Mrs. B until Alice returned.

True to her word, Dolores remained with Mrs. B even after her shift ended. While sitting with her patient, she noticed a light snow had begun to fall outside, so Dolores turned her patient's bed to the window so she could watch the snowfall. Soon after, Mrs. B's breathing became labored, and she reached for Dolores. The typical procedure at this point would be an intubation, but knowing Mrs. B's wishes, Dolores held Mrs. B's hand to soothe her. Mrs. B pulled Dolores

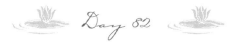

closer. Dolores cradled her patient, deciding to climb into the bed and wrap her patient in comfort and strength.

There they remained, nurse and patient, watching the snow snowflakes softly fall from the sky until Alice returned. That evening, Mrs. B peacefully passed away, with Alice and Dolores by her side.

In a time when it is easy to get caught up in the technology of providing health care, the compassion and caring that Dolores unselfishly provided reminds us all that sometimes the best intervention for our patients are not the tasks we provide—but rather that healing touch that comes from our hearts.

—Submitted by Diane McFarland, Dolores Kemp, and Marissa Putman, Inova Loudoun Hospital, Leesburg, VA

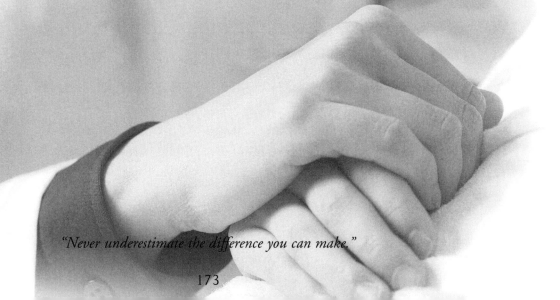

"Never underestimate the difference you can make."

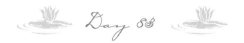

BEING THERE WHEN IT COUNTS

One of the main reasons I became an emergency room nurse was because I had a strong interest in injury prevention. As an emergency medical technician, I had seen many tragedies that could have been prevented if the people involved had only known how to protect themselves. Part of my job now, as an RN and injury prevention coordinator in the ER, is visiting high school classrooms to teach teenagers about injury prevention—specifically about not driving drunk.

High school students are one of the toughest and most important groups to teach. They often have trouble making good choices because they don't have much life experience to draw from. They think they're invincible and that their behavior never results in severe consequences.

About 15 years ago, during my program at one school, I gave each of the students a card to write down the names and numbers of two people they could call if they were stuck somewhere and needed help. The object was for them to carry these cards in their wallets to use in an emergency.

During the exercise, one of the students tentatively approached me and said, "Nurse Robin, I don't have anyone to call." This boy, whom I'll call "Rob," lived in a foster home, and he was afraid he would jeopardize his situation if he called his foster parents drunk. I took a good look at him and made a quick decision. "You can use me as your person to call," I said. I gave Rob the number of the ER

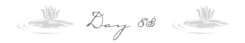

where I worked and told him to call that number if he was ever stuck somewhere and needed help. Even if I wasn't working, I told him, someone would help him.

A few months went by, and I didn't think much more about Rob—until the night I heard from him again. "You probably don't remember me," said this voice over the phone, "but you came to my school and talked about making healthy decisions. Well, I'm at a party, and I've been drinking, and I have no way to get home. You said I should call someone I trust. Can you help me?"

At that moment, there was only one thought in my mind: I have served my purpose on earth if I have reached one student. I have to help this boy. I told Rob I couldn't pick him up myself, but I would help him find a way home. I then called a cab company, explained the situation, promised them I would pay for the fare and sent the cab to take Rob home.

My coworkers were shocked I was paying a $40 cab fare out of my own pocket, but I had promised Rob I would help him. And there was no way I could break my word. He felt like no one cared about him, and I wanted him to walk away from this situation knowing that there's always somebody in his life who can help him explore options.

Rob initially wanted me to help him tell his foster parents why he had broken curfew and try to talk them out of grounding him, but I told him he needed to take responsibility for that himself. He asked if I was mad at him for being drunk. "Actually," I said, "I'm very proud of you. You were in a tough situation, and you had the presence of mind to think about the options you had before making a bad choice—getting behind the wheel drunk."

People make mistakes. It's how we deal with those mistakes that makes the difference. This situation continued to fuel my passion for prevention. The fact that my message got through to at least one student was very inspiring for me.

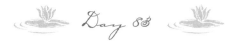

And when I received a letter from Rob thanking me for my help, I was gratified beyond words. I found that being there when it counts is truly what being in health care is all about.

—*Submitted by Robin Ihde, Community Memorial Hospital*

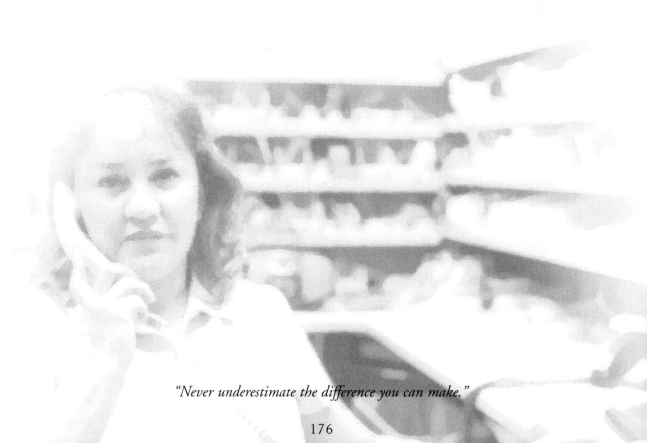

"Never underestimate the difference you can make."

SUPER VOLUNTEERS

Karen O'Brien and Belinda Brouillette are the ultimate volunteers. They pitch in whenever and wherever needed. Over the years, they have worked in play rooms, as baby holders, and in pastoral care. They have even taken on leadership responsibilities as well, as Karen and Belinda served as president of The Auxiliary to Texas Children's Hospital. But they truly demonstrated their value, and the value of all volunteers, when Texas Children's Hospital and the entire city of Houston responded to Hurricane Katrina.

Many children were transferred from hospitals in New Orleans directly to Texas Children's Hospital. Others, who had not been hospitalized at home, came to stay at Reliant Park, which is very near the Texas Medical Center. As time went on, many of them needed some form of medical care and so they came to our hospital.

Texas Children's opened a family support center where families who came to our clinics or Emergency Center could access resources to help them locate family members. We also stocked donated clothing, food, toys, strollers, diapers, and many of the other necessities of life that had been left behind. These items were offered to any family who had come to Houston to escape the devastation on the Gulf Coast.

Volunteers helped stock the center by going shopping, sorting the clothes, and dividing the toiletries into personal hygiene bags. Others helped in the center by making phone calls for families and helping them access resources such as the

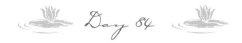

Red Cross, which maintained a database of families seeking other family members. Karen and Belinda helped out in all of these areas, but they didn't stop there.

They realized that some of the families came to the Emergency Center late at night and in the early morning hours. They knew that the Emergency Center staff was very busy keeping up with the medical concerns of the families and did not have time to try to meet the everyday needs of the parents and children who didn't need medical care.

Belinda and Karen decided that it was up to them to fill that gap. They came early, stayed late, and even spent several nights in the Texas Children's Emergency Center. They ran to the family support center to bring back needed items. They sat with children whose siblings were being treated. They talked and listened to parents who had left everything behind and who did not know if they had anything waiting for them at home.

The staff at Texas Children's Hospital provides superior medical care. There is at least one child who survived that horrible time only because she was treated at Texas Children's. But the staff also realizes that families have other needs and those who work here keenly feel the desire to help meet those needs.

Volunteers so often step in to fill that gap. As demonstrated by Belinda and Karen, volunteers often go above and beyond the call of duty when they perceive the need. I believe that those who were touched by Karen and Belinda in September 2005 took a little of their fire with them. Families were warmed by the flame of their concern. Staff members were inspired by their dedication. You don't have to receive a paycheck to be a Fire Starter!

—Submitted by Pat Dolan, Texas Children's Hospital

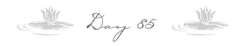

Above and Beyond

Pam Stone is one of those rare people patients never forget. She comes in contact with her patients in their homes as she serves their needs through her job with Medical Center Home Health.

Not only does Pam serve her patients' home health needs, she has a sharp eye for the other situations that exist in their lives. Once, while at the home of an elderly gentleman who lived alone, Pam noticed that his house needed a good cleaning. So what did Pam do? She stayed after hours and personally cleaned his entire house!

Pam's concern for her patients does not stop there. She keeps a mental list of other needs and while she meanders through yard sales, she picks up clothing, small appliances, and other items, and delivers them to her patients. She has even taken food out of her own freezer and prepared meals while caretaking in her patients' homes.

Pam touches the lives of her patients in practical ways, because she has the insight to see the actual needs. While many caregivers go about their assigned duties and then go home…Pam keeps looking. She has truly made a difference in the lives of many patients.

—Submitted by Linda Pledge, West Tennessee Healthcare, Jackson, TN

"Never underestimate the difference you can make."

The Real Story

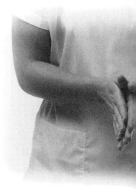

The woman who presented herself in our Emergency Department (ED) complained of a headache, but the bruises on her body told a different story. Working in an inner-city ED, I was becoming more and more aware of the symptoms of domestic abuse, and the answers I was getting from this patient did not fit her physical condition.

I gently questioned her about the various bruises and her home situation. My patient lowered her head, avoided looking straight at me, and kept denying there was anything wrong at home.

Before she left the ED, I took her aside. "I know you said you are safe at home, but if there comes a time when you feel you aren't, this ED staff is here for you," I said. "You come in, any time of day or night, if you need help."

I won't say I was totally surprised when, the next day, this patient returned to the ED, after having been beaten by her husband with a baseball bat.

"You were right," she said, "but I just wasn't ready to admit it."

I helped her obtain a protection from abuse order that day and had her escorted home by the police, who then searched for the bat used in the attack. Subsequently, her husband was arrested and convicted.

Sometimes our jobs include more than healing the sick. This was one of those times that helping a patient meant making sure she learned how to move from victim to survivor.

—Submitted by Barbara Versage, Lehigh Valley Hospital & Health Network

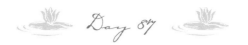
Making a Difference

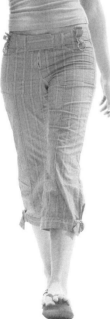

*I*n my job as a member of the case management department at Jennie Stuart Medical Center, I have seen how ordinary people can have great impact on the lives of others. No one fulfills this role more than my coworker, Pam Oliver.

Pam is known throughout the community, as well as our facility, as a caring hard-working advocate for patients and their families. Her knowledge of discharge planning and resources is outstanding, and her ability to make everyone feel at ease, along with her beautiful spirit, allows her to make friends easily. Her energy, sense of humor, and dedication are appreciated by her coworkers as well as her patients.

Twenty years ago, as the young mother of a two-year-old child, Pam was diagnosed with Hodgkin's disease. Despite painful diagnostic procedures and surgery, Pam continued to come to work through six weeks of radiation therapy. Pam was determined to fight. And, in the end, she was diagnosed as cancer-free.

Pam has become a leader in the community for the American Cancer Society, helping organize the Relay for Life events in two counties, raising thousands of dollars. However, Pam's dedication

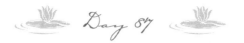

to the community does not stop there. She is a volunteer for Pennyroyal Hospice and was recognized as their volunteer of the year.

As a United Way volunteer, she has earned the coveted J. William Flowers Award for excellence and has served as treasurer for the local chapter of the Kidney Foundation.

Recently, Pam lost her beloved brother, when his plane, Comair Flight 5191, crashed in Kentucky. Despite this crushing loss, Pam has continued her service to improving the continuum of care for all her patients. She has worked not only as an advocate for our patients, but also as an advocate for the whole community.

Pam's hard work, determination and commitment to a better health care system has made our hospital and community better places to work and live. Pam's life exemplifies what health care is about—people who make a difference.

—Submitted by Louanne Young for Janet L. Myers,
Jennie Stuart Medical Center, Hopkinsville, KY

"Never underestimate the difference you can make."

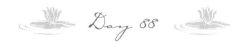

A Last Goodbye

I work in the Emergency Department as an emergency care technician. The one story that sticks out in my memory is about a little girl that we saw frequently as a patient. Due to a congenital heart defect, she suffered from cardiomegaly and a host of other medical problems.

One evening, our paramedics were called to a residence in Emmetsburg, Maryland, for a child in cardiac arrest. When they arrived on the scene, they found an unresponsive child lying on the front lawn. Her mother stated that they had just walked back from the neighbor's house, and her daughter was laughing and goofing off. All of sudden, she didn't hear her daughter and turned around to find her lying in the grass. At first, she thought that the little girl was just playing around. When she walked back to help her up she realized that she was unresponsive. The paramedics were able to resuscitate the child and transport her to the ER. While in the emergency department, the physician and nurses tried everything to maintain life but were unsuccessful. After several more attempts to stabilize the child, the doctors and family decided that there was nothing more to be done for her as she continued slipping away.

The ER doctor asked me to find a comfortable chair for the child's mother. I went to the maternity ward to borrow one of their nice wooden rocking chairs. The mother sat down in the rocking chair while the doctor and the nurse disconnected all of the life-saving equipment from the little girl's body. The

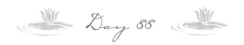

doctor gently picked up the little girl and placed her in her mother's arms. Everyone except the doctor left room and allowed the parents to hold their child while she gently passed away.

I was touched by such a caring and kind gesture on the doctor's part. It was important to allow the family some peace in their daughter's final moments. The Emergency Room staff is usually a group of tough individuals but we weren't too tough that night. In that moment, we were simply humans with a need to help a family when they needed it the most.

—*Submitted by Elisa Laughman, Gettysburg Hospital, Wellspan Health*

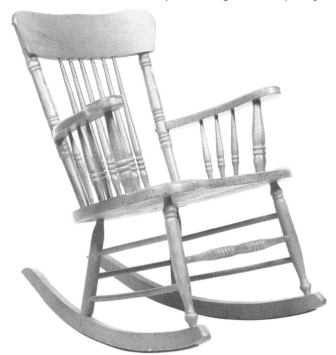

"Never underestimate the difference you can make."

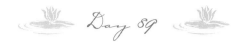

A Gift of Christmas Cheer

Having raised her family, Christa devoted her time and talent to Advocate Christ Medical Center as a volunteer. As a volunteer patient greeter, Christa's job consisted of visiting with patients and checking to see if she could help them learn how to operate the telephone, television, or the hospital bed. While visiting with a patient on December 21, he mentioned to her that he was being discharged to a nursing home. He asked Christa if she could find him a Santa hat to take with him. He explained to her that he thought the hat would be a fun way to break the ice in a new environment. Christa was unable to find a Santa hat around the medical center so she walked six blocks in the freezing Chicago weather to a Walgreens and purchased a hat with her own money.

—Submitted by Eileen Treacy, *Advocate Christ Medical Center, Oak Lawn, IL*

"Never underestimate the difference you can make."

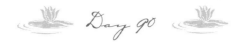

Above and Beyond the Call of Duty

You could say that Betty Lenoir is a physical therapist, but that would only be half the story. The other half of the story is that Betty is an extraordinary person who has responded to human need in the highest, most committed way—by bringing it home.

It was nearly three years ago when Betty met Ebony, a 16-year-old bilateral above-knee amputee. As the weeks passed, Betty began to learn of Ebony's personal story. Ebony was born with Malfucci's Syndrome, which causes severe deformities of her legs and feet. The doctors had often recommended amputations, but her mother refused, feeling it was not her decision to make. As a result, Ebony never learned to crawl, and she suffered through multiple infections—robbing her of a normal childhood. When Ebony was nine years old, her mother passed away and she was sent to live with her grandmother. Eventually, the doctors received permission to amputate her legs above the knee, and Betty came into Ebony's life as her therapist.

Through their involvement, Betty realized that Ebony had no wheelchair. She scooted around inside her house with an old office chair, maneuvered herself from her house to the car on a folding metal chair. No one at home was helping her with her home exercises, which were critical for walking with prosthetic limbs. Because of her many illnesses, Ebony also had frequent absences from

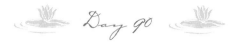

school. Rather than help her to catch up, the school just put her in a slower class, and Ebony continued to fall farther behind.

Ebony's situation tugged at Betty's heart. Personally moved by this child's special needs, Betty located a loaner wheelchair, and then worked to get her a brand new one. And she began to work very hard to get Ebony strong enough for normal activities. Betty began taking Ebony to community outings, and even got her involved with a wheelchair basketball team. Betty would drive to Ebony's home, take her to basketball practice, and then back home again.

Betty still felt as if it wasn't enough, and she wanted to help Ebony in a consistent way. After much contemplation and family discussion, Betty took the ultimate leap of faith and invited Ebony to live with her family in a foster-care type setting. Of course, the answer was a resounding, "Yes!"

Nearly three years have passed since Ebony became a part of Betty's family. She is now attending a private school through a scholarship and is walking on two prosthetic legs using only forearm crutches. A car has been donated to Ebony with hand controls installed, and Ebony is signed up for a driver training program. She participates in wheelchair racing, and has lots of fun traveling to various events with her newfound family to places like Oklahoma, Tennessee, and Mississippi. Ebony has enrolled for the Endeavor Games held in Oklahoma, wheelchair basketball camps in Illinois and Alabama, and an amputee camp in Nashville. Much of this is paid for with Betty's personal finances, but the joy as Ebony completes each new challenge is reward enough.

What began as an ordinary patient visit has blossomed into a mutually caring relationship that has greatly enriched both of their lives. Today, Ebony is a happy, active teenager. What Betty has given her goes far beyond increased physical strength for a more active lifestyle. Betty has given Ebony hope for her future, a

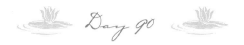

brighter outlook, and a caring, loving extended family. And for us, as health care employees, Betty has reinforced our belief that miracles really do occur here, every day.

—Submitted by Linda Pledge, *West Tennessee Healthcare, Jackson, TN*

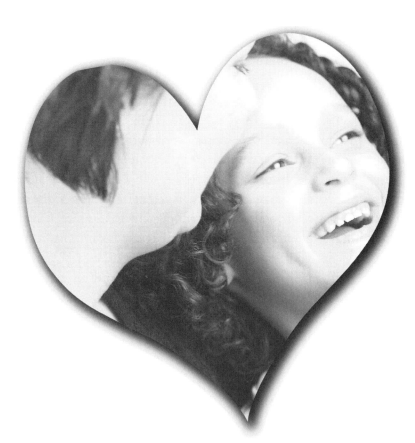

"Never underestimate the difference you can make."

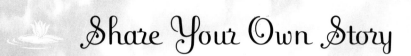

Share Your Own Story

Please share an experience that connected you back to purpose, worthwhile work, and making a difference. You are a big part of what's right in health care!

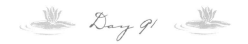

A GOOD SHEPHERD

An elderly gentleman was admitted to our residence at the end of his life. He was a car mechanic, loved to work on engines, and was always out in his garage tinkering on them. The neighborhood boys all knew him. One young man in particular had befriended him. I don't remember his name, but he was about 18-20 years of age. This young man would come to visit him, and every time, he would get teary-eyed.

One evening, I made a point to go into the room while this young man was visiting to see if I could help in any way. He started telling me all about the patient and how good he was at fixing cars. He said, "I liked going over to his garage. I felt that in a way, he was looking after me."

By this time, the patient was lethargic and barely responsive. He did not recognize or respond to his young friend. The young man started to cry and said, "He would always call me 'Shepherd,' and I just want to know why he called me that."

In an effort to console the young man, I said, "Well, what does the word 'shepherd' mean? A shepherd looks over his flock of sheep. So maybe your friend felt like you were watching over him."

The dying man, who was hardly even responsive, opened his eyes wide for just a moment and mouthed the words, "You are right." Then he drifted off again.

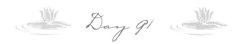

Of course, I was in shock that this dying man came out of a comatose state to confirm that indeed, he felt this young man was watching over him and that is why he called him "Shepherd." The young friend was just as amazed as I was, but he was also very comforted by that momentary response.

The next day, the patient died, with the young man, his shepherd, at his bedside.

—*Submitted by Marina Falzone*

"Never underestimate the difference you can make."

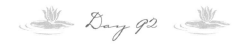

The Gift of Selfless Service

This letter, which was written by a grateful patient's wife, is a testament to the hospital staff and their tireless efforts on her husband's behalf.

Sometimes it is difficult to express the deep emotions you feel by simply using those two little words: "thank you."

My husband arrived on your emergency room doorstep with what appeared to be stroke symptoms. His speech was slurred and he had little use of his right leg and foot. Volunteer Diane quickly brought a wheelchair to assist us as Manuel helped me complete papers to satisfy the hospital requirements. Lori B. helped us with admitting and had us quickly on our way to RN Bruce and Dr. Bowers in the ER. A CAT scan revealed two hematomas, the result of a car accident when he had been rear-ended by a semi, which then left the accident scene!

Now...all of this might seem more routine for the ER area, but you also need to know we had just arrived in Tyler a week and a half earlier in a move from California...having not yet found medical care and barely knowing where the hospital district was located. The immediate care and concern we were given overwhelmed my husband, his mother (who moved from California with us), and me.

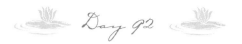

Surgery by neurosurgeon Dr. Jon Ledlie and Dr. Renfro, with care by Dr. Brian Pfieffer and his RN, Davey Hamilton, reassured us that we had been guided those many miles to this place. There are so many names I have tried to remember who comforted us along this journey, and I apologize for many I am unable to recall. Dana, Courtney, and Katie in the IMC, clinical liaison Karen Rose, Donna, the pre-op nurse, and the three surgical nurses, Debra, Debbie, and forgive me, one more whose smile I remember but not her name, as well as Dr. Daniels, the anesthesiologist.

While in ICU, precious Sam, along with Terry and Rayne, kept reassuring my husband (and us) that he was going to be fine. And on the sixth floor, Barbara, Aretha, and several more gave tirelessly of their time and comfort. Every place we turned, we found smiles and words of comfort to ease our fears and guide (not send) us to various locations in the building. To say this was a pleasant experience would be stretching it because of the circumstances. However, to say a difficult time was eased and made as pleasant as possible would be absolutely correct.

It was difficult to leave family and friends in California to make the move for a business opportunity for my husband, but we felt this was God's plan for us. May each of you know how grateful we are. Every corner we turned showed each member of your team believes we are all God's children and that treating others with kindness on life's journey is a way of showing His gift of love. May God continue to guide you as you serve Him by serving others.

—*Submitted by Cindy Kidwell, Trinity Mother Frances Health System*

"Never underestimate the difference you can make."

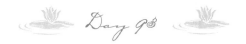

A MOMENT TO REMEMBER

What we do is so important and we can leave powerful impressions on the lives we touch. I was reminded of this a few weeks ago.

A gentleman came up to the unit with donuts and coffee for the staff. He explained to everyone that today was his 60th birthday and that before he could go to work or engage in any other celebrations, he needed to come and thank the staff of the oncology unit, who had saved his life.

The man had been a patient about five years earlier and recounted the gentle care he received and credited that care with his life as he knows it now. He explained to the staff that every day he thought of "the girls," as he called them, and wanted them to know his gratitude.

"I could not begin the day without the girls who saved me," he told the staff. "There is not a significant day over my life in the last five years that I haven't started out my day without thanking the angels."

Tears began running down his face and soon the whole unit was crying along with him. Everyone was overcome with his kind gesture.

Some of the staff who had cared for him remembered him as a patient. One such person was our unit secretary, who said, "All we did was our jobs, yet he feels he is alive because of our care and kindness. I can't believe he took the time to come here and thank us before starting his own day!"

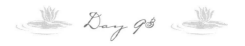

Day 98

This gentleman's kind gesture reminded everyone how important our profession is to the lives of others. "What a powerful profession we are in," Donna stated. "That is what it is all about! We sometimes forget, but it is moments like that that help to remind us and make it so very meaningful."

—Submitted by Linda Charlite-Ruiz for Donna Sherrill, Winchester Hospital, Winchester, MA

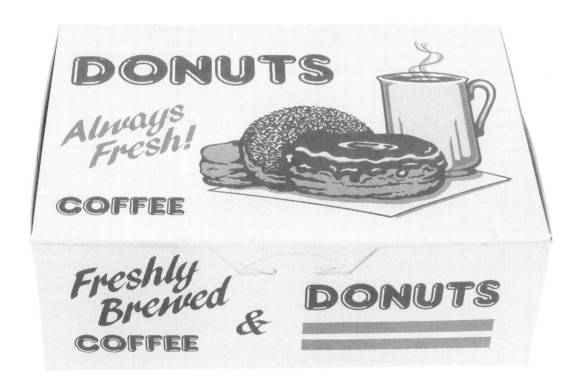

"Never underestimate the difference you can make."

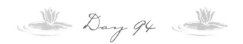

Above and Beyond— With a Smile

Carmen Reyes, catering associate at Overland Park Regional Medical Center in Overland Park, Kansas, always takes great care of her patients. In this case, she definitely went above and beyond her typical hospital duties.

Carmen had an 86-year-old patient who was crying when Carmen went to her room. When Carmen inquired as to why she was upset, the patient said that she did not have a ride home from the hospital because her family was busy. Carmen offered to take her home and then spent several hours helping her settle into her home.

Since then, Carmen has befriended this lady. Once or twice a week, on her days off, Carmen takes the patient on errands that otherwise the lady would not be able to complete. Most importantly, Carmen spends time with her. When her family did not step up to take care of the lady, Carmen did. The lady told Carmen she has come to think of her as an adopted grandchild and Carmen feels the same way about her "grandma."

The positive influence that Carmen has made in this woman's life by just being a friend shows that Carmen truly puts people first and will go to great lengths to make that happen. Carmen is a real asset to her team!

—*Submitted by Overland Park Regional Medical Center, Overland Park, KS*

"Never underestimate the difference you can make."

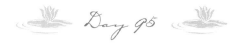

When Emergency Becomes Crisis

*T*here's a certain predictability about hurricanes on the Gulf Coast. When a storm enters the Gulf, you dust off your emergency management manuals. A couple of days later, you either breathe a sigh of relief because the storm's going to hit Pensacola or Brownsville, or you activate your emergency command system. Then, you assign sleep rooms for staff who will relieve the ones working now, arrange for emergency child care, lose power for a few hours, and, after the storm has passed, clean up the tree limbs.

That's what started to happen on Monday, August 30, 2005, in Baton Rouge, Louisiana. In fact, the senior staff at Woman's was breaking down our HEICS command center when it became clear that this was not like other storms. Five days later, our world had changed forever.

In the United States, we never really think much about having to evacuate whole hospitals—let alone a whole city of them. Hospitals are safe places where people are sheltered from harm.

We have all taken part in hospital evacuation exercises before. In fact, we recently developed a very complete plan for evacuation of our 90-plus-bed NICU.

We also knew the plan for the state and for our region for emergency preparedness. The way it is supposed to go, each hospital keeps the Office of

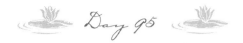

Emergency Preparedness in our region apprised of both our capacity and our needs. Everything is supposed to run through the Designated Regional Coordinator. Hospitals should not call each other to make independent plans.

The rising water in the city of New Orleans made the situation different. The breaks in the levees filled the saucer of the city, making all plans and drills obsolete, and isolating hospitals from resources and life support.

At first, we followed the drill: calling the Office of Emergency Preparedness and attempting to work through the staff there—when we could get through. Trouble was, Baton Rouge was not unscathed from the storm. Widespread power and phone outages included cell phones, pagers, towers, and networks. The 70 miles between Baton Rouge and New Orleans seemed like 700.

One of every ten calls went through. We knew we would be needed to help, but could not get through to find out how. Then we received a call from another hospital. It was clear the system wasn't working for the evacuating hospitals, either.

We decided that it would make more sense for Woman's Hospital—with our capacity for NICU infants and high-risk moms—to take over coordination of the evacuation of neonates from New Orleans. After all, our neonatologists know the neonatologists there, and an evacuation plan for a two-pound preemie is different from one for an eight-pound well baby. We could assess acuity and triage far more efficiently through direct contact with the physicians working in our sister nurseries in New Orleans.

So, a neonatologist and two vice presidents hopped in a car and drove over to the state OEP. In the bullpen made up of 40 or so carrels representing state, federal, and private agencies, we tracked down Dr. Jimmy Guidry, the state health officer, and told him what we had in mind. His response: "God bless you!"

From that moment on, contacts between neonatologists and administrators allowed 121 babies and over 200 moms to be rescued. By ambulance, helicopter,

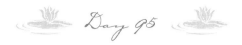

and boat, a vital lifeline developed between New Orleans and Baton Rouge that provided for efficient and effective evacuations of this important subpopulation.

Not one of these hospitalized babies died.

The staff in the hospitals in New Orleans were absolute heroes. Physicians, nurses, respiratory therapists, pharmacists, and others worked for days in temperatures exceeding 100 degrees, with no electrical power and limited—if any—supplies, drugs, food, and water. Staff went without. Patients were handbagged for hours, carried up and down stairs, and fanned by hand. Staff slept—when they slept at all—on gurneys, sofas, and floors.

Because babies and families were being separated, it quickly became necessary to establish a center for coordinating family communication and reuniting family members. Hospital administration offices, staffed by the area's administrative assistant, the strategic planning coordinator, the patient relations coordinator, the hospital's interior designer, and others, were pressed into service.

Heartbreaking phone calls, desperate stories, and thousands of contacts later, all babies received by Woman's, and many other facilities, were reconnected. Communications were both critical and difficult. Typical of Woman's Hospital and our culture, frequent communications to staff and physicians, by every medium available, allowed us to pull together to do what was needed. Email, phone, posted memos, daily briefings of the medical staff, and word of mouth to staff kept people informed, grounded, and motivated. The difficulty came because every technology available to communicate with the outside world failed regularly. Internal SpectraLink® phones were reliable and became invaluable.

This was an extraordinary experience, for the organization and for the individuals who make it up. More than one of us has expressed gratitude that we were in a position to be able to help. What we did as individuals and as an organization will prove to be a life-changing experience for many of us.

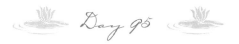

We have lots of work to do. Health care in Louisiana will change, and we will be part of that change. What we are committed to is the principle to use this experience—horrible and hopeful, enervating and energizing—to learn as individuals and as an organization. We have an unprecedented chance to make conscious decisions about the future and new opportunities to achieve our mission to improve the health of women and infants.

—*Written by Jamie Haeuser and Stan Shelton, Submitted by Karen Clarke, Woman's Hospital, Baton Rouge, LA*

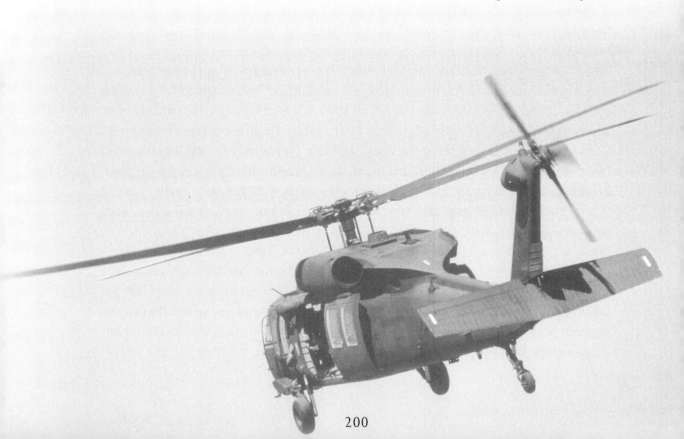

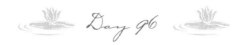

Lessons in Life

My work at a nursing home facility has brought me into contact with many different types of people, but there is one woman I will never forget. Her name was Lois, and she was an elderly, country woman who was quite sick and dying of kidney cancer.

I worked the 3-11 p.m. shift and would often go in and sit and talk with Lois. She and I became good friends, and it was because of her that I often looked forward to going to work. Lois was 76 years old and had a daughter but did not have a good relationship with her. She was lonely and enjoyed talking to me about her life, children, and her late husband. She spoke of her regrets as well as the good times.

My daughter had to do an interview for a school project, and Lois consented to do it. My daughter made a little book with a photo of Lois and highlights of Lois's life story. We gave it to Lois once it was finished, and she cried.

One day, Lois began to feel really bad. She went to bed and became unresponsive. I knew what it meant—Lois was dying.

I did not have to work the next day but as time passed, I had this overwhelming urge to go back to the residence and see Lois. When I got there, Lois was still unresponsive and rapidly breathing. She was alone in her room— no family there at the bedside. I walked in the room, sat on her bed, and grabbed her hand and stroked it.

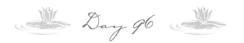

"I'm here now, Lois," I said. "It's okay. You don't have to be afraid. It's okay to die," I kept repeating to her. After a few minutes, Lois took a deep breath, then stopped. I stared at her, waiting for another breath, feeling the tears rolling down my cheeks.

She breathed once more, and as she did, I saw what appeared to be white smoke coming out of her mouth, like someone blowing smoke rings. In that moment, I felt her spirit was leaving her body. I just held on tight to her hand and continued to cry. Then I pushed the call light for the nurse on duty.

When the nurse entered the room, she realized Lois was gone and called her family. Her daughter and son-in-law came and collected her belongings and thanked me for being Lois's friend.

Yes, I was Lois's friend but it was not a one-way street. Lois had been a friend to me, too. She had taught me never to judge a book by its cover. Lois may have looked like a plain country woman, but she was a spiritual person who had a lot to share about life and what it means to live a good life as well as die a dignified death. I will never forget the lessons I learned from my friend and patient Lois.

—Submitted by Marina Falzone

"Never underestimate the difference you can make."

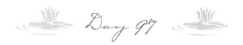

A Light of Hope

Mel Legari, the cancer services liaison in the Dyson Center for Cancer Care, joined Vassar Brothers Medical Center on June 5, 2002. The words of a former patient, gleaned from a Press Ganey survey, describe her perfectly: "Mel Legari…is my angel. This lady could make the devil smile. She gave me hugs when I really needed them. She was there to listen and she was there to help. I absolutely love her."

Mel was honored in December with our Nurse of Distinction Award. Mike, a patient from the Infusion Center, was one of the people attending the ceremony. Mike had met Mel at his first treatment, where he acknowledged a lifelong fear of needles. Mel inserted the needle, and he said he had not felt a thing, so Mel assured him she would make sure it was the same for each treatment.

Mike was 44 when he was diagnosed with head and neck cancer. Mike dreaded his treatments; he was dehydrated, in pain, unable to sleep or eat, and becoming increasingly depressed and unable to cope, physically or emotionally. He was ready to give up. Mel was there for him every step of the way. She provided him with honest, straightforward information and was there as an advocate, giving suggestions for pain control alternatives. She offered support not only to Mike but also to his family. Most of all, Mel gave them hope. In Mike's words, "She was there when I was ready to give up. She was a light and made me want to come in to finish my treatment."

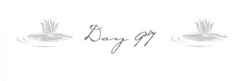

The day after she received her Nurse of Distinction Award, Mel cashed the check, called Mike to the Infusion Center and gave the money to him. She told him to do something nice for his family—take them out to dinner, buy a nice Christmas gift.

Mary Luvera, director of oncology services, was there to witness Mel's generous gift and sums up the moment well. "Mike was speechless. He didn't want to take it and she insisted. He hugged her so hard, I could see his arms trembling and tears in his eyes," Mary relays. "That is what nursing is all about."

—Submitted by Vassar Brothers Medical Center, Poughkeepsie, NY

"Never underestimate the difference you can make."

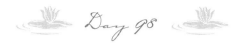

Reaching Out to the Lost and Forgotten

The following letter was sent to Eleanor Cochran, clinics director, St. Mary Medical Center, Long Beach, California, in regard to the services offered at an ambulatory clinic.

My name is Randy Roach. I am now in my 34th year working as a journalist for Channel 7 Eyewitness News here in Los Angeles. And it is my distinct pleasure to write this letter about a group of heroes who work for you at the Family Clinic of Long Beach.

In my spare time away from work, I try to reach out and help homeless people and others desperately in need. As a veteran newsman, I know firsthand about the plight of the homeless in their neighborhoods of suffering. I have won eight Emmys and 19 nominations from the Television Academy, many of them for my documentaries about the homeless, for which I spent days, weeks, and even months on skid row—an eyewitness to what is tragically the most vivid symbol of inner-city poverty in the country.

The Family Clinic of Long Beach has become a beacon in the harbor of hopelessness for several formerly homeless people I have rescued off the streets in recent months. After securing housing for these disadvantaged men, I was able to obtain Medi-Cal for each one of them.

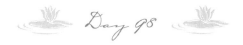

And that provided us with the opportunity to seek primary health care at the Family Clinic of Long Beach.

I have seen firsthand the compassion and tireless dedication of the clinic's staff members, who are nothing less than civic treasures. Quite simply, their enthusiasm is infectious. And time after time, I have watched this team reach out to those who have been abandoned with a life in chaos, confusion, and a resume of humiliation. Medi-Cal may pay the bills but what this clinic team offers in return is priceless.

I would like to single out Dr. Angela Tang and Dr. Eva Kreye for being the primary physicians in these cases. They are nothing less than miracle workers, who believe that for anyone to achieve, they must first be given the opportunity to try. And it is refreshing to see these two valuable community assets take the time to light a candle in the darkness of life for the helpless who were trapped in despair.

The well-deserved praise doesn't end there. Ms. Cochran, I've held but one job over more than three decades—in one pressure cooker of a stress-filled environment. I know quality when I see it. At this point in my career, I better. And the work ethic of medical assistants Rosie Amezcua and Angie Zendejas, along with Dr. Shannon Reider and Dr. Israel Hernandez, is second to none.

The staff members at the Family Clinic of Long Beach have taught me one valuable lesson…that life is indeed a gift that should be celebrated each and every day. And by reaching out to the lost and forgotten and giving them a chance, these heroes are proof that there are no limits to what the human spirit, guided by God, can truly achieve.

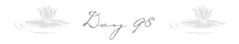

In closing, I would like to share with you a benediction that symbolizes the heart and spirit of this wonderful clinic. "May God bless you with tears to shed for those who suffer from pain and rejections, so that you may reach your hand to comfort them and turn their pain into joy. And may God bless you with enough foolishness to believe that you can make a differencc in this world, so that you can do what others claim cannot be done."

If I can be of further assistance, please don't hesitate to call me. My late father and mother taught me that when someone goes far beyond the call of duty, I should always take time to say "thank you," and that is why I'm writing this letter.

Signed,
Randy Roach

—Submitted by Eleanor Cochran, St. Mary Medical Center, Long Beach, CA

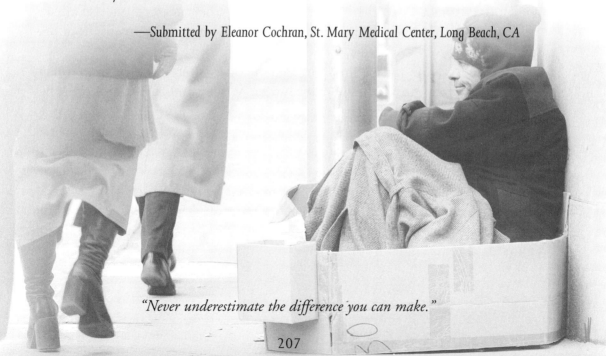

"Never underestimate the difference you can make."

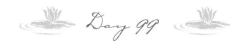

Care Without Boundaries

Adrienne London, a case manager at Vassar Brothers Medical Center, is one of those rare people who intuitively knows what patients might need—and she is there to guide them through difficult times.

"I want to thank you for all the kind things you did for me," one such patient wrote. "Going in there and not knowing anyone, I was scared. And then I met you, thank God. You're an angel that was sent to me...I'll never forget you."

This particular patient was so terrified of hospitals that she had never even gone to a doctor's office. When she arrived at Vassar, her breast cancer was already in its late stages. Adrienne literally followed her through her treatment, from pre-surgical testing to the recovery room.

Adrienne has the innate ability to meet people where they are emotionally and help take them to where they need to be. When someone has no one, they find they have Adrienne, heart and soul.

Anyone who knows Adrienne will agree that she is a woman of many words, as it would take many words to describe her: genuine, strong, insightful, and positive.

Adrienne goes where angels fear to tread. Each person reacts to grief in his own way, and sometimes caregivers may become a target of a distraught patient or family member. Invariably, Adrienne always finds a way to give support.

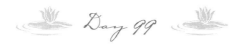

There are no boundaries to Adrienne's willingness to go above and beyond, as demonstrated to a couple from Israel. Just before Yom Kippur, the husband suffered a heart attack, ending up in our CCU. Adrienne arranged for the wife to accompany her to Yom Kippur services and welcomed the woman to her home for dinner with her family.

The stories are endless. Adrienne's many professional clinical contributions, from cancer support groups to guided imagery to crisis support for staff, are well recognized and appreciated. What seems to be her most outstanding quality, however, is Adrienne's ability to be where people need her, just when she is needed most.

—Submitted by *Vassar Brothers Medical Center, Poughkeepsie, NY*

"Never underestimate the difference you can make."

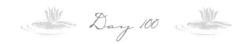

HEROES AROUND US

ilitary heroes are all around us. Veterans of World War II, the Korean War, Vietnam, and the Gulf War, and those who served in the United States military during peacetime quietly grace the hallways at Sumner Regional Health Systems' facilities every day, exhibiting a loyalty and commitment to teamwork often found only in the armed services. Some work as volunteers, a few patrol hospital campuses as security personnel, others distribute correct equipment and supplies, and still others work with patients to perform various diagnostic tests.

Add "performing neurosurgery" to the list of veteran duties at Sumner Regional.

Dr. Marshall Watson, a neurosurgeon and a Major in the United States Army Reserves, was called up in late July, giving him approximately three weeks to temporarily close up shop and report for duty.

"I joined the Reserves during the war," Dr. Watson said. "I knew full well the possibility of being called up. It's difficult to put a practice on hold and restart it, but doing this was important to me."

Germany's Landstuhl Regional Medical Center, Europe's definitive military hospital and the largest American military medical facility outside the United States, served as Dr. Watson's clinical home for three months. While practicing at this hospital, Dr. Watson treated injured soldiers from Iraq, Africa, and

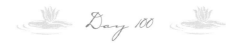

Afghanistan. This hospital took in all casualties and injuries from the War on Terror. Most of the soldiers Dr. Watson treated suffered gunshot wounds and improvised explosive device injuries, plus other typical injuries such as herniated discs and broken bones. He treated not only American soldiers but also other coalition forces.

One injury Dr. Watson became all too familiar with was isolated gunshot wounds to the neck.

"Snipers in Iraq have gotten very good at finding that window below the helmet and above the body armor," Dr. Watson said. "We saw a lot of wounds of this type in our hospital."

In one case, Dr. Watson's patient made news in the U.S.

"A soldier was shot in Iraq," he explained. "It was a head shot and went straight through the head. In October, *The New York Times* ran a photo of a bloody hand holding a bullet. That bullet was the one that had gone through this soldier's head. We did surgery on him in Germany; he was flown back to the U.S. and is recovering today.

"The neurosurgeons serving in Iraq are fabulous," he continued, noting that in all of Iraq, the military employs two neurosurgeons, and Africa and Afghanistan have none. "This guy survived because of the neurosurgeon who worked on him initially."

As one can imagine, the time for transporting a person from these battle zones to Germany can be extensive. Dr. Watson believes that, even with traumatic injuries, soldiers are able to survive because of their ages and fitness levels.

"The body can take an astounding amount of trauma when you are young and healthy," he said.

Not every situation turned out so well.

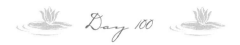

"I remember telling a British family that their soldier, who was shot in the neck, was brain dead," Dr. Watson relayed. "Another soldier had just gotten married before going to Iraq. He was injured by an IED (improvised explosive device) and lost almost all the blood in his body through his leg wound. He was brought to Germany in bad shape. His wife was also active duty military, and she and his family ultimately decided to withdraw care. He was buried in Texas."

Still, almost every single soldier who comes through the doors at Landstuhl Regional Medical Center is anxious to get back to his or her unit.

"Maybe not universally, but close to universally, the soldiers want to be back where they were," Dr. Watson said. "I treated one such soldier in particular. An IED had gone off in his face between the two frontal lobes of his brain. He was a Master Sergeant. He didn't want to go back to the U.S.—he wanted to go back to his unit. Another 21-year-old soldier was shot by a sniper in the back of the neck. He said to me, 'Doc, all I ever wanted to be was a Marine Recon and now I can't. Why am I even living?' You just give them whatever you can."

Despite the challenges of packing up his practice, being on a different continent from his family, and staring death in the face each day, Dr. Watson realizes that he could go through all this again in about a year. Still, he claims his own 90 days of deployment are a flash in the pan compared to that of some other recruits.

"As inconvenient and unpleasant as it was for me to leave my family and practice, it was nothing compared to what those soldiers do," he said. "They are gone away from home for 12-18 months, sometimes even longer. What they sacrifice and what they go through is far beyond anything I have done."

—*Anonymous Contributor*

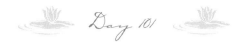

A Very Special Birthday

$\mathcal{E}$ddie Golden works in Food Services at Methodist University Hospital. Recently, one of Eddie's fellow associates, Elaine Ervin, was hospitalized in University Hospital. Her birthday fell on a day she was in the hospital, and her family gathered in her room to celebrate. Eddie was delivering food trays and realized that Elaine was celebrating her birthday in the hospital. He took it upon himself to go out and get an ice cream cake so that Elaine and her family could have a special celebration. During an extremely difficult time, his thoughtfulness, positive attitude, and wonderful smile meant the world to Elaine and her family. It is for this extreme act of kindness that Eddie Golden was presented with a Miracle in Motion Award.

—Submitted by Ruth-Ann Hale, Methodist Le Bonheur Germantown Hospital, Germantown, TN

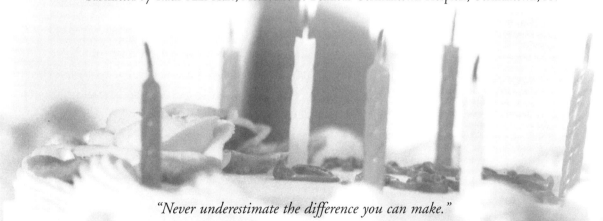

"Never underestimate the difference you can make."

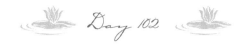

Support in Difficult Times

Chaplain Karen Gorski was paged to the emergency room on January 21st to provide support to the family of a baby who was brought in—an apparent victim of SIDS. He was one day short of being two months old. The infant's mother and both sets of grandparents were present. The baby's father was in the military and the Red Cross was in the process of contacting him.

Barb Sitarski, one of the facilitators of Heart to Heart, the hospital's support program for families who experience an infant or perinatal loss, was also contacted. Even though it was Barb's day off, she came in.

One of the important elements in providing support to these families is to collect as many "mementos" as possible. With the family's permission, Barb cuts a lock of the baby's hair. Whenever possible, Barb will also make a mold of the baby's hand and foot.

When Barb arrived in the emergency room, she informed Chaplain Karen there appeared to be no more alginate, the substance used to make foot and hand impressions. Because the medical examiner was on the way to pick up the baby, Barb and Chaplain Karen didn't have much time to make the impressions to later give to this family. Barb recalled the substance is the same as that used by dentists for impressions, so Chaplain Karen proceeded to contact a dentist who might be willing to provide some alginate.

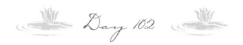

The dentist Chaplain Karen contacted was more than happy to help and refused payment for the needed material. In the meantime, Barb was supporting the family, sharing information about what was going to happen next, some of what they might experience emotionally, and more about the Heart to Heart support group.

When Chaplain Karen arrived back in the emergency room, Barb explained that she was going to take impressions and then gently took the baby from his mom's arms. She brought the baby back later, wrapped in a handmade quilt, so mother could have a few more moments with her baby.

The medical examiner arrived, and a nurse informed the family it was time to say their final good-byes. Barb gave the mom a memory box (hand-painted and donated by a local artist) with a lock of hair, ink prints, and hospital band inside. She was also given the baby's quilt. Finally Chaplain Karen and Barb gave her a stuffed bear, donated by Sierra's Bears. Mom held everything tightly to her chest.

The compassionate care and support that Chaplain Karen and Barb demonstrated to this family certainly made a difference during a most difficult and emotional time. However, this is but one example of the caring services they provide through the Heart to Heart program.

—Submitted by Tonia Campbell,
Henry Ford Wyandotte Hospital, Detroit, MI

"Never underestimate the difference you can make."

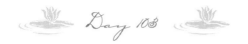

A Blessed Life

The following compelling letter was sent by a grateful family to the nephrology and dialysis teams at CHAM.

We are approaching, next month, the one-year anniversary of having our son, K., in your lifesaving care. K.'s first birthday is next week; however, it is a special milestone to mark with you, with a little celebration. Without your collective expertise, aggressive philosophy, and dedication, we suspect we'd lack a reason to be so joyous and grateful today.

There are, we believe, many challenges and tribulations ahead. We don't take success for granted, but we also don't stick our heads in the sand and hope that science and faith will take care of everything. We overlay our own experience, philosophy, and parental instincts on the care you provide. This is not always easy for you all, we know.

Yet, our critical and special partnership with you is continuing to provide every last little advantage mortals can add to K.'s chances for a healthy and fulfilling future. So as we consider with awe the miracles that allow us all to stand around a smiling, smart, and absolutely fat one-year-old this month, we also ascribe K.'s relative health and his prospects to your collective care.

Please celebrate one year of blessed life with us by enjoying these accompanying treats, in honor of this special, most fortunate boy.

—*Anonymous Contributor*

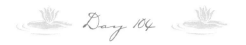

International Health Care Relief Efforts

*T*wo of our nurses have traveled the world helping other people and their communities. As part of Mercy Ships International, John Dobrie, RN (PACU), spent two weeks sailing the coast of Africa on a floating hospital. He joined other nurses and doctors from around the world to provide medical care and surgical procedures to communities that do not have access to medical care.

Another nurse, Susan Sanborn, worked with the World Medical Mission in providing relief to the victims of Hurricane Katrina. As an active member of her church, Susan has traveled with World Medical Missions to places like Rwanda and Saipan, providing medical care in areas so remote that no water or electricity was available. Both John and Susan show true volunteerism at its best.

—Submitted by Patricia Lavin, Good Samaritan Medical Center

"Never underestimate the difference you can make."

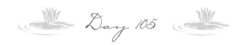

Making a Difference:
The Breast Health Center

Following is a story narrated by Breast Health Center Nurse Bonnie Edsel, RN:

Nancy just got the kids on the bus Monday morning, and she rushed to the Mammography Suite before work for her routine mammogram. After the routine four films were processed, the specially trained mammography technologist informed Nancy that the radiologist would like a few more pictures of the left breast and a sonogram. Suddenly this very composed wife and working mother of three felt the panic rise in her throat. What's wrong? Did you see something? The radiologist informed the nurse that Nancy had a very small, 8mm spiculated mass in the left breast suspicious for cancer. The nurse was on-site to answer Nancy's many questions, reassuring her that they would have a preliminary diagnosis in as little as 30 minutes. The nurse called Nancy's referring physician to obtain a prescription for a sonogram and a possible fine needle biopsy.

Our unique breast imaging services are staffed by a dynamic interdisciplinary team, including dedicated breast imagers, pathologists, referring physicians, surgeons, specially trained technologists, and registered nurses, all coming together to provide the women of Long Island with the most timely, modern, and compassionate care for breast disease.

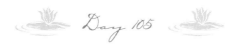

The patient had her spot films and was brought into the sonography room. A nodule was visualized in the upper outer quadrant of Nancy's left breast; the patient consented to fine needle biopsy. Following the procedure, the four slides were brought immediately to the pathology lab. Within 15-20 minutes the pathologist was on the phone with the radiologist confirming that the nodule was suspicious for cancer. The radiologist called Nancy's referring physician with the results. The nurse joined Nancy in the radiologist's office, where she was told that the small nodule was indeed suspicious for an early cancer. The nurse reassured the patient that the nodule was small and that with early detection comes good prognosis. The patient was told that her referring physician recommended a surgeon. Nancy concurred and an appointment was made for her three days later. The nurse asked if there was family or a friend to call. Nancy asked us to call her husband; he arrived at the suite within 20 minutes. While the nurse proceeded to answer questions for the patient and her husband, the clerical staff prepared copies of reports and films for the patient to take to her surgical visit. The patient was assured that the nurses in the Breast Health Center would follow her every step of the way. The patient was given discharge instructions and a phone number to call with any questions or concerns.

Four days after her surgical appointment, Nancy met with the Breast Health Center nurse. She was given a blue bag with the inscription "Gift of Health and Inspiration" that was donated from one of the local Breast Cancer Coalitions. It contained many useful, practical items for education, relaxation, and recovery after surgery. On the day of surgery, the Breast Health Center nurse met the patient in the Ambulatory Surgery Unit and accompanied her to the Operating

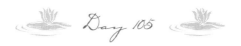

Room. The role of the Breast Health Center nurse at this time was to support the patient. Holding the hand of a frightened patient as she goes to sleep under anesthesia is often the most comforting and appreciated unique practice of our care. Nancy finished chemotherapy and is in her third week of radiation. She attends support group meetings, where she finds a safe place to share her story with other women who know what she's fighting against and what they're surviving together.

The Breast Health Center is partnered with the American Cancer Society in programs such as Reach to Recovery, Look Good Feel Better, and Making Strides Against Breast Cancer Walk. We are also partners with the Witness Project of Long Island and the Women's Health Partnership. Together we provide mammograms and diagnostic work-ups for low-income, uninsured women in New York State. We work closely with the local Breast Cancer Coalitions, West Islip, Babylon and Islip Coalition, to best serve the individual needs of the community.

—Submitted by Patricia Lavin, Good Samaritan Medical Center

"Never underestimate the difference you can make."

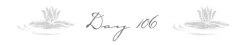

Tending to the Needs of the Entire Family

A dramatic example of nursing independent judgment occurred on Sunday, May 8, 2005, when a terrible tragedy struck a local family and their precious eight-year-old daughter. While riding on the back of a bicycle, this little girl was struck by a car. Upon arrival to our ED, she was in full arrest and was sent to the PICU. The young girl was in grave condition and was rapidly declining. The nursing staff of the PICU, along with the staff of pediatrics, worked heroically to try and save her life. With her family standing by watching, the nursing staff made sure that both the patient was cared for and that also the needs of the family were addressed.

During PICU ICC rounds the next morning, the nurse made referrals to the child life specialist to provide assistance to the little girl's sibling and to pastoral care for spiritual guidance and support for the family. One of the pediatric nurses sat with the family and explained everything that was going on to try and save this little girl's life.

As her father stood watching the nurses and physicians working valiantly to save his daughter's life, he expressed his amazement at all that they were doing. When neurosurgery and pediatric neurology examined her, they pronounced her to be clinically brain dead. Again, nursing was there at the family's side for support and to answer any questions.

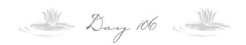

The father approached the nurses about donating his daughter's organs. The nursing staff set everything in motion and notified the New York Organ Donor Network. The staff worked feverishly to keep this little girl alive so that her organs could be retrieved. The Organ Donor Network arrived that night and the process began. For the next two days, the nursing staff, in conjunction with the physicians and the Organ Donor Network, worked to turn this family's horrible tragedy into the gift of life to honor their wishes.

Nursing arranged to have a room set aside for the large extended family. They also provided a comfort cart, with food and drinks readily accessible to the family as they maintained a constant vigil at the girl's bedside. Nursing provided reclining chairs and seating to accommodate the family so that they could grieve and say their good-byes. Jennifer McLaughlin, NP, RN, Neurosurgery, was a huge support to the patient, family, and nursing staff during this difficult and emotional time. Her knowledge, caring, and compassion provided a beautiful light for the family and the staff during this horrible time. On May 10 the little girl was brought to the OR for organ retrieval and on May 11 many families woke up with a new beginning.

The nursing staff of Peds/PICU worked tirelessly, exercising independent judgment, caring, and compassion to honor the wishes of this little girl's family. The nurses supported and cared not only for the patient but for her family and for each other. Out of this terrible tragedy this little girl and her courageous and gracious family changed many lives, including those of the nursing staff who cared for them.

—Submitted by Patricia Lavin, Good Samaritan Medical Center

"Never underestimate the difference you can make."

Amazing Dedication

Norma Nawroth is a staff nurse in the Kettering Medical Center Network. She would prefer we didn't draw so much attention to her, but her compassionate work in the Southview Hospital maternity unit is deserving of special mention.

Norma joined Grandview Hospital in 1963 and moved to Southview with the maternity unit in 1998. She has always worked with mothers and their babies. Her special gift is the Bereavement Program. Norma organized it, trained her coworkers in this delicate ministry, and shared her knowledge with Emergency Room personnel at both Southview and Grandview Hospitals.

Norma developed the Comfort Care package that helps grieving mothers deal with the difficult loss of a baby. Most importantly, Norma will sit in the room with these mothers and help ease their suffering. She will come in on her day off to personally deal with a situation. She keeps in contact with the patients once they return home.

Her supervisor says Norma is amazing…and her coworkers agree!

—Submitted by Sherri Herrick, Kettering Medical Center Network

"Never underestimate the difference you can make."

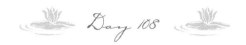

Giving Back

When I came to work this Monday morning, I found a basket of beautiful silk flowers in front of my office door. I thought, *how nice* and read the card: "Thank you for all you've done for our mother over the years. The Miceli family." I thought, *how kind of them to thank me.* Their mom, a patient of mine for almost 20 years, had been in and out of the hospital over the last several months and over the years had endured a number of serious illnesses—heart failure, diabetes, bowel obstruction, chronic dialysis for kidney failure and many infections, below the knee amputation of one leg and a forefoot amputation on the other side. She had rallied many times, like a cat with more than nine lives, but during this admission her condition had spiraled downward with fading hope for recovery.

When I saw the flowers, I didn't yet know that over the weekend she had died. In a few moments, my associate Dr. Vetrone came into my office and told me something I will never forget.

"In the end, Mrs. Miceli was very clear," explained Dr. Vetrone. "Everyone, all her children and close family members, were around the bed when she told them to stop dialysis and the medication for her blood pressure support."

Dr. Vetrone continued, "On her deathbed, she made me promise to tell you how much she appreciated all that you have done for her over the years and how

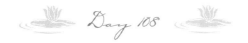

she knew that if it hadn't been for you, she would have died much earlier, and to say thank you."

It took a little while to realize the impact that these last words had on me. In fact, it really struck me only as I was sharing the story with our chaplain, Bonnie. I thought to myself, *This is really it. This is why I became a doctor. To be able to reach out my hand and make someone's day, year, or life a little better, a little more cared for, a little more guided, a little safer, a little happier, a little more comforted, a little more meaningful, and—hopefully—to make it a little longer.* Everything was clear.

—Submitted by Barbara B. Loeb, Good Samaritan Hospital, Downers Grove, IL

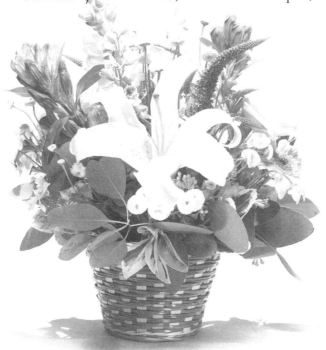

"Never underestimate the difference you can make."

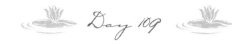

The House with the White Picket Fence

*T*here are some people who enter your life for a brief period of time and leave an indelible imprint upon your life, and most importantly upon your heart. One of those people is Jean Tibbitt, a beloved hospice nurse. For anyone who knows Jean, it is a blessing to have her as a part of your life. You are doubly blessed, if when you reach the crossroads between Earth and the hereafter, you have Jean at your side as your hospice nurse.

Jean is one of those unassuming individuals through whom God can shine the light of Christ's love into even the darkest of souls, and she does so naturally and effortlessly. Throughout her 19 years of service, she has reached out with an undying commitment to touch the lives of those patients and families who are living with the realities of a terminal illness. Jean is gifted with genuine warmth that exudes the love of Christ envisioned by the Sisters of Bon Secours at their inception when the Sisters provide care in the home. Jean provides more than good help to those in need.

This past summer, in the middle of an exhausting August heat wave, Jean ministered to the needs of a young woman, "Terri," who had been admitted to hospice with terminal endometrial cancer. Jean found Terri living in impoverished conditions in a dilapidated trailer without air conditioning, hot water, or electricity. She realized that this ailing woman was living without the basic necessities that so many of us take for granted.

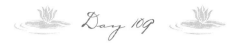

Jean took it upon herself to see that this young woman's needs were met. As usual, Jean went above and beyond the call of duty. Terri was extremely self-conscious of the large tumors growing out of her body. Out of her own resources and on her own time, Jean made sure that Terri had beautiful nightgowns to help her retain her sense of femininity. Jean's sensitivity and generosity helped to restore a positive self-image at the end of Terri's life.

Jean noticed that this young woman of faith had an old and tattered Bible that was literally in pieces. As a gesture of shared Christian faith, she bought Terri a new leather Bible with hopes of continuing to encourage her in her journey with Christ as she lived out her last days.

The lack of air conditioning coupled with the intense heat wave of August left this young woman's trailer feeling more like a broiler oven than a home. Terri's deplorable living conditions greatly distressed her and she expressed deep shame about her surroundings. Unfortunately, her family did not see the need to keep the trailer fit for human habitation. Jean did not take "no" for an answer, and she inspired a difficult family to do some housekeeping for the bedridden patient.

Jean secured an air conditioner for Terri only to find out that there was a danger with faulty electrical wiring. Not to be defeated, Jean bought a big fan to try to cool the trailer down. Before each visit Jean purchased some of Terri's favorite beverages and snacks, whatever she thought would calm Terri's nausea and give her strength to get through the heat. Jean even remembered to bring doggy biscuits for Terri's beloved dog.

On one occasion Jean asked Terri what she would wish for if she could have anything in the world. Her dying wish, Terri shared, was to live in a little house with a white picket fence around it where everyone was nice to each other. While Jean could not buy Terri the house with a picket fence, she did her best to make Terri's actual living situation as pleasant and peaceful as possible. Jean purchased a beautiful comforter with a matching sham to brighten Terri's bed. Through the

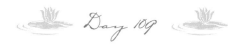

efforts of Jean and the hospice chaplain, the family rallied to support Jean in lending spiritual, emotional, and physical support to all those involved with Terri's care. This support from Jean continued after hours and on her days off.

In the end, Terri died with a smile present across her stilled face. It was a smile that perhaps lent itself to a reality that Terri was in a better place, in her little house with the white picket fence where everyone was nice to each other.

—Anonymous Contributor

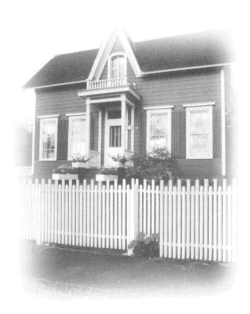

"Never underestimate the difference you can make."

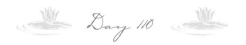

The Smile That Will Last Forever

I volunteer my hands and heart at Covenant Hospice in Pensacola, working the magic of massage therapy on both staff members and those they care for. On this particular morning, I entered the room of a woman who lay on the bed curled into a fetal position. Her face was contorted, and she was moaning in discomfort. She appeared to be about 90, but was only 41, so racked was she by

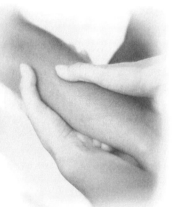

the cancer that had consumed her body. Using the softest possible strokes on her face and head, my hands then moved on to her shoulders, seeking even the smallest degree of comfort. Her breathing became more rhythmical and her face began to relax, a good sign as I had learned from my years of experience. I began to work on her right arm and hand and asked her softly if I could please have her other arm. Extending her arm, she rewarded me with the most radiant smile I have ever received from another human being. I continued with the soothing strokes as she began to sleep peacefully.

I learned the next day that her family did not make it in time. They were comforted by the knowledge that she was relaxed and peaceful, and that she had blessed me with that final radiant smile.

Am I making a difference in the lives of others when I volunteer? I hope so, but most importantly for me, those I help make a difference in mine.

—Submitted by Clara Brosnaham, Covenant Hospice, Pensacola, FL

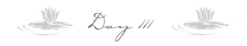
THE THANKSGIVING STORY

"E" is a 37-year-old female who was diagnosed with adenocarcinoma of the nasal pharynx ten years ago. She has been a patient to the Palliative Care Service where I work since November 2004, so I was notified when she was admitted to the hospital for pneumonia one week prior to Thanksgiving.

E is married and the mother to three young children. Her husband was out of work at the time, and E was concerned with feeding and providing for her children, not with celebrating the upcoming holiday. As Thanksgiving approached, I received word from the Community Relations Department that the local Holiday Inn was offering to give away a five-night stay and free breakfast for a needy family. I immediately thought of E. Since she was feeling better and her recovery from pneumonia was well underway, it was safe for her to be discharged.

When the offer was extended, E and her husband agreed to take the children to the Holiday Inn for the five-day stay. Knowing E's financial status, I knew the family couldn't afford to buy hotel food for five days, so I contacted local restaurants in search of help. When I explained to them what the Holiday Inn was doing, they gladly stepped in and helped out. One restaurant provided Thanksgiving dinner and gifts for the children. The staff from mammography collected and donated $250 to offset the family's expenses. Everyone was very

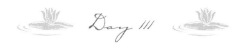

moved by the experience. E was feeling great after her unanticipated vacation, and for a brief time, life was almost normal.

E is in decline now, and her family continues to be supported by the interdisciplinary team. Social work continues to address the family's economic and medical equipment needs. Hospice provides respite for E's husband and the palliative care physician helps to monitor her pain. Thanks to all the good Samaritans in our community, this is a story that won't soon be forgotten.

—Submitted by Patricia Lavin as narrated by Eileen Roberto, Good Samaritan Medical Center

"Never underestimate the difference you can make."

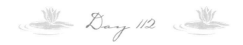

Heart of Gold

On December 23, 2005, Johnny Foster, pot washer at Decatur General Hospital in Decatur, Alabama, went to his director's office because he had something on his mind. Johnny said he had been up all night, thinking about the kids who would be spending Christmas in the hospital and he wanted to do something special for them. When Johnny stated that he planned to buy them gifts, the director responded that she would gladly give him money to help with the purchases. He replied that if he didn't have enough money with him, he would let her know later.

As Johnny carried the food carts to the floors, he stopped on pediatrics to ask a nurse exactly how many kids would be spending Christmas in the hospital. The nurse told him six.

Later that morning, Johnny came into the food and nutrition department carrying a stuffed animal for each of the kids. For Christmas, the children received a gift from Johnny and so did Johnny's coworkers who discovered Johnny has a heart of gold.

Johnny's kindness continues. If a coworker is admitted to the hospital, Johnny Foster will be the first visitor—arriving with a balloon or a stuffed animal and his infectious chuckle. Johnny's kindness is always greatly appreciated.

—Anonymous Contributor, Decatur General Hospital, Decatur, AL

"Never underestimate the difference you can make."

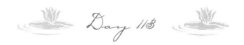

Exercising Compassion with one of our own

Johanna Mirabella worked in the nursing department for over 30 years as a nursing assistant in numerous units throughout the hospital. Johanna was a single mother and overcame many obstacles in her life, including breast cancer. Johanna had a love of animals and a special passion for dogs, as demonstrated through the love and care of her own two puppies.

Johanna had a strong belief in the therapeutic effects of pet therapy. When the Nursing Research Committee was formed, she contacted the chair of the committee to inquire about starting an EBP workgroup for pet therapy. Johanna did a thorough and exhaustive search of the literature and engaged the assistance of a registered nurse from cardiology to partner with her on the possibility of a pet therapy program. Johanna and the cardiology nurse worked with Dr. Rich from Molloy College to critique the literature and to form a team to evaluate whether the best practice initiative would meet the needs of our patient population. Johanna also enrolled the geriatric nurse practitioner to join the team, and they selected the advanced care of the elderly (ACE) unit to pilot the initiative. Meanwhile, during Johanna's focus on a pet therapy program for our geriatric population, her cancer came back.

She never mentioned to the EBP team the incredible odds she fought against every day to return to work. Then one day, she had to take a medical leave. Ultimately, she was admitted on 4 North with metastasized breast cancer to the

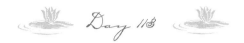

brain. Her mental status waxed and waned, but through it all, Johanna wanted to see her dogs.

According to the hospital's infection control guidelines, dogs were not allowed into the building. However, Johanna kept asking for the dogs, and the nurses on 4 North knew they needed to make it happen. The nurses contacted Pat Hogan, the CNO. Pat listened to the request. She knew Johanna well because of her efforts over the years to realize her dream of a pet therapy project. Pat knew how much Johanna's own dogs meant to her and sought to make her wish a reality. Thus, with the CNO's permission, Johanna's dogs came to visit her on 4 North one weekend night. Johanna was very lucid that night; she was happy to see her trusted friends. Johanna passed away soon after. Her program is now a reality administered once a week on our geriatric unit with wonderful outcomes for all our patients who participate.

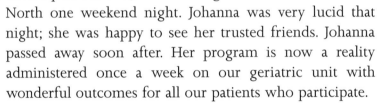

—Submitted by Patricia Lavin, Good Samaritan Medical Center

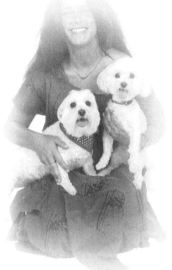

"Never underestimate the difference you can make."

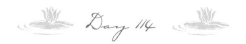

The Right Fit

A typical day for the Ellen H. Lazar Shoppe on Fifth is one in which we have the opportunity to provide renewed hope for our clients. By creating the new Shoppe on Fifth, a very special oncology boutique for people with special needs, Hackensack University Medical Center has made a commitment to make life beautiful again for women, children, and men who are experiencing or have experienced cancer in their lifetime.

There are so many stories that would be appropriate for a book about what's right in health care, but let me select one that truly reflects our focus on providing new hope.

One day we had a couple who appeared to be quite anxious. I asked them to come into the private fitting room so that we could discuss their concerns. The young woman spoke softly and asked if she could be fitted with a prosthesis that would allow her to feel whole and normal on both of her breasts. I assured her that she had come to the right place, and that we would do everything we could to help her feel whole again.

During the fitting her husband never left the room. When I felt that I had a good fit with the prosthesis, I took her garment and twisted the back as tight as I could. Out of the corner of my eye, I saw her husband's eyes get very big. I told him to stand behind her and close his eyes and embrace her breasts to check for symmetry. I then asked him to embrace his wife, and he did. Suddenly, tears

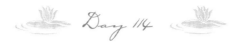

began to flow in the room. I had simply helped this woman feel normal again, but that act meant the world to her. It was great being able to help in such a special way.

I would like to close with a quote from Dr. Bernie Siegel that I often think about in my work: "Dress yourself for work and be aware of the weave and texture and fabric of your life. And how that has prepared you for your journey, and should your garments need to be repaired, remember that they can be repaired continuously with love."

—Submitted by Constance Niclas, Hackensack University Medical Center,
Ellen H. Lazar Shoppe on Fifth,
Hackensack, NJ

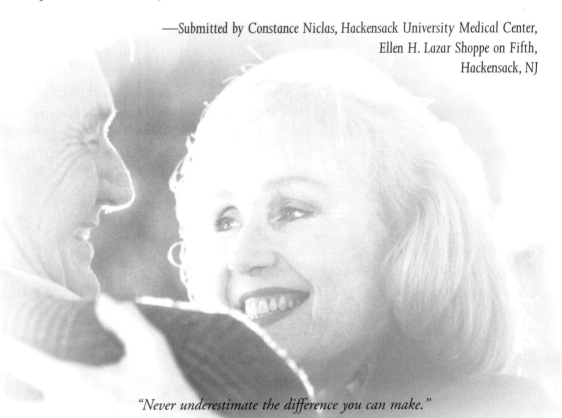

"Never underestimate the difference you can make."

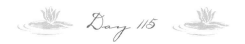

Senior Appreciation Day

The Senior Appreciation Day was instituted under the leadership of Kathy Gallo, geriatric nurse practitioner, and the Division of Geriatrics seven years ago. It began as a small event and has grown to have an average attendance of approximately 200 community seniors. Held in GSHMC Conference Center, Senior Appreciation Day provides a fun, healthy, and informative day for our senior community.

Each event is planned around pertinent, relevant themes for seniors. Past topics have included fall prevention, driving and the older adult, and medication safety. This past April, our focus concentrated on memory. With a theme of "Maintaining Your Brain," the day featured discussion, lectures, and interactive activities designed to address unique aspects of memory problems. Presentations included helpful tips on preserving cognitive abilities, earning Senior Appreciation Day designation as a White House Conference on Aging event.

This health fair is a collaborative effort between all disciplines in the hospital. Balance and gait suggestions, nutritious refreshments, mini therapy sessions, and giveaways abound. Nursing comprises the largest component of volunteers, as nurses man tables to provide free services such as blood pressure monitoring, glaucoma, diabetes, and cholesterol screening, as well as other innovative sessions and information.

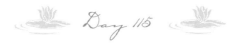

Local businesses and community experts share information about vital resources available to older adults of all functional and cognitive levels. Guest speakers offer educational insight, enlightening the audience about the theme, which this year was chosen based on our biannual newsletter, "Seniority: The Art of Aging." Good Samaritan is visionary in developing and supporting programs that reach out to our seniors. Nursing has embraced this population and is working to provide cutting-edge, geriatric-specific services to help people to not only live longer, but to live well.

The 2005 White House Conference on Aging was held in Washington, D.C., in October. The conference is intended to make recommendations to the President and Congress to guide national aging policies for the decade ahead. GSH's Senior Appreciation Day and Health Fair were among the events presented at this conference in 2005.

—Submitted by Patricia Lavin, Good Samaritan Medical Center

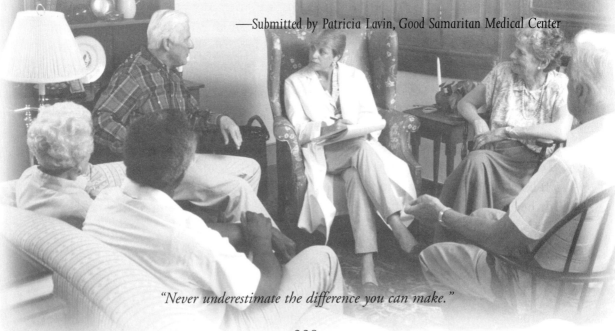

"Never underestimate the difference you can make."

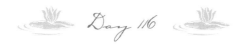

THANKING DAVE

This is a letter I sent to our CEO about the difference he made in the life of one of our hospital volunteers:

August 23, 2006

Dear Jim,

I had too much to say to fit into a thank you note, so it had to be a letter. As you know, one of our volunteers, David G., passed away recently. During his short time here, barely a year, he became quite a celebrity.

In the fall of 2005, Dave was recognized for an Above & Beyond story involving taking flowers to a patient he didn't even know. When I found out about the incident, I forwarded you the information. Dave received a thank you card from both of us…this is where it begins.

Shortly after receiving his thank you notes, Dave came to my office. In a very choked up voice, he explained that he had worked for Huron Valley Steel for over 20 years and Target for over 10 years and not once had he ever received a thank you note.

He said, "I've been volunteering here for six months and I get a thank you from the CEO." At the time, he told me he had framed both thank you notes and hung them in his study.

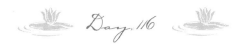

In January of 2006, Dave was one of the recipients of our Excellence Awards and was acknowledged during Excellabration. He was so humbled by the whole experience, and his wife and family attended the celebration.

Dave was beginning to have some health problems and shortly after that went on a leave of absence from his five-day-a-week volunteer position that he loved. During his illness, he kept calling and telling us that he was coming back. As his illness progressed, he had his wife keep us posted.

At Dave's funeral service, his dear friend, his brother, and the pastor all mentioned Dave's "job" volunteering at HFWH and how he couldn't wait to get well and return. His brother talked about the pride he felt seeing his brother's picture in our lobby. A few weeks later, his widow, Judy, came to my office to donate the $500 gift card that Dave had received as part of his award. She said he never felt comfortable keeping it and wanted to give it back himself. She said, "Do something good with it." The gift card was donated to Helping Hands to assist a rehab patient with her diabetic medication.

Jim, why am I reminding you of all this? Because if you had never come here, none of this would have happened. Dave ended up getting more recognition at the end of his life than he had ever had. Your Studer program, your accountability in implementing it, and the way you walk the talk with the volunteers enabled us to give Dave, a wonderful man, the recognition he had probably deserved his whole life. I am very grateful to you. There are benefits of a program like this that will never be measured on a survey.

Gratefully,
Carol Bridges, Director, Volunteer Services

—Submitted by Carol Bridges, Henry Ford Wyandotte Hospital, Wyandotte, MI

"Never underestimate the difference you can make."

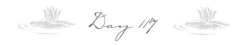
Ministry of Prayer

Recently I began a journey as a volunteer lay minister in our chaplain's office at Frye Regional Medical Center in Hickory, NC. It's been an amazing experience. Each day the challenge comes in not knowing what the morning's visits will hold for me. Many times there have been wonderful surprises, and I hope that I will always remember these special moments. Here are a few of my favorite moments that I think help show what's right in health care:

I have a routine that I use each time I enter a patient's room. I always introduce myself and then explain that I'm coming from the chaplain's office to see if there is anything we can do for them during their visit at the hospital. That's where the similarities in my visits with patients end. From that point, each patient is different.

After introducing myself one day, a female patient indicated to me that she was in a confused state. She was being discharged the day we met, and she lived all alone. She told me that she didn't feel well enough to stay alone and didn't want to impose on friends for help. She explained to me that she was trying to decide what she should do. As luck would have it, a volunteer job of mine is calling Bingo every Friday evening at an assisted living residence, which is located near this hospital. I explained to the patient that at the residence they do respite care, which would be perfect for her situation. I explained the program to her,

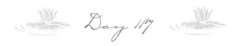

and she asked, "How do I get in touch with them?" I picked up the phone and had her talking with the right person within minutes. She was extremely happy with the way things turned out, particularly with the fact that the price would be cheaper for her at the residence than if she were to hire someone to take care of her. For me, it was a wonderful experience of being in the right place at the right time. I was so happy to be providing help to someone so early in my journey as a chaplain.

A few days ago, I entered the room of a new mom. The new mom was lying in bed with her new baby in her arms. On the other side of the baby was a little guy, probably about two years old, on the sofa was another little guy, probably about four years old, and over beside him was the father. It was great being in a room where everyone was smiling back at me. What a precious moment in time! "What a precious family," I said as I introduced myself. They told me they didn't need anything, but I asked if I could offer a prayer of thanks for them before I left. They graciously accepted. After the prayer, I congratulated the mom and dad and spoke to the little sons. After that I asked the name of the baby. Imagine my surprise when the mom answered "Katherine," and, looking at my ID badge, said, "And we're spelling it the same way as yours." "How wonderful," I said. I spoke to the boys, and told them I had two older brothers who were always very good to their sister. I felt the Lord had given me a gift that day. It was wonderful being in the presence of that beautiful family and their new baby daughter with whom I shared a name.

On another day I was assigned a lady in the Heart Tower. After chatting and praying with her, she asked me to please come back again later in the day. Since she appeared to be so lonely, I told her I'd come before I went home for lunch. Before I left she said, "Bring me back something." After my other assignments

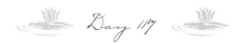

were completed, I searched the gift shop for an idea of something to bring back. I found a happy angel card with a nice verse inside the card. I decided if I put it on her tray table, it would cheer her up during the afternoon. I signed it, "From your new friend, Katherine," read it to her, and then set it where she could see it. I am so glad I was able to spend a little extra time with her that day, as sadly, two days later I read her obituary in the newspaper.

On another day, I visited with a Catholic woman. Originally, one of the other members of our chaplain's team had been assigned to see her, but the patient specified to this team member that she'd like someone to visit her from the Catholic Church, and that she'd like to receive the Eucharist. When our chaplain read this on the patient's chart, he called me to see if I was available to visit this lady as I am Catholic and do hospital ministry for our church. I was glad to do it. In visiting at her bedside, she could speak to me only in a tiny voice, which trailed off, as she appeared to fall asleep. As I stood there, I offered a prayer for her. She opened her eyes and told me she'd heard the prayer. She seemed to be acting strangely, and the nurses explained to me that they were trying to stabilize her condition. They told me they suspected she was diabetic and was perhaps going into a coma. While I was at the nurses' station, I called our church directly and told them the seriousness of the patient's condition. One of our priests came up and took care of her spiritual needs before she lost consciousness. I visited her the next day. Fortunately, she had received the medical help in time and eventually made a full recovery.

I truly enjoy and am deeply grateful to be doing this ministry. I pray I may be an effective instrument of God's love wherever He desires me to be. The joy with which He fills my soul is an unforgettable sign of His presence in my life!

—Submitted by Katherine Cuzzone, Frye Regional Medical Center, Hickory, NC

"Never underestimate the difference you can make."

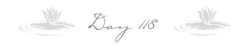

Why Nursing Is Such a Special Profession

After 22 years of nursing, I know there could never be any other profession for me. One moment in particular in my nursing career stands out for me to this day. I had a very special moment when a patient, whom I had cared for two years prior, and her husband found out where I was working and came back to me to say, "Thank you."

This patient and her husband have made a difference in my life, and I'd like to share their story to help make a difference in yours, too. I was the nurse manager of a 30-bed intensive care unit. One very busy afternoon, we received a call from MHW and the cardiac cath lab to say that an emergent code heart was coming over and was extremely sick.

The patient, a woman, was about 56 years old. She and her husband were shopping in Publix when her husband went to the deli to get chicken wings for lunch. When he came back to his wife, he found her collapsed and lying on the floor next to their cart. He had seen CPR on TV so he yelled for help, checked her airway, and started CPR with the assistance of fellow shoppers.

His wife had a cardiac arrest. She was defibrillated and resuscitated on-site, intubated, and transferred to MHW, where she was stabilized and then transferred emergently to MRH. The doctor in the cath lab worked on her for quite awhile. She was in cardiogenic shock, and an intra-aortic balloon pump was placed. My clinical manager at the time on nights welcomed the patient's husband to the ICU

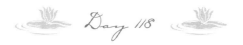

and told him that we would do everything we could, but that his wife was in extremely critical condition.

The next day I met the family on my rounds in the ICU. Mrs. Z, the patient, was not responsive. She remained not responsive for the next few days and was exhibiting all the signs of a patient who had suffered an anoxic event. To be honest, my nurses and I did not think she was going to survive. And, if she did survive, we felt she would have very little quality of life.

Her whole family gathered at her bedside with a pastor who led them in deep prayer. As I rounded, I found them praying. My simple words to them were, "You all are doing the right thing—just keep praying." They prayed for the next few days and slowly her body started responding to all the therapy. We weaned her off all the machines, and about one week later, miraculously, she was out of bed and responding neurologically.

After about six months passed, I left my nurse manager position and transferred to MHP. I received a phone call from Mr. Z. He had remembered my words of encouragement and had called to say, "Thank you." He told me his wife was alive and doing well. She had started a rehab program and was on her way to recovery. I also got to speak to the patient. I had goosebumps! I could not believe this patient had done so well.

After another year had passed, Mr. and Mrs. Z called and said they would be in town (They live up North, but their children live down here). They wanted to take time out of their visit to come to see me. I could not believe what I saw when they arrived. Mrs. Z was walking, had lost 100 lbs., and the only deficits she suffered as a result of her heart problems were short-term memory loss and balance problems.

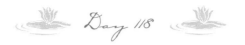

They hugged me and said, "Thank you." It was the most heartwarming moment. Mr. Z told me that he was grateful to have his wife. He said they would have never survived without the devout belief they have in God.

I share this story with the hope that never again will a health care worker give up on a patient. Keep talking to your non-responsive patients; you never know what they hear. The power of family, love, prayer, and will are what I believe kept my patient alive. To me she is a miracle.

—Submitted by Elizabeth Reed, Memorial Healthcare System, Hollywood, FL

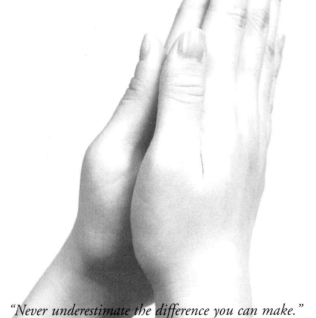

"Never underestimate the difference you can make."

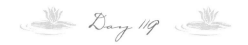

Nurse Lifesavers

*T*he following event occurred after a major hurricane in October 2005. The staff nurse involved and the CNS for oncology were awarded the Lifesaver Award for the Memorial Healthcare System in 2006.

While making walking rounds at the change of shift one day, the nurse was introduced to a lovely female patient who had a history of multiple myelomas. She was admitted just prior to the arrival of Hurricane Wilma with a diagnosis of back pain, rule out cord compression.

The patient was kept on strict bed rest to minimize damage to the spinal cord. The day following the hurricane, the primary physician requested a neurosurgical consult. The neurosurgical consult examined the patient and recommended emergency radiation therapy as primary treatment. He chose this recommendation due to the morbidity and mortality associated with neurosurgery. Unfortunately, due to the power outages that ensued during the storm, radiation therapy had not yet been initiated.

After morning rounds the patient began to complain of a heavy feeling in both legs. Knowing that an impending, progressive paralysis is associated with decrease in motor function, the nurse placed "stat" calls to the primary physician and neurosurgeon. Also, aware that bladder function is a late sign of spinal cord compression, the nurse asked the patient when she last voided. She stated that it had been almost twelve hours. The nurse recognized that this was a sign of

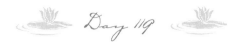

neurogenic bladder, and the nurse immediately catheterized the patient for a significant amount of urine. After this, frequent neurological vital signs were initiated, and the patient was continually assessed for further changes.

Realizing that the communication systems had been rendered inoperable following the storm, the direct care nurse suggested to the clinical manager that she contact the command center to initiate emergency communication with the physicians who had been involved with this patient. The CNS located the director of oncology services to determine the status of the radiation therapy (RT) services regarding the need for emergency services.

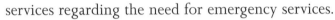

The CNS was able to contact the RT department, located in an adjacent city, and spoke with the radiation oncologist regarding the emergent need. Arrangements were made for immediate transfer and treatment.

At that moment in time, the nurse was able to reach the involved neurosurgeon and discussed the current nursing assessment with him. The nurse was asked to keep the patient NPO (nothing by mouth) for possible surgery. The neurosurgeon came to the unit and further assessed the patient. Unfortunately, he found that her spinal cord compression was progressing. Within minutes, the patient was on her way to the operating room for emergency neurosurgery.

As a result of sound nursing clinical judgment of this nurse and interdependent practice, the patient received the care she needed and regained neurological function.

—Anonymous Contributor, Memorial Healthcare System

"Never underestimate the difference you can make."

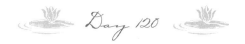

Shining Star

Everyone knew that Shirley Hughes was a special employee, but on July 6 her dedication and commitment became apparent to the whole community.

Shirley's supervisor was called away from her post to answer the phone. Shirley was calling to explain that her home had been lost in a fire the night before. Thankfully, no one was hurt.

"Take all the time you need," her supervisor said, "and let us know how we can help." But Shirley protested, "No, no, I was not calling to take off. I just wanted to make sure I could come to work without my uniform." Every item Shirley owned had gone up in ashes, including her uniforms, shoes, and her ID badge.

A few hours later, Shirley arrived, shy smile still there, eyes swollen from tears, her head held high. Immediately, the food service department began helping with clothing and money for Shirley and her family.

The Morrison team at Gadsden Regional is fortunate to have such a wonderful, dedicated associate working there. Shirley is no less than a shining star in her department. For Shirley's outstanding service, she received the Morrison Healthcare Food Services "2006 People First Award."

—*Anonymous Contributor, Gadsden Regional*

"Never underestimate the difference you can make."

Share Your Own Story

Please share an experience that connected you back to purpose, worthwhile work, and making a difference. You are a big part of what's right in health care!

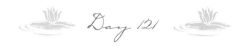

A Journey Home

In the summer of 2005, we had a patient admitted to the oncology unit with a diagnosis of lymphoma. A Colombian woman in her late fifties, the patient was uninsured, not a resident of the United States, and had no family here in Florida. She was employed by a couple who owned a nearby restaurant and she cleaned their home to pay for her room and board.

As "Ms. R" became increasingly ill and spent more time in the oncology unit, the staff grew close to her. There were various meetings regarding her treatment referrals and care, which included RNs, social workers, oncology physicians, and clinical resource managers (CRMs).

On their days off, many of the direct care nurses provided her transportation to her treatments. The family she worked for found a distant relative living in New Jersey. Through this relation they were able to contact her family in Colombia, who then flew her daughter to the United States to visit her ailing mother. When it became evident Ms. R was not responding to treatment, the oncology unit formed a collection fund called the "Send Ms. R Home" collection. The unit raised enough money to send Ms. R back to Colombia. The day before she left, many of the direct-care nurses, pharmacists, CRMs, and patient care assistants spent the evening with Ms. R. The day of her flight, two of the direct-care nurses from the oncology unit took Ms. R to the airport. Two weeks later, her

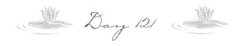

family contacted the oncology unit to let us know she had died peacefully at home.

The nurses are committed to assisting families and patients in achieving their goals through the continuum of care. Palliative care is a nursing intervention that was used to assist the family. In this instance, the patient and family desired her return to Colombia so she could be surrounded by her family and die in peace. The nurses were able to assist them in achieving that goal, making a dying woman's journey a little bit easier.

—*Anonymous Contributor*

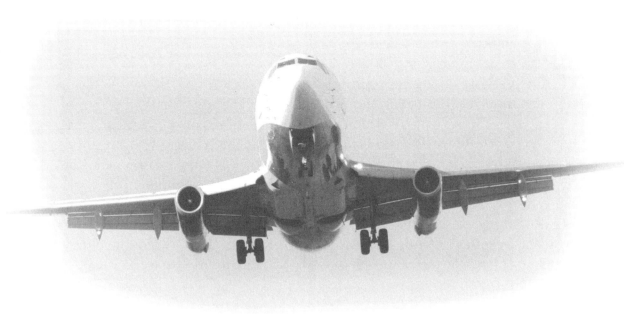

"Never underestimate the difference you can make."

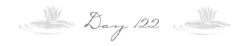

Ceremony of Remembrance

On June 25, 250 people attended the first annual "Ceremony of Remembrance" held at Vassar Brothers Medical Center (VBMC). Each person attending was there to acknowledge someone special who touched his or her life for an all too brief time.

Each year, more than 40,000 families across the country suffer a fetal demise. In the past, health care providers typically treated this loss clinically, often ignoring or downplaying the emotional aspects of this intensely personal loss. Thanks in large part to Ann Critelli, VBMC handles such losses in a different manner.

Ann understands the tremendous sense of despair experienced by mothers after the loss of an infant. Fifteen years ago, Ann delivered a full-term baby girl, but was never able to hold her. All she has to remember the life of her child is a poor quality Polaroid photo, and the cold memory of an ill-prepared staff who were uncomfortable caring for her after the birth of her stillborn daughter.

Following this painful experience, Ann became an advocate for parents who suffer a fetal demise, working to set a new standard of care. After 11 years of offering support to bereaved parents on a volunteer basis, Ann was hired as the perinatal bereavement coordinator at VBMC, a position funded by a grant from the March of Dimes.

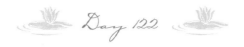

Although Ann's position is not full time, she is available 24 hours a day via pager. She contacts each family who suffers a loss and offers support. She visits families in their homes, attends them through labor and delivery, helps make funeral arrangements, and attend funerals. She listens, she cares, and she makes a difference.

After a baby's death, parents most often seek some acknowledgement of that child's life. Ann encourages the family to bond with their infant and create some memories. She works with other organizations to supply "memory boxes" to hold precious mementos, such as a birth certificate, wrist bands, foot/handprints, locks of hair, etc. Other groups donate tiny dresses and bonnets for the infants.

In addition to offering individual support, Ann helps facilitate HANDS (Help After Neonatal Death through Sharing), a monthly support group, and she has started a second support group called Moving Forward.

Ann's dedication and sensitivity have made a tremendous difference in many families and how they cope with such a devastating loss. The bereavement work she does offers comfort to parents left behind to deal with life—and moving forward. At the Ceremony of Remembrance, quilts lined the front of the room, with each block containing a message to a baby who was loved and missed. The ceremony is a tribute to each tiny life Ann has helped parents acknowledge.

—Submitted by Vassar Brothers Medical Center, Poughkeepsie, NY

"Never underestimate the difference you can make."

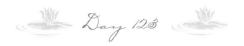

Monsignor Edmund Klimek: A Canticle to Care

*P*atients and visitors at Sacred Heart Hospital in Eau Claire, Wisconsin, greatly admire the expertise and brilliance of the facility's physicians and employees. Every day, they witness firsthand how the hospital's employees save lives, provide exceptional care, and deliver service that is ranked in the top one percent in the nation. This care makes Sacred Heart Hospital, an affiliate of the Hospital Sisters Health System, an exceptional place of hope and healing.

Among those who offer hope every day is Father Edmund Klimek, a priest who lives on-site. In 2007, he celebrates 39 years of pastoral care ministry at Sacred Heart Hospital. For 37 of those years, he was simply known as "Father Klimek" until Pope Benedict XVI bestowed the Papal Honor of "Chaplain to His Holiness" with the title "Monsignor." Not even the Pope was able to change several generations of tradition, as most people still request to see "Father Klimek."

Following Christ's example, Father Klimek continues to faithfully serve the sick at Sacred Heart Hospital. He frequently walks the halls and is always ready to go above and beyond what is required or expected. For some families, Father Klimek has ministered to three and four generations. He quietly goes about his work with joy, and his respect for the dignity of every human life is evident to patients, their families, and hospital staff. With a glint in his eye, he says, "No matter where we work at Sacred Heart Hospital, we're all a part of a team. Every

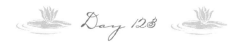

level of our care, from Maintenance to Maternity to Medical Records, is rooted in the belief that every person is a treasure, every life a sacred gift, every human being a unity of body, mind, and spirit."

Father Klimek truly sees the face of Jesus in those he serves. Reflecting on the work of a pastoral care chaplain, he commented, "It is more than tossing a rope down into a well to help someone out. It's actually climbing down there and being present with them. It's loving and being with people in the best of times and the worst, always being able to see Christ in them, treating them as Christ, and seeing great dignity in each individual." Sometimes pastoral care is not just his words. He once sat quietly in the corner of a room as a grief-stricken husband wailed and yelled and pounded the floor for 45 minutes after the death of his young wife. Father Klimek knew that what this man needed was silence, presence, and unconditional acceptance of this style of grieving.

"The words, 'There is Hope Here,' greet all who pass through the hospital's doors," commented Father Lawrence Dunklee, Director of the Center for Spiritual Care. "Hope is a fundamental component of the Hospital Sisters' Franciscan Mission: to give light to those who are in darkness—no matter if the darkness is due to illness or despair. We do this with joy, one of our core values, and with a strong connection to our hospital mission, vision, values, and purpose. This constant connection to purpose enables every employee to do great things in the health care trenches."

—*Anonymous Contributor, Sacred Heart Hospital, Eau Claire, WI*

"Never underestimate the difference you can make."

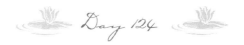

Health Care Heroes —
Extraordinary Stories of Caring

At Columbus Regional Hospital, our employees often go beyond expectations to show compassion and concern for patients and their families. Recently, C., the mother of our patient, K., expressed her appreciation for Cheri Wildridge, her daughter's nurse.

C. tells us that, from the beginning, Cheri and all of the other nurses took great care of K. However, she is most thankful for Cheri's kindness when her daughter's condition changed, requiring immediate surgery. C. was very frightened so Cheri stayed and comforted her long after her shift ended. C. wrote, "Even though Cheri's shift was over, she stayed with me and my daughter. Her presence helped me to relax and trust that my daughter would be all right. She even included my daughter in her family prayers. Cheri did a great job all day and could have left at the end of her shift, but instead gave her personal time to my daughter and me. We will never forget Cheri and all the nurses on Tower 6."

Cheri's actions demonstrate how our staff members demonstrate an extraordinary level of caring and compassion for those we serve. We salute the exceptional example they set for all of us.

—Anonymous Contributor, Columbus Regional Hospital, Columbus, IN

"Never underestimate the difference you can make."

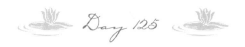

Memory of Chuck

One morning, my husband Woody and I rose before the sun to make our way down to a favorite place of ours—Laguna Beach. We sat on a boardwalk bench as the sun ascended. We watched as several men of all ages walked out onto the sand to form a circle of one. Two of the men played guitar as a chorus of beautiful voices sang praises to God. Beholding grace, I felt the ocean breeze cool upon my face. I gazed as seagulls were drawn in close to the circle only to soar off with my thoughts, flying high on the winds of time.

A memory of Chuck, a recollection of my distant past, flew in and descended upon my heart. For more than a year, I visited Chuck twice weekly at Huber House, a residential home for men with AIDS. As his nurse, I assessed his condition, drew his blood, educated him on treatments, and monitored his responses. As his friend, I listened to this gentle young man speak of his hopes and dreams. I recalled fondly that Chuck realized his dream vacation to the Bahamas.

Sadly, his family had abandoned him due to homophobia and fear of AIDS. I accompanied Chuck as he tried to make sense of his illness and find meaning in his life. He gradually moved through all the stages until finally, the end drew near.

Chuck transitioned to an inpatient hospice facility in Laguna Beach where he could receive full care. He was discharged from our home care service and I needed to say goodbye. That weekend, we drove down to Laguna. Woody took

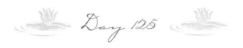

our two young boys to the beach, while I visited with Chuck. He was in that in-between stage, semi-comatose and unable to speak. I let him know I was there and sat quietly holding his hand. A caregiver came by and delivered a letter. She asked if I would read it to him, as they were just too busy. It was from a relative of Chuck's that happened to be a priest. Reading that letter to Chuck was one of the most profound experiences of my life. It was an outpouring of forgiveness, reconciliation, and love. Overcome with emotion, I continued reading as tears streamed down my face. After a while, I kissed Chuck and bid this sweet gentle soul farewell. I left in awe of the miracle I had just witnessed. God had placed me there at just the right moment so that I would become the messenger of His love.

Sitting on the boardwalk bench, I listened to the rhythmic in and out breath of the ocean's tide. The sun began to poke its head above the hills, greeting us in a radiant glow of warmth and light. The sky glowed iridescent with pastel hues of blue and pink, reflecting the beauty of Chuck's gentle spirit in the shimmering gray of the sea's fluid movements. Grateful once again, we took our leave.

—Submitted by Elizabeth Wessel, St. Joseph Health System, Home Health Network, Orange, CA

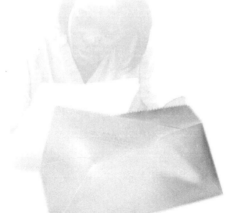

"Never underestimate the difference you can make."

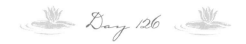

THE STORY OF JIM

My name is Pam Paul, and I am an oncology home infusion nurse. I first wanted to perform home health after working for a gynecological oncologist for three years. Whenever my patients had a crisis, such as pain or dehydration, it was the home health nurse to the rescue. When my patients were too sick to come into the office or when they began to move towards heaven, it was the home health nurse who acted as our eyes and ears. They were the nurses who developed relationships even when they knew it may last only a few months. They were there to hold my patients' hands as they took their last breaths.

Seven years ago, I joined the "troops" and I have enjoyed the challenge. We administer chemotherapy, hydration, antibiotics, and growth factor. I am even certified to administer packed red blood cells from the hospital. The clinical skills we learn are only part of the story. Jim's story exemplifies the power of home nursing.

I saw Jim for approximately six weeks. Jim had advanced throat cancer and could not swallow anything. He tried to suction himself constantly to be able to talk without choking. He had a gastric tube for food and a percutaneous inserted central catheter (PICC) line for hydration. His wife was a tireless workhorse and took great care of him, but she was overwhelmed with his symptom management. He did have good pain control, but he was not sleeping well. First,

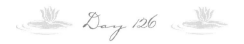

we tried atropine drops with limited success. Then we tried Phenergan with codeine and experienced great results.

I continued to see him weekly for PICC dressing changes, and, for a few weeks, he was stable. I continued to try to talk directly with Jim, but he would not make eye contact until about my fifth visit. It was a small gesture, but we had a conversation and he finally looked at me.

The next week he was complaining of shortness of breath and the physician ordered oxygen to relieve his symptoms. I brought the pulse oximeter out to determine the proper amount of oxygen. This took some time. We were up to three liters and he was still at 85 percent saturation. His wife looked at Jim and said, "I have to go pick up the kids at the beach, but I'll only be gone 10 minutes." Jim looked at me and then at his wife and said, "Go, Pam will take care of me." I told her not to worry and not to hurry. Again, she looked at Jim and again asked if he was sure. With a small smile, he repeated, "Pam will take care of me." We worked on the oxygen at five liters, his saturation was only 90 percent, but it was the best I could do.

I had ordered a mask and planned to reassess the next day. Jim died that night at 3:00 a.m. He was surrounded by his family, and his wife was grateful that it was painless and peaceful.

Those six words, "Pam will take care of me," are the reward for my commitment to home nursing. There is nothing more powerful than having a stranger trust you with his or her life. I give a lot to my patients but they always give it back tenfold. I encourage anyone who wants to make an intimate difference with patients to become an oncology home health nurse.

—Submitted by Pam Paul, St. Joseph Health System, Home Health Network, Orange, CA

"Never underestimate the difference you can make."

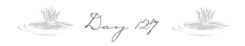

A Nurse's Story...

Each of our patients has a story to tell. One of our team's chronic debilitating rheumatoid arthritis patients has an incredible story. She touches all who see her, including me.

Our nursing staff would see this patient each week. Every time we saw her, she was either in her bed or in her electric wheel chair. She suffers from a severe hand deformity, and requires special silverware and plates in order to eat. The first time I heard her get out of bed, I heard bones cracking so loud, I wasn't sure if she was okay or not.

About six months ago, I saw her when she came in for her regular visit. I was tired and it showed on my weary face. She looked at me as I came into the room and told me that I forgot to open my gift. Confused, I looked at her and asked what she meant. She explained that God gives me the gift of joy every day and today I forgot to take the bow off and open it. My eyes filled with tears as I realized the depth of her words. Before I leave for work each day, I take a moment and try to mentally open my gift.

That lovely lady has continued to slowly debilitate. She can no longer safely get out of bed and move around. One day, I stopped by to see if I could help a fellow nurse as she performed a procedure on the patient. I sat on the side of the bed and held her hand while she talked and vented. She told me that she wished her husband could do the one thing that I was doing at that moment, sitting,

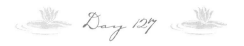

holding her hand, and listening. She told me I was not just a nurse, but that my nursing was a ministry.

She was hospitalized just a few days ago, and her husband will no longer be able to care for her in their home. Her biggest concern was whether she would still be able to see her favorite nurses while in her assisted living facility.

Like many others in the middle of my life I have found the job I know I am supposed to be doing. It is reinforced every day that I have the privilege of serving our community.

—Submitted by Barbara Turnblom, St. Joseph's Home Health, Orange, CA

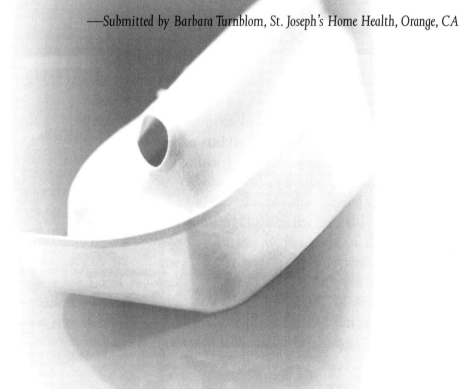

"Never underestimate the difference you can make."

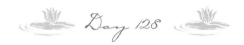

Fried Shrimp and Fancy Coffee

*I*n Human Resources, we touch patients' lives indirectly through the services we provide to employees and the caregivers we hire. However, we seldom have the opportunity to touch a patient's life directly. When we can, it's a wonderful gift. One day near Easter, my coworker Sarah and I were dining at O'Charley's after work when a gentleman beside us started to make conversation with us. He told us that his little girl was a patient at our hospital. She had undergone multiple plastic surgeries to correct a facial deformity and he said St. Francis was the only hospital he and his wife trusted enough to help her. He and his family had traveled to St. Francis from their home in Florence several times for the surgeries and it had really taken a toll on them. He told us that he and his wife had been sleeping in their daughter's hospital room for sometime. We also learned that his wife really loved "fancy coffee" and that his little girl's favorite food was fried shrimp from the West Ashley Crab Shack. That day we insisted on paying for our new friend's food and asked him if he would mind us stopping in to visit the next morning at the hospital. He was thrilled and immediately gave us their room number.

That same day we contacted the Crab Shack and asked the manager for a gift certificate for the family. He gladly complied, thrilled to help with such a great cause. Next we went shopping and bought an Easter basket filled with all kinds

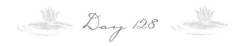

of candy. Finally we picked up a nice package of espresso for our friend's wife, plus enough bagels, pastries, and muffins for everyone.

When we entered the little girl's room, she was lying in bed surrounded by her stuffed animals. The man and his wife were also in the room, looking completely exhausted. We told the little girl that the Easter Bunny had stopped by our office and told us that her favorite restaurant was the Crab Shack and he wanted us to deliver a gift card and some other surprises just for her. She was grinning from ear to ear and whispered something in her father's ear. He told us, "She wants to have her picture taken with you." Sarah and I had our picture taken with this beautiful child a few minutes before we left. I wonder if they could see the tears in our eyes when they had their film developed. Although we may never cross paths with this family again, it felt so good to have been able to make a very difficult time in their lives a little brighter.

—Submitted by Pennie Peralta for Deborah W., Bon Secours St. Francis Hospital, Charleston, SC

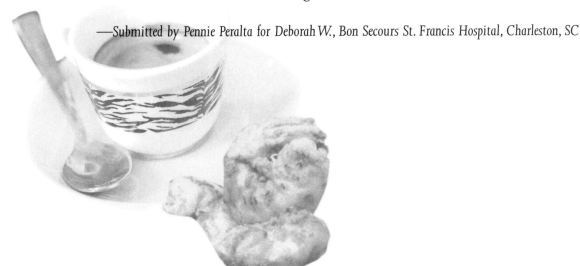

"Never underestimate the difference you can make."

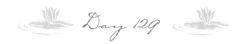

True Team Spirit

*T*hree nursing units exemplified true team spirit in action when caring for a family that fell victim to a motor vehicle crash. That day our staff displayed excellent quality of care, nursing leadership, and in particular, interdisciplinary relationships.

A young mother fastened her two young daughters into their car seats and proceeded to run errands as she would any other day. However, three blocks from home her car was broad-sided by another vehicle.

Within minutes, the mother and her two-year-old were on their way to the nearest hospital for stabilization of their injuries. The five-year-old was transported to Hackensack University Medical Center (HUMC) and was crying upon her arrival—a great sign, as it indicated that she could breathe. The nurse manager notified the children's father. He let her know he was on his way, and, when he arrived, she escorted him to his oldest daughter's bedside. As she explained to him his child's status, the sound of a helicopter hovered in the distance. His other daughter would land momentarily and would join her sister in the Pediatric Intensive Care Unit.

Meanwhile, the mother was still at a different hospital and in critical condition. There she underwent emergency surgery and was transferred to HUMC the following day. Finally, all family members were in one hospital.

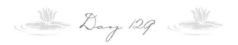
Quality of care and nursing leadership were well demonstrated throughout this entire process. The nurse managers, APNs, and staff nurses, as well as the physicians, child life specialists, social workers, and pastors all pulled together to ensure that the most urgent care could be given to everyone involved.

Through it all, multiple family members kept vigil at their loved ones' bedsides. As time progressed, it became clear that their mother simply could not

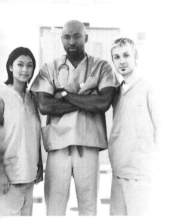

pull through. She was eventually pronounced brain dead. A group of nursing staff helped orchestrate a special visit for the children and family members as a final goodbye to their mother, sister, daughter, and wife. The ICU room was re-designed to look like a bedroom through the eyes of a child. Their grandparents, aunt, and uncle, watched as the children presented their mother with pictures they had drawn and sang songs for her.

Though it was a devastating situation, this beautiful goodbye validated the love everyone felt for this woman. Her husband made the ultimate act of kindness and allowed her organs to be donated to patients desperately awaiting transplants. She gave a 66-year-old woman a new kidney. The other kidney went to a 22-year-old mother of two children. All transplant patients are reportedly doing very well.

While working together to provide the best possible care for this family, these medical units also cared for each other. The SICU nurse manager arranged a session to assist the staff in the healing process that would ensue for everyone involved. These three nursing units demonstrated that individual nursing units do not and cannot work in isolation. In coming together, they were all able to do their best to serve and support their patients to the best of their ability.

—*Submitted by Lisa Iachetti, Dianne M. Cheer, Denise Crustsa,*
Hackensack University Medical Center, Hackensack, NJ

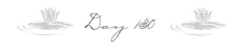

Dedication Infused with Passion

Willis Williams, a team member who has touched the hearts and lives of countless associates, customers, and clients, displays his commitment daily through his passion for food and dedication to his profession.

Willis is the first to work and the last to leave. When issues arise, he travels great distances on a moment's notice and will not quit until the job is completed.

A member of the culinary team, Willis is rarely heard. Instead, he is seen in the field, getting the job done. Willis can be found in the kitchen, working on the front line with chefs, managers, and associates, ensuring proper hands-on training. His overall goal is to guarantee that excellent quality food products are served daily.

Anyone who knows Willis can attest to his passion for food and his dedication to training, to making the staff the best they can be. People from across the country will inquire about Willis, as his reputation is truly legendary within the food service industry.

Willis provides an example that gives everyone something to strive toward—excellence, dedication, and passion for his profession, as well as service to patients, caregivers, and associates.

—Anonymous Contributor

"Never underestimate the difference you can make."

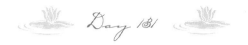

PRINCESS ROOM

*F*or obvious reasons, September 11th holds memories of fear and sadness for most of us. But this past year, the date gained even deeper sorrow for me and a family in my practice. On that date, I had the unfortunate task of having to break the news to a mom and dad that their six-year-old daughter had cancer.

The situation rapidly became worse. Upon further evaluation by the oncologists, this beautiful young girl's cancer was determined to be metastatic, widespread, and untreatable.

When I visited her at Dartmouth Medical Center, I found her scared and in pain—and her family was reeling in a pain of their own. It was difficult to embrace the depth and breadth of the sadness and helplessness that I felt. Medically, there was nothing I could do to help.

I wanted to find some other meaningful way to help, so I coordinated the patient's Make-A-Wish Foundation wish, which was to have a "princess room." I even helped drywall areas of her new room, mudding and taping to get the space ready in time for her return home.

I checked in with the family every few days by phone, and periodically stopped by their house in the hope I could comfort the family as well as myself. I let the family know I was available to help them at any time—night or day. Any

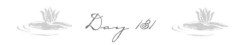

time spent in their assistance seemed insignificant compared to the life-altering journey this family was enduring.

Yet, the family showed unbelievable courage in the face of personal tragedy. Upon learning of the truly hopeless diagnosis, her mom stated that now she knew why God had sent her to them—to show her six years of love, to help her know God, and to comfort her in her suffering. Talk about teaching us, humbling us, showing such faith and strength amidst adversity…they continued to show genuine concern for all those around them even during their trials. The family was an inspiration to the entire community with how they handled their daughter's illness.

Almost two months to the day from her diagnosis, while preparing to give a lecture at a conference, I received an urgent page that she had just died. Within the hour I was at the family's house, assisting the family with preparations. I had the honor of holding her while her dad bathed her and moved her to put on the princess dress her mom had brought to dress her in.

The CD I made for her and her family early on in her illness (a CD that became her "favorite") had the following "line" notes:

> This CD is my attempt at telling a story, a story of a little girl, so loving, so loved, who touched many people's lives. My hope is that listening to these songs may be among the ways you keep [your daughter] alive in your hearts. This music is my attempt at a tribute to her life, as well as her and your courage in bearing her cross…my prayer to [her] and to you.
>
> Love, Bill

She died the day before I was leaving for the conference, a commitment I could not easily change. Somehow I think she didn't want me at her funeral. My role in her life and death was done. I did, however, have a tribute that was played for her family at the funeral—the song, "I Wish," by a friend, Sean Forrest (a song he wrote to help deal with his wife's miscarriage):

"I wish I could have held you in my arms, to feel your gentle breath upon my heart. But that's okay 'cause I know the Father holds you oh so near and our Blessed Mother rocks you to sleep as Jesus whispers in your ear: rock-a-bye my baby, don't you shed a tear. I'll take care of your mom and dad, so don't you have a fear. My promise is true, that's why I died for you, and they will see you once again. So pray with Me child for your mom and dad so we can help their hearts to mend."

Her mom, as part of her tribute to Taylor, had these words to say:

"To the most amazing pediatrician in the world, Dr. Bill Storo, who gave us 24/7 access, picked up medication in the middle of the night, who kneeled by Taylor's bedside at 11:30 at night and sang her to sleep, who assisted in the construction of the 'princess room,' who made Taylor the most moving CD, and who shared his strong faith with us along our journey. As soon as Taylor hit Dartmouth, Dr. Bill's work was done—little did we know in Dr. Bill's eyes, his work had only just begun. We will forever be touched by his deep love for Taylor."

Obviously, I was touched by this family more than they could ever know. Even in our helplessness, we can make a difference. It is sometimes when we can only do so little, that we can do so much.

—*Submitted by Dr. William Storo, Dartmouth Hitchcock Concord, Concord, NH*

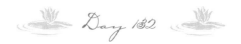

Beyond the Call of Duty

At Columbus Regional Hospital, our employees often go beyond expectations to show compassion and concern for patients and coworkers. Recently, Dan Spartz, Director of Emergency and Pulmonary Services, was listening to the ambulance scanner from his home around 5 a.m., when he heard a call go out at an address in his neighborhood. Feeling certain it was a coworker, Rich R., who needed help, he rushed over.

That morning, while bending over, Rich's hip become displaced. Rich couldn't move and was in extreme discomfort. Dan stayed with Rich and his wife while they waited for the ambulance to arrive. He kept everyone calm and reassured them that everything would be fine.

When the ambulance arrived, Dan assisted the paramedics by moving furniture out of the bedroom and helping them get Rich into the ambulance. Before he left, Dan placed the furniture back into the bedroom.

Rich says that "Dan is an exceptional person and neighbor and he truly lives the Columbus Regional Hospital motto of care, respect, and service. He truly did go beyond the call of duty. Dan, a sincere thanks to you for your help and compassion."

Dan's actions exemplify the extraordinary level of caring and compassion our staff members provide to those we serve. We salute the exceptional example he has set for all of us.

—*Anonymous Contributor, Columbus Regional Hospital, Columbus, IN*

Everyday Excellence

While she was on break one day, Macara Zalenski, NICU, read an article in *The Oakland Press* about a photographer who provided free services for terminally ill children.

The article featured Erin Drallos, who founded the American Child Photographers Charity Guild, an organization of more than 700 photographers across the world who volunteer their time and services to take pictures of terminally ill babies and children.

A few weeks later, she had a patient who she had cared for a lot and bonded with. "I didn't expect that she would live through the week," says Macara.

"I called the photographer over the Fourth of July weekend and didn't really expect to hear anything."

The photographer came in the next day and took photos of the baby for the family.

"She took the most amazing photographs for the family," says a coworker. "Macara did this out of the kindness of her heart because she wanted the family to have those photos."

Macara's manager and colleagues agree that it's her everyday excellence that makes her so special. "She spends so much time outside of her job duties reading stories, playing music, holding or rocking the babies, putting bows in their hair, giving them warm baths, and just being kind." says a coworker.

"She's a model for others," says another.

—*Submitted by Lisa Kozemchak, Beaumont Hospitals, Royal Oak, MI*

Wedding Bells and Hospital Halls

In the spring of 2006, we had a 50-year-old gentleman that came into our facility and ended up having a very extended stay. The staff got to know not only the patient but his fiancée as well. We didn't know that the wedding day was quickly approaching until the day before the actual event.

He was still our patient at this time and wanted to know if there was any way that we could help with his wedding. We offered him the use of our chapel, which he declined due to his condition.

To help make it a day to remember, one of our staff members bought a wedding cake on her way into work. We set up streamers and wedding bells from a prior wedding shower for a staff member, and we decorated his doorway.

His future in-laws were in attendance, along with a justice of the peace. The staff joined in just outside the doorway. Our unit photographer took lots of pictures to help preserve this very special time in our patient's life.

We had cake and ice cream for the family party along with plates, napkins, and Diet Sprite for the wedding toast. We even left the decorations up for a few days and not only the staff but other patients joined in wishing the happy couple congratulations.

Three days after the wedding the patient and his bride left our unit with many thanks for helping their dream of a nice wedding come true.

—Submitted by Deborah Peterson, Florida Hospital Memorial Division Ormond Beach,
Ormond Beach, FL

"BYE FOR NOW"

"It is not what you serve; it's how you serve it," she said.

"But Joyce," I interrupted, "we are only eating a sandwich with a few chips. I'll just use the foil it came wrapped in."

"Jane, my mother always said that it's not what you serve; it's how you serve it. Now sit down and eat."

I sat down in the chair that reminded me of my great-grandmother's kitchen set. It's the kind of chair that deflates an inch or so when you settle on it, the kind that sticks to your skin like cotton candy.

I glanced around at the elegant table setting. A silver plate displayed a pile of chips; my soda was poured into a shamrock glass from one of Joyce's trips to Ireland. The paper towel was folded as if it were silk linen.

This woman, I thought to myself, has given me friendship, shared her knowledge and taught me the importance of compassion—without even knowing it.

It all began when I was assigned to a new house. I was never fond of venturing into a new patient's home because I never knew what to expect—a grumpy old man, or a lonely widow whose husband passed away ten years ago and who still wears black everyday…faithfully.

According to my schedule, her name was Sara and she was listed as a mobile patient who needed assistance with physical therapy and personal care. I was

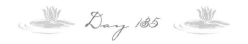

assigned three days a week for a period of two hours. I parked my car on the side of her house, which was in my own neighborhood. I entered the side door as the instructions stated and climbed the creaky wooden stairs to the second floor.

Before I could knock, a petite woman greeted me. I introduced myself with a smile and silently classified the 90 pounds or so standing before me as one of the "cute ones." Her name was Joyce and she was Sara's sister.

"Sara," Joyce called in a soft voice. "The new aide is here." She brought me into the sitting room where Sara was awaiting my arrival. She said, "It's a pleasure to meet you, Jane."

My scheduled time with Sara passed very quickly that day. I was on my way out when Sara turned to me and said, "Thank you for coming, Jane. I really enjoyed our visit today." I was astounded when she thanked me. No patient had ever said that to me before.

I replied to her, "You're welcome. See you Friday morning at 10. Goodbye!"

As I walked over the scatter rug that divided the kitchen and dining room, Joyce stopped me for a moment.

"Jane," she said, "Please don't say goodbye. Goodbye is too long, usually forever! 'Bye for now' works better, don't you think so?" I had to agree.

My visits with Sara and Joyce began to resemble a hobby rather than a job. Over time, I became used to their lifestyles. A sister named Harriet frequently came by to take Joyce shopping. Harriet and her husband James watched out for Sara and Joyce. James took out the garbage every week while Harriet took Joyce to one of her favorite stores. I got to know the oldest sister just as well. Her name was Gertrude and she was the only sister who had children. Sara and Joyce took great pride in the nieces and nephews!

Within a year, unfortunate circumstances developed and Gertrude passed away. Sara developed pneumonia and her health declined rapidly. The virus took control of her internal system and late one evening, she, too, passed away. My health also dwindled after I suffered a lower lumbar sprain accompanied by severe spasms. As a result of this accident, I could no longer be a home health aide.

As I worked on strengthening my back, Joyce and I would routinely meet for lunch. I didn't want her to feel alone due to the loss of her sisters. I knew Harriet and James would check on Joyce each day, but I still felt that she needed me as much as I needed her. I was glad to be there for her "my mother always said" stories. I was the grandchild she never had.

Everyday issues were becoming more complicated for Joyce. She needed my help, my opinion, and my guidance. While my back healed, I started working as an emergency response technician. As soon as I learned what a personal emergency response system was, I contacted Harriet and Joyce and asked to meet with them at one o'clock that afternoon.

As I did upon my first visit several years earlier, I climbed the creaky wooden steps again and quickly discovered Joyce was not very receptive to the idea of a response system.

"Jane, I don't want one of those things," Joyce said in her stubborn Irish accent. "I can get along just fine."

"Now Joyce, hear Jane out," Harriet interrupted. "Joyce, think of how many times you have slipped on those scatter rugs placed all over the pine wood floor.

How often have you caught yourself before falling to the ground? What is going to happen if you fall and can't get up to call for help?" The two women discussed the situation and finally, Joyce agreed that she may benefit from the unit. From that day forward, she never took the chain off of her neck.

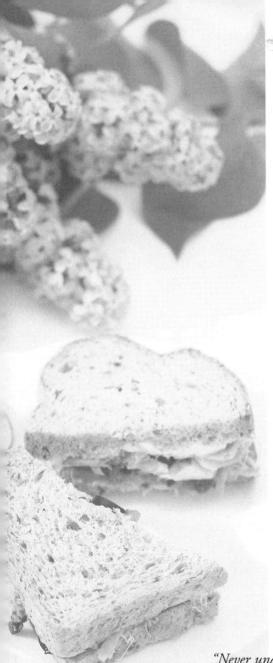

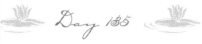

My phone rang very early the morning of my birthday. Assuming it was a wrong number or one of my friends calling to tease me about being a year older, I rolled over and closed my eyes. The phone rang again almost instantly. This time, I answered it. It was the emergency response service center. Joyce had used her system for the first time and was being transported to the hospital.

As I rushed to get dressed, I called the emergency room. The receptionist transferred me to a doctor. "I'm sorry, but…"

Joyce was gone.

I was there to help Joyce, but she had a tremendous impact on my life, as well. She inspired me and I learned so much from her. Sometimes we are sent to help others and we are the ones who end up learning.

Dear Joyce: thank you so much, and—"bye for now."

—Submitted by Jane E. Gagne,
North Shore Medical Center, Salem, MA

"Never underestimate the difference you can make."

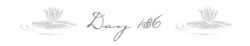

Care Before Computers

I have been in nursing since 1985, beginning with an assistant job and working my way up to completing my BSN and, finally, beginning an MBA with a Health Care Management Specialty. I was offered the opportunity to be the director of nursing in July 2006 at a brand new hospital—Oak Tree Hospital at Baptist Northeast. I was thrilled because this was such an exciting and rare opportunity for me. One of my jobs as director of nursing was to interview and hire new nurses and assistants that would take care of the first patients that came through our doors. I had never before been in the position to make ultimate hiring decision and frankly, I was very intimidated by this task. But, I knew what type of facility and environment I wanted to create, so I decided that I would assess both skills and candidate attitudes and go from there. My goal was to find employees who displayed caring, compassion, and a true desire to do what was right for our patients.

One of my first interviews was a woman named Melissa Jamiel, or Missy. This vivacious young woman was from a small town and had very few computer skills. Though I loved Missy's lovely personality, a large part of her job would require advanced computer competency, and Missy's experience with computers was limited, to say the least. I told her that I definitely wished I could hire her, but was concerned about her lack of computer skills, especially in the initial start-up phase. I didn't want her to feel as though she was incompetent in any way,

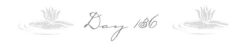

and I was uncertain that we could devote the time that would be needed to help her gain the skills that she would have to master. I told her that I would be calling her to fill a position in the next round of hiring, because I didn't want to put her in a situation where she would be frustrated and unprepared. Missy agreed that her computer skills would be an issue, and I told her that I would be in contact in the next couple of months.

Within a few weeks, I received a call from Missy, who stated that she wanted to work for me immediately and did not want to wait for the next round of hiring, so she had signed up for a four week computer class and wanted to know if this would be enough for her to get hired now. My initial response was "Wow, what initiative!" This was exactly the kind of employee that I was looking for. So Missy joined our initial staff, and has proven to be one of the best assistants I have. She pays attention to detail, and her goal is always to do things right. We both laugh because her computer skills are still not the greatest, but they certainly are better than they were before.

But this is not the end of the story. Shortly after I hired Missy, we received a patient who had a chronic blood disease that left her with little immunity to fight infection. After a few weeks, it was evident that her suffering would soon be over. When she passed away, our staff suffered and cried along with this woman's very large family, feeling our own grief almost as acutely as they did. Only afterward did I learn just what an extraordinary person Missy truly is.

Tina, the RN on duty that day, came to my office to share what Missy and Marcie, another new assistant, had done. Missy knew that this patient had an aversion to hospital gowns. After she passed, Missy took the time to dress the woman in her own pajamas. She wanted to make sure the patient looked as close to what she would have wanted as possible. The patient also loved to wear her vanilla scented lotion. Missy massaged this woman's hands with her lotion and then placed her carefully in her bed. Once she removed all the excess medical equipment from the room, Missy invited the family in to view their loved one as they remembered her. She went far out of her way not only to honor the patient the way she would have wanted, but she also tried to do all she could to comfort the grieving family as well.

I went out to find Missy and Marcie to tell them what a great job they had done and how impressed I was that they had taken the time to take such extra special care of a lady that had meant so much to all of us. Missy, who looked a little bewildered, replied that she did not do anything at all, only that she knew that the patient would have had a fit if she knew that Missy had put a hospital gown on her! I laughed and walked away, thinking that I almost let this dedicated employee get away, simply because of a lack of computer skills. To me, the caring she exhibits daily means more to me than the most experienced computer guru ever could.

—*Submitted by Krista Van Bever, Oak Tree Hospital at Baptist Northeast, LaGrange, KY*

"Never underestimate the difference you can make."

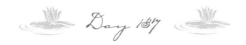

Miracle in Haiti

*I*am a member of the senior management team at Cheshire Medical Center/Dartmouth-Hitchcock (CMC/DHK) in Keene, NH. My background in health care has spanned four decades, including serving as a medical corpsman in the Air Force, working as a respiratory therapist, and working as a physician assistant associated with one of Boston's major teaching hospitals. Health care has been an important part of my life for a long time.

Dr. Douglas Keene, my personal physician, coworker, and friend, travels regularly to Haiti with medical teams to conduct health clinics for some of the world's most medically underserved people. Teams arrange for their own expenses, take time off work, and buy medications needed by the clinics. I was encouraged by Doug to put on my rather dusty physician assistant hat and join a team he was taking to Haiti in October 2005. It was a trip that had a huge impact on me—one I will never forget.

Haiti, a Creole and French-speaking nation of about eight million people is only a 90-minute plane ride from Miami…but it is light years away. Haiti continues to increase its population at an incredibly rapid rate, despite having one of the world's highest infant mortality rates and a total life expectancy of only 51.6 years.

Our medical team of six flew into Port Au Prince, the capital of Haiti, on a Saturday afternoon in October. Chaos ruled at the airport and my first

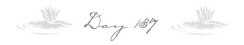

impressions of Haiti were customs agents helping themselves to the medications we brought for our clinics and hundreds of men jostling one another for the opportunity to carry our bags. Pushing and fighting was common in the frenzy to capture a small tip.

We were met by our host, Ed Amos, a physician assistant who worked with us at CMC/DHK before he relocated to Haiti as a missionary.

The clinics we held were generally assembled in simple cinder block missionary schools, orphanages, or churches. Most were in inner-city neighborhoods in Port Au Prince. One of the exceptions was Lelette, a small fishing village about two hours out of the city.

We held our clinic in a cinder block building with a dirt floor, holes for windows and doors, and a tin roof. I am sure it was where the village's goats, pigs, and chickens had slept the night before. Curious children of every age and size stood in the doors and peered through the windows, silent sentries watching everything we did as we set up the clinic. It was hot and very busy and we were due to see about 150 patients that day. Three of us were working as "providers" that day, two people were registering patients, writing down complaints and taking temperatures and blood pressures, and the rest were working in our makeshift pharmacy.

It was early in the afternoon when a woman brought in a baby girl with hydrocephalus, which causes an infant's head to become enlarged due to a build-up of cerebral spinal fluid in the brain. If left untreated, hydrocephalus causes brain damage, seizures and mental retardation. Corrective treatment is a surgical procedure where a shunt is put into the brain to drain the cerebral spinal fluid. This procedure, as far as anyone knew, was not available in Haiti, and if it was, it

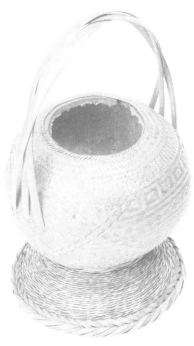

would be too expensive for this woman to pay. Besides, medical treatment in Haiti is only available if one pays in advance.

Prospects looked dim and all of the team was disheartened with the thought of having this beautiful child, named Betchara, regress to a diminished neurological state caused by brain damage.

In December 2005, Ed Amos, the physician assistant and missionary who was our host in Haiti, sent a newsletter with photos to his friends and supporters, telling the story of Lelette. What follows is a condensation of Ed's account of how treatment was provided for little Betchara.

In Haiti, because no one can afford surgery, children such as Betchara are discards. They are left to die by their parents on garbage heaps or in the "abandoned baby ward" at General Hospital.

Betchara's mother, Marie, wasn't going to do that to her baby. She lived on the shore of a lake that provided free fish for the catching and good neighbors who were able to share their rice and beans. Thank God for the medical team that visited four weeks ago.

Before our team left, I found out that a surgeon was coming to Haiti to perform shunt surgery for 17 children. Of course his schedule was full, but I insisted that Betchara was the perfect candidate. After one simple phone call to the States, our wonderful surgeon said that this was just the type of kid he wanted to operate on. She was a child with the potential for a full recovery and a normal

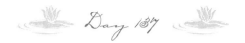

life. He said he would certainly do the surgery. All we needed to provide was a pre-op physical and a CAT scan.

Tom, my fellow teammate, left me with a donation to help those in need or to buy medicine. I thought Betchara was qualified so there was no reason not to run out to her village and get her. Of course her mom knew nothing about what was to happen. My interpreter and I arrived at the village one week before the surgery was to be performed. Mom and baby would need to come with me immediately if Betchara were to have a chance at a normal life. As we talked, a crowd gathered. Soon, the whole village was there. Villagers volunteered to take care of Betchara's sisters and brothers and told her mother not to worry. Before they left, the entire village gathered for a large community prayer. I could not hold back my tears as I watched Marie crying for her baby and the answer to the prayers only a mother could pray.

Karen, a great gal from Canada with a real heart for handicapped children, had arranged for Betchara's physical and the CAT scan, and provided a place for mother and child to stay while they awaited surgery. So off we went to Karen's house.

A few days later, Karen called to say that Betchara was running a fever and might not be able to have the surgery. Well, contrary to U.S. treatment standards, I loaded her with amoxicillin. Her fever broke.

The surgery was performed on November 21, and I'm pleased to announce that Betchara did very well. She was a candidate for a new procedure called a ventriculostomy, sort of an intracranial shunt without tubes that need replacing. If all works well, and there's no reason to think it won't, our little friend's head will shrink to normal size, she will have no seizures, and will escape any risk of mental retardation. In other words, she will be able to grow into a happy and healthy young woman.

—Submitted by Tom Link, Cheshire Medical Center/Dartmouth-Hitchcock, Keene, NH

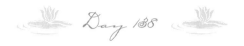
Bringing Families Together

The Oncology Unit received a patient, J.W., who recently had been diagnosed with Burkett's Lymphoma, and was treated previously at another South Florida Hospital. He came to Memorial Hospital West (MHW) at the request of his friend, an employee of MHW.

Eventually, J.W.'s trust in the care and practice at MHW grew and during his readmissions, he became part of the family of caregivers in the unit. Most recently, while in remission, he was hospitalized for a final round of chemotherapy. During his stay, he experienced a reaction to the therapy and was placed on a ventilator and transferred to ICU. The staff and the friend noted that J.W. had no family visiting. As it turned out, J.W. had not alerted his family to his most recent treatment.

The staff, as well as J.W.'s friend, recalled several conversations they had with J.W. about his family, so they worked to locate them in Coffeyville, Kansas. Arrangements were made for his parents to fly in to visit him.

On arrival, a staff member of the Oncology Unit met them at the airport and brought the parents to MHW to visit J.W. The parents could not afford a hotel stay during Super Bowl week, so the nurse manager of the Oncology Unit hosted the family at her own home during their visit. The same employee that picked the parents up drove them to the nurse manager's home and gave them instructions on how to return to MHW.

This is just one example of what is right in health care and why most of us are in it.

—Anonymous Contributor

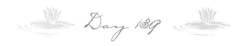

Blessings in Hospice

"*I*n the last hours of life, there is the same expectancy at death that there is at birth. The times when I've gone on a vigil, I see the patient going out of the physical and into the spiritual. For me, it is as important as the beginning of life."

These are the words of Beverly Nelson, a vigil hospice volunteer. She has just spoken them in a public restaurant in a shopping mall where busy people are going about their lives. It might seem a little strange to be talking about this in the middle of a bright Sunday afternoon where life is vibrating from every corner. But for a hospice volunteer this is shoptalk, and not unusual at all.

When the hospice coordinator calls, Beverly said, it doesn't matter what time of day it is because she knows she is needed to help the patient make the transition from the physical to the "non-physical." She meets the patient in the place where clinical medical practice ceases and a different kind of care emerges.

"It's just a very special time," says Beverly, a time when she can be in that space alone with the patient. "Both of us are present with the same intention and awareness of what's going on—the entire process of dying. I'm there to help them get that completed. I'm assisting that."

As a hospice volunteer, Beverly is picking up where the physicians and nurses leave off, even in a hospital setting. Many hospital staff and insurance claims processors may wonder if it is appropriate to have patients dying in hospital rooms, if it can be avoided. To a hospice volunteer with no agenda however, the

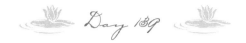

hospital room is just one more place, among many, where one goes to meet a dying patient.

At Jordan Hospital, where Beverly has been a vigil volunteer on three separate occasions, she has found it helpful to turn off the institutional lights and use a table lamp for lighting, accompanied by soft music playing on a portable radio. This way the patient doesn't have to be disturbed by the sights and sounds of a busy hospital that normally focuses on living, getting well, healing, and finding a cure. "This provides a different feeling," Beverly said. "We need to help nurses understand that an atmosphere of comfort and peace is the only focus that we have right now. We need to integrate our efforts, so the patients can be comfortable."

Beverly's recent experience has been devoted primarily to vigil hospice—attending to the dying in the final hours of life. Many hospice volunteers stay with a patient from the time they are enrolled in hospice, sometimes with the patient for six months or more as they progress through the final days and weeks of life, as opposed to the final hours. In these cases, hospice is both inside and outside the professional health care setting. It is obviously and clearly beneficial. A vigil volunteer program is quite different. You could say it extends care for the patient well past the boundaries traditionally set for a clinical practice of any kind.

But what of those last hours? In what way can those hours be attributed to health care?

Studies show that doctors and nurses do not give up easily. For them, it is hard to see death as anything more than failure, though they see it every day. Hospice vigil volunteers who come into the clinical environment and private homes, do, without question, extend health care by literally "keeping watch" while others in the field really must move on and attend to the living.

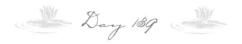

"When I go to a patient," Beverly says, "it is generally at 2 a.m., when no one is there. The family is absent, because they can't be present for one reason or another, so I have that special time to connect with patients in a way that I really feel is a kind of 'labor' or 'laboring' to get out of their physical being. When I try to describe this, people just don't understand, it's so hard to describe."

Hard to describe, yes, but incredibly rewarding, Beverly says. "I know the families always say how grateful they are for what we do, but I get so much more out of the service than they can ever know."

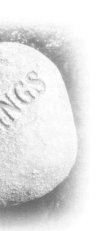

With her own technique and her own way of being with a patient, Beverly says, "There is a blending of spirits," where she can connect with the heart and mind of the patient, who is almost always non-verbal and medicated to control pain and discomfort and to make their passing as comfortable as possible. At Jordan Hospital, now the steward of Cranberry hospice in Plymouth, Massachusetts, health care takes on a new dimension by extending its programs, facilities, and staff to include the hospice and palliative care movement. By doing so, Jordan has enlarged the meaning of health care and has taken a step toward helping those at the end of life find some measure of comfort and support in dying—where all of the measurable progress is invisible, inward, and a matter of the heart.

"People wonder why we do this work," Beverly said. "'Isn't it depressing?' they want to know. No it's not, and it brings me to a place of gratitude every single day. It changes the way you see things and enriches your life in a way that you can't even describe. It's like seeing everything in Technicolor."

—Submitted by Karen Foster, Cranberry Hospice, Plymouth, MA

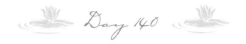
The Bed That Never Was

It was November 2006, in the ETD, and as usual it was notoriously busy. A young man named J.P. came into the triage area and sat down. Another headache, I thought, how many is that today? I have one too!

As J.P. went on to describe his symptoms I was getting suspicious that this may be more than just a headache. I triaged him and into the abyss he went. Later my suspicions were confirmed as I learned that the pain he had described was a tumor.

J.P. was a vital young man who had recently been in the military. This was not the news he expected to hear. The ETD MD had contacted a neurologist and scheduled a neurosurgeon to see J.P. An Emergency Department (ED) doctor on staff, who had recently undergone brain surgery for a similar diagnosis, talked to J.P. and gave him hope that he too could achieve his goal of living a long life and having a family.

That night as usual, the hospital was packed and J.P. spent the night in the expansion area of the ED. A colleague of mine named John cared for him. John was also a former serviceman and they spent all available free time talking about the military and where they had been stationed. In the morning, there were still no beds available and I wandered back in to take over for John.

John left and J.P. and I continued to talk about Japan where he, John, and my son were stationed. We developed a rapport with each other, and he requested I

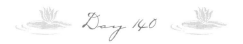
help him get rid of his boredom. I gladly put him to work putting stickers on empty charts while he waited for his family to arrive from Florida. Around midmorning, some of his family arrived, and we talked for while about what J.P. could expect post-op and where he would be placed after surgery. The surgeon came to talk to J.P. and his family. He told them it would take place that afternoon.

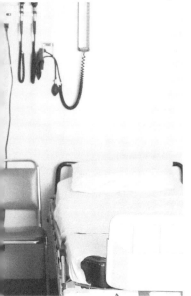

J.P. was scared. Fear was evident in his face. We sat for some time and just held hands while his family went to give information to his mother.

Next J.P. was assigned a bed and a room with a view, phone, and a TV bigger than a postage stamp! I came in to tell him his bed was up, only to hear him say, "No, I want to stay with you here in the ETD until I go to surgery. I don't want to go there. I feel safe here." Deep inside I was really flattered, but I said, "What? Are you nuts? People are waiting for beds and you have one!" J.P. said, "Give it to them, I don't want to go." I had been in this ETD for 18 years, and many patients had said they would like to stay to watch how the ETD works, however this was the first time I had ever had a patient downright refuse to go to a bed. I called my supervisor and informed her of the request. We cancelled the bed and it was given to another waiting patient.

My shift was almost over and the OR called and said they were coming for J.P. He and his family were scared and I could feel both fear and courage when we embraced. He left that day and went to the OR. I heard that the surgery went well and that he had a good recovery. J.P. came to the ETD last month. He was visiting friends. He asked for me, but I was off work. I felt good knowing he asked for me, but the best thing was that he was here, here just visiting friends.

—*Submitted by Kim Mattes-Szucs, Hackensack University Medical Center, Hackensack, NJ*

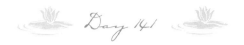

Everyday Angel

We admitted a very sweet elderly patient who takes care of her mentally challenged son. When we admitted her, we got a two for one bargain because her son is constantly by her side. This patient was pending discharge but her only concern was whether she could get her son to his doctor's appointment and then to find a rehab that would accept them both.

Crystal interacted with the patient and her son frequently, and she volunteered to take the son to his doctor's appointment. His mother expressed her gratitude to everyone within earshot. She told me she knew there were many angels in this hospital watching over her and her son but that she was so grateful that she finally got to meet one personally. Crystal does a great job every day. Her compassion toward our patients goes well beyond the call of duty. Thank you, Crystal. You are highly respected!

—Submitted by Pat Travis, Methodist Health System, Dallas, TX

"Never underestimate the difference you can make."

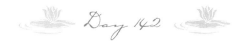

A Lesson Learned

Jeff was 35 years old and dying. He had been diagnosed with lung cancer five months earlier. This was his third hospitalization. The year was 1973, and I had been a nurse for almost a year. This was before hospice and many more people died in the hospital then than do today. We did primary care nursing back then, and I was Jeff's primary nurse. This meant I cared for him during each admission.

It was a Saturday at 11 a.m. when Jeff's visitors appeared. I had already cleaned Jeff four times from diarrhea and vomiting. First the vomiting would start, then the diarrhea. Jeff was deteriorating. The chemotherapy and radiation had been relentless.

I turned when I heard the door opening, and in came four of Jeff's "buddies" from the Fire Department. "Hey Jeff, you still alive, man?" one of them quipped. I felt my face flush at how disrespectful this guy was being. I finished straightening the room and left to check on my other patients. I was very upset at the lack of respect these "buddies" were showing Jeff. The poor man was dying and they were making jokes!

Later that evening, Jeff had a talk with me. "You seem upset, Randa," stated Jeff. I explained to Jeff that I thought his friends were out of line. Jeff enlightened me. "Randa, you and I both know I am dying. What is wrong with having some laughter on the way out?" Hmmm, I had not thought about that.

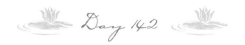

The next night we talked for a long time about quality versus longevity and how people react to death in their own way. I was letting it sink in when I looked out the door of Jeff's room and saw his four buddies. This time they all had shaved heads like Jeff's!

"You still breathing?" one chirped, and Jeff's face glowed with a big smile! The four came in and popped the top off a beer can and gave it to Jeff. The man, who had not kept solid or liquid food down for several days, took a swig of the beer! (By the way, he kept the beer down!)

For the next week, Jeff's buddies would come to see him with a six pack. I put a sign on the door stating "STRICT ISOLATION DO NOT ENTER." I could hear laughter and music and knew in my heart this was the best medicine for Jeff.

Jeff died about a week later, on my day off. I will never forget the lessons this man taught me. Bravery, compassion, dignity, and laughter should be a part of every care plan.

—Submitted by Randa Harrison, Osceola Regional, Kissimmee, FL

"Never underestimate the difference you can make."

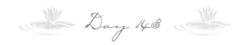

A Place to Belong

We are fortunate to have many dedicated and caring volunteers at Columbus Regional Hospital. Carolyn Souza recently encountered a young man while volunteering in the Emergency Department. After first refusing any assistance, the young man finally confided in Carolyn that he was homeless and needed a place to stay. He had been abandoned by his mother, didn't know where his father was living, and had no one else to contact. His mobility was limited due to severe birth defects, he had no money and only the clothes he was wearing. Carolyn and the Emergency Department staff made several calls to the local shelters, but were unsuccessful in finding accommodations. Knowing that she had to do something to help this young man, Carolyn and her husband took him to a local hotel and checked him in for the night. Carolyn returned the next day to make sure he had a good breakfast at the hotel and then took him to the drug store to purchase basic toiletries. She then drove him to various other organizations looking for housing assistance. She was finally able to secure an additional three days in the hotel through Horizon House.

Then, Carolyn began trying to locate his family and, with the help of an acquaintance, was able to find the boy's father. Once contacted, the boy's father immediately came to pick him up. Carolyn continues to talk with the young man

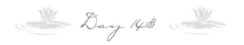

weekly. Thanks to Carolyn's help, the young man is doing well living with his father, has applied for Social Security and is interviewing for jobs.

Carolyn's actions demonstrate how our volunteers demonstrate an extraordinary level of caring and compassion for those we serve. We salute the exceptional example they set for all of us.

—*Submitted by Columbus Regional Hospital*

"Never underestimate the difference you can make."

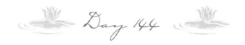

Support During Difficult Times

At Columbus Regional Hospital, our employees often go beyond expectations to show compassion and concern for patients and their families. Recently, Gina Gengelbach, a social work therapist, purchased a pre-paid phone for a patient that had become very ill and had no phone access. The patient and her companion were financially strained and living in poor conditions with no water or electricity. When she stopped by to deliver the phone, the patient's companion told Gina the patient has experienced a bad night. Gina went in to check on the patient and recognized she was in the process of dying. She informed the patient's companion that it was time to call hospice. Gina stayed with the companion to calm and counsel him while they waited for hospice to arrive.

Vickie Lowney has also been involved with the couple throughout the patient's illness. Vickie helped the patient and companion apply for Medicaid and food stamps. She has attended appeal hearings and provided food and emotional support. Vickie and Gina have worked tirelessly to support this couple through all their financial concerns and they continue to support the patient's companion with his medical and financial needs.

Gina and Vickie's actions demonstrate how our staff members provide an extraordinary level of caring and compassion for those we serve. We salute the exceptional example they set for all of us.

—*Submitted by Columbus Regional Hospital*

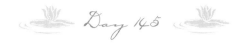

"Safe Within the Walls of Mercy"

riday morning started out like most days except for the palpable awareness of the Joint Commission on Accreditation of Healthcare Organizations'(JCAHO) in-house presence; it was day three of the surveyor's visit in Fairfield.

About mid-morning, I received a page from the Emergency Department requesting me to visit with a patient's mom in room 8. As I went into the ED, I instantly recognized Mrs. G. from her multiple visits here with her daughter who had recently died. As we reminisced about her daughter, the JCAHO physician survey team walked into the unit. Immediately, Mrs. G. wanted to know who these "important folks" were. Upon explanation, she asked if she could speak to them about the care we provided to her and her family.

She promised to keep it short as she knew that the surveyors had work to do. She just wanted them to know about the care people receive here on a daily basis and over a long period of time, as compared to what the survey team would see in their brief exposure. It was what she said after that that touched my heart and the hearts of those around her.

Mrs. G. explained that she had been here many times over the past few years with her beautiful, young daughter who had died of cancer; at all hours of the day and night, seeing many different physicians and multiple care providers on the various units. Each time, the entire family had been treated with a sense of

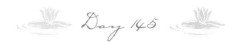

welcome, respect, compassion, and expertise unlike any other experience she had had at any other hospital in the greater Cincinnati area. "In fact," she said, "the only time I felt my daughter and family were safe and protected was when they were within the walls of Mercy. From the big CEO to the folks who clean the rooms, they treated us like we were family."

In the midst of her loss and grief, Mrs. G. felt the need to reach out and say "thank you" to those who cared. She said it again this Friday as she had said it each time she was here. Thank you, Mrs. G.

—*Submitted by Lynda Savelli, Mercy Hospital Fairfield, Fairfield, OH*

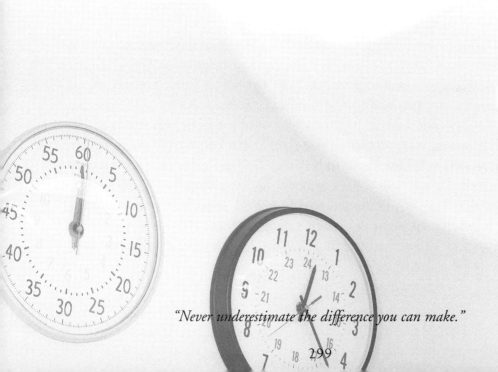

"Never underestimate the difference you can make."

299

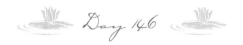

The Special Wedding

This is a story about medicine, a marriage, a mother, and a daughter's wish to have her mother at her wedding. It was July and unseasonably hot, when Darlene, 66, was hospitalized at the Aurora Medical Center. Darlene was battling stage IV high-grade non-Hodgkin's lymphoma, a cancer that originates in a patient's lymphatic system. She had been in and out of remission three times before, and doctors gave her a stem cell transplant in April. It was thought that the procedure provided plenty of time for Darlene to regain her strength and attend her daughter's July wedding.

In June, Darlene's health began to worsen and tests found lymphoma cells in her spinal fluid. Now hospitalized with a reservoir installed in her head so that chemotherapy treatments would go directly to her spinal fluid, the treatments became too much for her body to withstand. Darlene's doctor told her that further treatments would have to be postponed until her body was stronger.

Six months earlier, when Darlene's daughter Dawn had started planning her wedding day, she expected her mom to be there. Darlene always had expected to be there as well. Dawn had always wanted her wedding to be something different. She decided on a summer wedding held outside. As the wedding approached, it became apparent to Darlene's daughters that their mother was not going to be able to attend the wedding. On the Monday before the wedding,

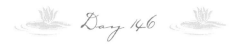

Darlene's daughter called Aurora Medical Center and talked with Betty Franz, a social worker, to ask for help.

Within 10 minutes, Betty called her back with a plan. The hospital offered their gazebo in the healing garden located behind the medical center for the ceremony. Unfortunately the weather was predicted to be in the upper 90s so it 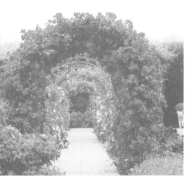 was decided the ceremony should take place in the hospital atrium. The staff on the third floor medical unit jumped into high gear to make this wedding wish a reality, as they knew the wedding inside the hospital meant Darlene would be able to attend. Nursing staff helped Darlene get ready, right down to applying just the right amount of make-up and lipstick to make this "mother of the bride" look and feel good. At times it was hard to see who was more excited, Darlene or the nurses taking care of her.

As the big day approached, hospital staff members decorated the atrium and one staff member volunteered to sing at the ceremony. Valerie Stevens, the hospital chaplain offered to perform the ceremony.

On Saturday, July 15, 2006, beneath a flower-draped arbor in the Aurora Medical Center atrium, the very first wedding was held at this facility. More than 125 guests, staff and family members watched as the most special person arrived just minutes before the bride herself. Seated in the front row, in a wheelchair and wearing a protective medical mask, Darlene watched her daughter marry the love of her life. Hugs, tears, and lots of keepsake photos were shared as a mother's and daughter's wish for this day came true. Darlene's health care team and the hospital staff knew that they had more than just medicine to offer. They gave a wonderful and lasting memory. On July 21, 2006 Darlene succumbed to her illness and passed away.

—Submitted by Colleen Wisnicky, Aurora Health Care / Aurora Medical Center, Milwaukee, WI

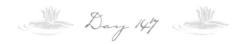

Memory Boxes

*T*he emptiness felt with the loss of a child is beyond measure. What can be said? What can be done to begin the process of healing? This was the challenge accepted by a group of staff nurses from Labor and Delivery and NICU. Partnering with the Pastoral Care staff, a task force was initiated and charged with developing a perinatal bereavement plan.

The first initiative was to standardize the delivery of care to affected families. The objectives of the group were to acknowledge with respect the life of the child and provide the family with something tangible to sustain the memory of the child. The idea of a memory box took shape.

The contents of the box, which was to be presented to the family at the time of the loss, included footprints of the deceased infant, a prayer, and a sympathy card available in English and Spanish. The nursing staff purchased a 35-mm camera to take a black and white picture of the infant for the family.

With enthusiasm growing, the pediatric nursing staff joined the group and a committee was formed. Feeling that there was still more work to do, the committee decided to ask administration for a standing memorial dedicated to the memory of the lost infants.

The guilds of Good Samaritan contributed to the funding of our Babies and Children Memorial Garden, a lovely sanctuary available to all bereaved families.

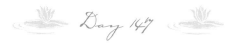

The members of the committee organized an initial dedication of the garden—all families who had lost a child in the last five years were invited to attend.

The perinatal bereavement initiative continues to evolve over time. Most recently, nurses in NICU and Labor and Delivery developed a comfort care protocol to address the palliative care needs of pre-viable infants born alive.

—Submitted by Patricia Lavin, Good Samaritan Medical Center, West Islip, NY

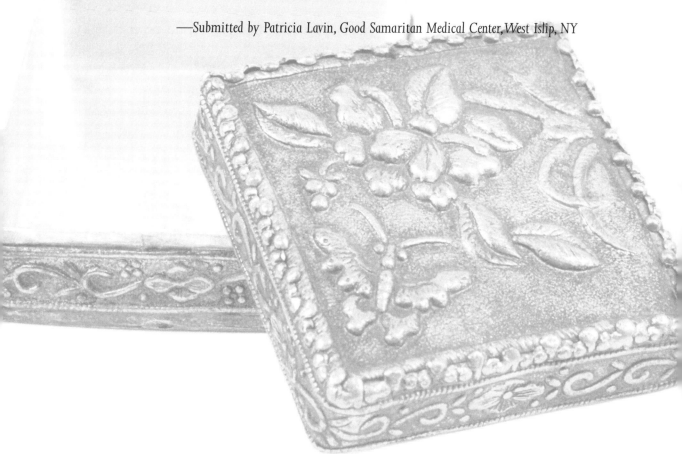

"Never underestimate the difference you can make."

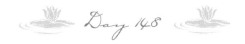

Filling Baby's Prescription

Employees at Columbus Regional Hospital often go beyond expectations to show compassion and concern for patients and their families. Recently, Gayle Wilson, patient registration team leader, received a call from a young mother asking if Medicaid had assigned a number to her baby. The baby was only a week old and needed a prescription filled. The young mother had no money to buy the medication and the pharmacy would not fill the prescription unless the baby had a Medicaid number.

It often takes 30 days to assign a Medicaid number to newborns, so a number had not yet been assigned. Gayle took the mother's phone number and told her she would call her back shortly. Gayle called several individuals asking for advice on how to help this young mother, but was unsuccessful in finding a solution.

Marita Burton, centralized scheduler, arrived to relieve Gayle from her shift and became aware of Gayle's efforts to find assistance for the newborn. Marita and Gayle decided to pool their money together to buy the prescription for the baby. Gayle drove to the pharmacy and delivered the money to cover the cost of the prescription. She then called the young mother and told her the prescription was paid for and she could pick it up at the pharmacy. The mother was not expecting such an act of kindness and was overcome with gratitude for Gayle and Marita's help in her time of need.

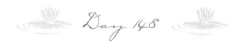

Gayle and Marita's actions demonstrated how our staff members provide an extraordinary level of caring and compassion for those we serve. We salute the exceptional example they set for all of us.

—*Submitted by Columbus Regional Hospital*

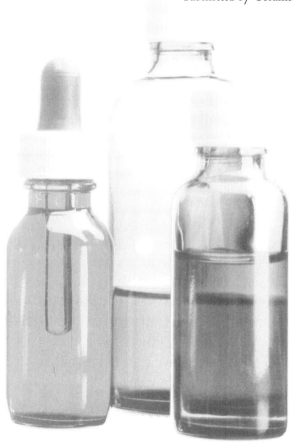

"Never underestimate the difference you can make."

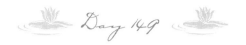

TAMMY

When "Mrs. Smith" came to Beaumont with her husband, she had already been to two other hospitals and was anxiously waiting for doctors to finish a procedure and diagnose her husband. At Beaumont, she met Tammy Oja, an Operating Room scheduling clerk.

"I was very alone, anxious and exhausted," says Mrs. Smith. "I met a very compassionate and caring young woman, Tammy, who went way beyond the call of duty to comfort me and reassure me that the doctors would do everything in their power to help my husband."

On her break, Tammy took Mrs. Smith with her to the dining room to make sure she had something to eat, and then took her back to the office to wait for the results from his procedure.

That evening, Mrs. Smith received news from the doctors that her husband's condition was not good and that he needed additional testing.

"By this time, Tammy's shift was over, but instead of going home, she came to the waiting room and stayed with me until my husband went back into ICU," said Mrs. Smith.

Tammy helped her write down the information the doctors had given her and stayed with her in the ICU.

"I understand that Tammy is raising her family and going to school to become a nurse," Mrs. Smith said. "She will be a great addition to the field of medicine. She is truly an asset to the hospital and should be commended for her excellence."

—Submitted by Lisa Kozemchak, William Beaumont Hospitals, Royal Oak, MI

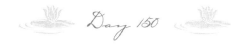

"The Christmas Room"

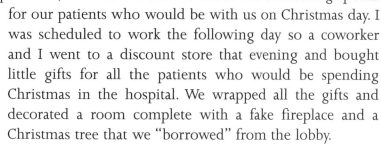

*T*he events in this story happened many years ago at a V.A. Hospital. It was Christmas Eve, and one of my patients had a "pass" to leave for 24 hours so he could go to his son's house for the holiday. His son came to visit, bringing his dad's Christmas presents with him. I told the son that his dad could spend Christmas Eve away from the hospital and that his father was really looking forward to going home. His son refused, stating that he would not take his dad home because he might wet the bed. I tried to explain ways to prevent this from happening, but the son still refused, saying his dad was just "too much trouble" to take home.

I decided that I hadn't done the greatest job in the "communication with family members" department, so I decided that we should do something special

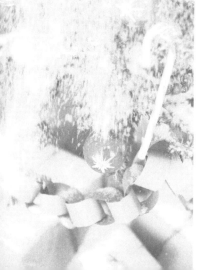

for our patients who would be with us on Christmas day. I was scheduled to work the following day so a coworker and I went to a discount store that evening and bought little gifts for all the patients who would be spending Christmas in the hospital. We wrapped all the gifts and decorated a room complete with a fake fireplace and a Christmas tree that we "borrowed" from the lobby.

The next morning we transferred all of the patients, including those who had to stay in bed, to our "family

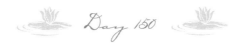

room" for Christmas dinner. We passed out gifts, sang carols, and kissed each patient on the cheek "under the mistletoe."

I will never forget this day, my first Christmas as an RN. I will always remember the smiles and joyful tears of my patients. This is what "caring" for my patients is all about!

—Submitted by Sandy Rush

"Never underestimate the difference you can make."

Share Your Own Story

Please share an experience that connected you back to purpose, worthwhile work, and making a difference. You are a big part of what's right in health care!

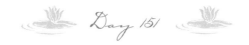

A Place for Carol

As the manager of marketing at the Marian Living Center at The Assumption Village in Austintown, Ohio, I learned firsthand from one very special resident what an important life-changing—even life-saving—event moving to assisted living can be for my elderly residents.

I had been working for two years with Carol and her son, trying to get her admitted to our 48-apartment assisted living residence. I had toured several times with Carol and her son and built a great relationship with them both. Despite the fact that her son was encouraging her to move to our assisted living residence, she simply couldn't make a final decision about what would be best for her.

One day, while we were still stuck in the process, Carol's son was diagnosed with terminal cancer. He decided not to tell his mom that he was dying to save her the worry, and he passed away soon after his diagnosis. Before he passed, he made me promise that I would speak with his mom and encourage her to come live at The Assumption Village.

I continued to build a relationship with her, but she simply couldn't make a decision. She was afraid to leave the house she had lived in for 40 years—the home her husband had built, the home where she had raised her son. Her son had made all of her decisions for her before he passed, and she just couldn't picture the rest of her life now that he was gone.

One night after work, I received a call from Carol. She asked me to come over to her house. I knew she didn't have anyone else and felt that I should help her in any way possible, so I went. When I arrived, I found her with a bottle of sleeping pills on her table and tears in her eyes. She was very upset. When I asked her about her fears, she said she wasn't sure where her place in the world was now that both her son and husband had passed. The house represented her ties to them, and they were ties that were going to be difficult for her to break. She also expressed her concerns about the transition and how it would be handled.

To my great pleasure, she decided to move to our facility after our meeting. To ease her worries, I made sure that we took care of all of the details. We arranged to have her power of attorney to handle her finances, hired movers to pack and move her things, and help her get settled into her new home. I noticed that once there was a plan for her in place she was actually excited about the move.

Not too long ago, Carol told me that the night she called me she had also called several other facilities asking for help. She said they only offered to give her brochures and more information when what she really needed was someone to talk to about her worries and fears. She said that she felt God was telling her she would make a decision one way or another that night—either she would end her life by taking the sleeping pills or she would make the decision to move to the Village. She is a big believer in signs, and she felt that my coming that night was a sign that The Assumption Village was the right place for her. After hearing this, I felt so blessed that I was able to be with her in her time of need. It was a humbling experience that taught me why my work here is so vital.

I continue to see Carol regularly. Now one of our happiest residents, she enjoys the socialization and new friends that she as made at the Village. Most importantly, she says she knows she isn't alone anymore and can see that she can live a happy life even though her husband and son are no longer with her.

—Submitted by Kristine Mariotti,
Marian Living Center at the Assumption Village, Austintown, OH

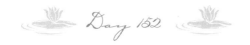

Vermell

At our facility, nurses have to be on call on the weekends, and at the hospital, on-call nurses respond only to urgent and emergent cases. We let staff members decide whether they want to take on cases that aren't urgent or emergent on these weekend shifts.

One weekend, Vermell, a friendly, warm woman who had been nursing for many years, got a call from a physician who wanted to do a procedure on a Saturday. The doctor explained to Vermell that the case wasn't urgent, but that the man who had just survived a battle with cancer was planning to go on a cruise with his wife, and that without this procedure, he wouldn't be able to go.

Although she had other plans, Vermell felt it was more important that she come in and help take care of this patient. On Saturday, when it was time for the procedure, the doctor told the patient that while Vermell didn't have to come in that day for this case, she wanted to do it so that he could go on his cruise. Vermell of course said she was happy to do it, and told the patient that she hadn't had any plans for the day anyway.

Vermell, who is always great at comforting the patients, struck up a conversation that eventually led to gardening, one of Vermell's passions. It came out that Vermell had planned to go to a garden show that day because she was in search of a certain kind of lily for her garden at home.

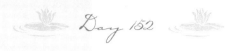

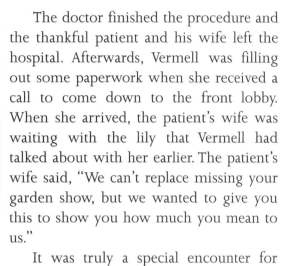

The doctor finished the procedure and the thankful patient and his wife left the hospital. Afterwards, Vermell was filling out some paperwork when she received a call to come down to the front lobby. When she arrived, the patient's wife was waiting with the lily that Vermell had talked about with her earlier. The patient's wife said, "We can't replace missing your garden show, but we wanted to give you this to show you how much you mean to us."

It was truly a special encounter for both the patient and Vermell. To this day, she still has the flower planted in her yard.

—Submitted by Tillie Balliet,
Roper St. Francis Healthcare, Charleston, SC

"Never underestimate the difference you can make."

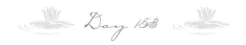
A Mother's Daughter

As a nurse practitioner for Kaleida Healthcare, I work at Herman Badillo Bi-Lingual Academy in Buffalo, New York, to provide at-risk children with medical care that they may not receive otherwise. We find that, after children get their initial vaccinations, many parents are unable to take their children back to the doctor because of the high costs of health care. Through working at schools, we help fill in the gaps that exist in health care for these children. Our routine exams have helped children in many ways. We've discovered vision problems, dental problems, and cases of scoliosis that may have otherwise gone unnoticed. These early interventions help prevent all kinds of problems, and provide the children with care that can ensure they stay healthy.

During one routine physical, I was fortunate enough to meet a very special young patient. I was examining an eight-year-old girl who told me that she didn't get much sleep at night because of her sick mother. She told me that her mother had lupus and, in order to take care of her mother, she spent her nights sleeping in a loveseat at the foot of her mother's bed. This ensured that she would easily know when her mother needed her in some way. This child had had several absences, and we discovered that on nights when she didn't get any sleep she would often skip school the next day to get the rest she needed.

It was imperative that we help this young girl and her mother so a social worker and I went to the little girl's house. The child's aunt, her mother's identical twin sister, opened the door and explained that her sister not only had lupus, but

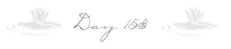

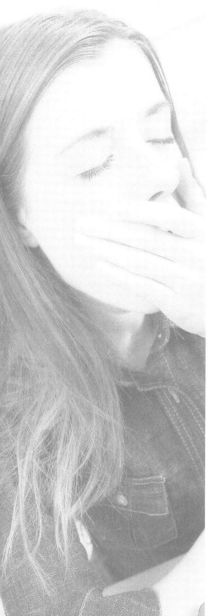

also suffered from arthritis that left her in so much pain she was completely bedridden. She said they had been trying for some time to get into housing that was wheelchair accessible because on good days the young girl's mother was able to get around via a wheelchair.

We explained to the little girl that it was okay for her to ask for help and to be a little girl. She didn't need to take on the adult responsibility of caring for her mother. The social worker and I worked together to find a solution. The girl stayed in the house with her aunt and mother, and eventually, we were able to get them into wheelchair accessible housing. We adopted the family for Christmas that year to further help them along.

Unfortunately, the young girl's mother passed away. After an understandably difficult time after the death, I am happy to report the young girl is doing well. She is an honor student and attends a charter school for children who excel at science and math. She is such a special young girl, and I was so happy to be able to be a part of her life. She impressed me very much as not once did she complain about taking care of her mother. She simply felt it was the right thing for her to do. The children I work with never cease to amaze me, and this particular young girl will be someone I will never forget.

—Submitted by Margo Villagomez, Kaleida Health

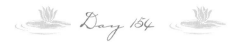

Maria's Story

*A*s a night charge nurse at a Family Birth Center at an Oregon hospital, you never know what is going to happen during your shift. One quiet evening at the Center, my fellow staff members and I found ourselves involved with a tragic story. On this particular night, we only had one patient in labor, and she was nearing delivery. I was with the doctor and the patient when one of my coworkers came in and announced that another patient had just arrived and was saying that she needed to push. My coworker asked that I handle the new patient's case, and I said that I would.

The patient ended up touching all of our hearts that night, her story so unbelievably sad. The patient's name was Maria. She was only 13 years old and was 33 weeks along in her pregnancy. After her examination we determined that she was fully dilated and in labor. We set up a room for her and started to get ready for the delivery.

We were having a lot of difficulty communicating with Maria. She was from Mexico, and her family was part of a small indigenous tribe with its own language. Her family spoke a little Spanish so we knew it was extremely important that we get a translator to the hospital as soon as possible. I called a translator and even though it was late at night she agreed to come right away.

Through the translator's conversations with the family we learned that Maria had been through a very traumatizing situation. Her pregnancy was the result of a rape and now this young girl was going into a pre-term birth.

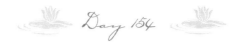

Because there was only one doctor at the Birth Center, we had to call in the on-call doctor. On this night, it was Dr. Huang. Known as a "straight shooter," Dr. Huang doesn't show much emotion with regard to his patients, but at the end of this night, I was very impressed with his ability to handle the situation and with the amount of caring he showed to Maria.

Our hospital is a level one hospital that cares for well babies and babies born after 35 weeks. Because Maria's baby was going to be born outside the scope of care we provided, we called in a transport team that would take her to another hospital which could better handle the pre-term baby.

The fetal monitor indicated that the baby's heartbeat was strong, but when Dr. Huang monitored Maria later, there remained only a faint tremor of the heartbeat we first heard. We all suspected the worst and the ultrasound confirmed that the baby had died. Maria's already tragic story had taken another turn for the worse. Dr. Huang delivered the stillborn child. But Maria wasn't out of the water yet. We discovered that she was preeclampsic, and as a result, she was bleeding heavily.

While Dr. Huang was treating Maria, we were able to talk with the family. We asked if there was a priest we could call to come and comfort them during this time. They said there was, but we were unable to reach him. Our chaplain came down to comfort the family and help them deal with this horrible situation.

Together, we all did our best to comfort Maria and her family. The chaplain and translator stayed with her and her family until it was time for her to be transported to another hospital. I was so proud of Dr. Huang who stayed with Maria until her transport despite the fact that he had had little sleep the night before and could have easily gone home as he was not on call. He stayed because he knew the importance of continuity of care for his patients and he saw that because he was fluent in Spanish he could be a huge help in the situation.

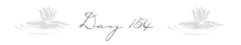

Weaving together medical care with spiritual comfort is never easy. We realized in this situation that it was necessary for Maria to receive both in order for her to truly receive the care she needed.

That night I was in awe as my colleagues worked together seamlessly in order to care for Maria. The chaplain later told me that he was very impressed with the way we worked together to care for Maria and show her the compassion she needed. I'm always proud to be a part of the Family Birth Center, but on that night as we came together to help Maria, I was grateful to have the opportunity to help someone who desperately needed great health care. I was so glad that we were there to provide it for her.

Even though we had all been through a tragic event that night, each of the nurses left feeling good about the care we were able to provide. We had enough help from the doctors and other staff and were able to learn a lot. By providing quality health care, we were able to find the positive in a tough situation.

—Submitted by Judith Lienhard

"Never underestimate the difference you can make."

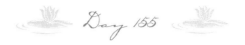
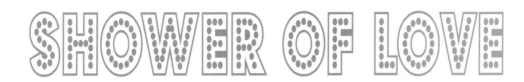

SHOWER OF LOVE

*L*ast year, my boyfriend was admitted to the Intensive Care Unit of the Southern New Hampshire Medical Center, the hospital where I am also employed as a nurse. A courageous guy, he has a rare neurogenic dystrophy and wasn't supposed to see his 20th birthday. Today, he's still going strong at 41!

During his 30-day stay in the ICU, he was being treated for pneumonia. While he was intubated, his tracheal tube became crimped, and he wasn't able to get the air he needed. As a result, his doctor had to perform a tracheostomy.

After his procedure, the ICU nurses were fantastic and my boyfriend was working hard to recover. Despite being in a wheelchair and mostly bedridden, he moved around as much as possible and was trying very hard to work his way off of the ventilator.

I realized that in all of his hard work for recovery what he really needed was a shower. In my experience, I had learned that showers can be very therapeutic for patients, particularly for those who have been stuck in their room for a long period of time.

I made it my number one priority to find him a shower somewhere in the hospital. There was one in the ICU department but it wouldn't accommodate his bulky wheelchair. I found a big shower on the fourth floor of our hospital, but the nurses thought it was too risky to take him so far away from the ICU. I finally

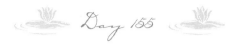

found a shower located in the pediatric ward, which happened to be the same floor as the ICU.

Once a location for the shower was found, my boyfriend's doctor had to write an order for the shower and when the doctor got the call, he said, "The guy on the ventilator? He's fighting pneumonia and has a new tracheostomy!" He was amazed that he was up for it.

After that everyone pitched in to make the shower possible. Our environmental staff came in and sanitized the shower. The ICU nurses helped run the proper tubes he needed. I stayed by his side the whole time and everyone cheered when he returned, fresh from his shower. I learned that sometimes doing the best thing for a patient isn't always easy or convenient for anyone involved. But we all realized what a positive experience it can be for a patient, when everyone works to give him the care that will heal him physically and emotionally.

—Submitted by Mary Beth Miller, Southern NH Medical Center

"Never underestimate the difference you can make."

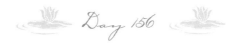

A Special Call

It's not often that I get a call at 10:30 at night. So when I picked up the phone recently, I was a little suspicious of who I might find on the other end. I would never have imagined the conversation I was about to have would become one of the most memorable moments in my career as a seasoned pediatric nurse, but it was.

The voice on the other end said, "I have been looking for you for so long." A little taken aback I told the lady I was sorry, but I would have to ask who she was. She said, "You may not remember me, but my baby died the day after Christmas in 1985." And instantly for me the memories returned.

On the day after Christmas in 1985, I received a call on an inside line at St. Mary's Hospital where I worked. When I answered the call, the worried voice on the other end of the phone said, "I think my baby is dead." The woman was calling from the Holiday Inn across the street from the hospital. I asked for her room number and told her that I was going to hang up to call 911. After making the 911 call, I immediately went to the hotel and room 218. I can still remember the room number today.

When I saw the baby, I knew that he had indeed died. He was 11 months old and suffered from multiple congenital anomalies. Instead of having the mother face the sight of her child being carried away on a stretcher I asked the paramedics to let me carry the baby to the hospital. I wrapped him up, and with

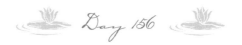

the paramedics, walked over to the hospital. I took the child to the morgue and for me the story had ended there. For his mother of course, it would never end.

Now on the other end of the phone was baby Tim's mom. She asked me if I really remembered. I told her that of course I did and recalled to her that they had a tiny Christmas tree on a table in the hotel room. I discovered that she had one question she had been wanting to ask for 18 years. She asked me where I had taken Tim once we got back to the hospital. Not wanting to give her the visual of carrying her child to the morgue, I told her that I had taken him to the Emergency Room so that they could examine him. She told me that she had thought about me every day for 18 years. She explained that she could remember me wrapping Tim up and going out the door but after that her memory becomes very vague. She said she needed to talk to me to find out where I had taken Tim. I think that little detail of the night was keeping her from finding any closure over the death of her son.

After many "thank you's" our conversation came to an end. Before hanging up the woman asked me if I was still working as a nurse. I told her that I was. And she said, "How blessed everyone is." Just before Christmas I received a note from the woman. It read:

> I hope you have a very Merry Christmas. One of my greatest Christmas joys this year is to be able to send you this card. I have thought about you every day for 18 years. Thank you again and again. Enclosed is our favorite picture of Tim.

I talked about our conversation to everyone at work for a week. It blew me away that I had had such an impact on one person, and it made me think about

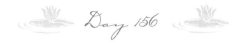

all of the other people I had helped over the years. It was so reassuring for me to discover the value and worth that nurses can have with patients. I was so proud to be doing what I do.

Since the Christmas time note, I haven't heard from Tim's mom. I hope she was finally able to get the closure she needed. I will never forget that phone call though. It was by far one of the most moving moments in my nursing career.

—Submitted by Pat Dwyer, St. Mary's Hospital

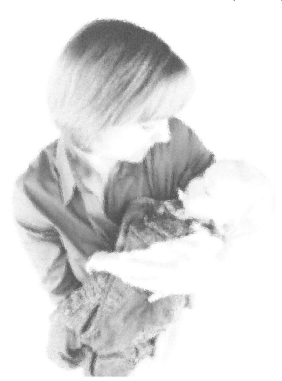

"Never underestimate the difference you can make."

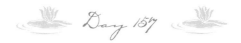
A Mother's Gift

Connie was a 42-year-old dialysis patient who had been in our long-term acute care hospital twice for several months each time. She had had one leg amputated due to diabetic neuropathy and was with us because the stump continually needed revisions due to repeat infections. This time, the outlook was grim. Connie was a single mom of very modest means who had two children for whom the staff provided a very generous Christmas. The staff also celebrated her son's birthday last month with a party at the hospital.

Last night, Connie's dialysis shunt clotted. After two attempts to fix the situation the nephrologists gave Connie the news that she would be unable to receive dialysis anymore and that she would not live much longer. With that news, Connie began to work diligently on embroidering two pillowcases so that each of her young children (ages 9 and 11) would have something to remember her by. It was heart wrenching to pass her room and see her busy with such intensity and purpose. She was literally fighting against the clock. Her only request was that she be allowed to travel from our facility in Indiana to her brother's home in Tennessee. She wanted to go to her brother's home to die since, if they were there, her brother could raise her children.

Once our President gave permission for our small hospital to charter a plane to move Connie, a very finely tuned plan developed within minutes. The case manager mobilized everyone, found a hospice that would take Connie (no small

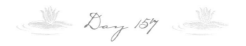
feat on Good Friday), and within a very short time we had a plane ready to take her the next morning. Our chaplain obtained a video camera so that she could make a film for her children to keep since they would be following in a car driven by a friend. Her friends were called, and they came to say goodbye. Our pharmacist worked with the physicians and friends at outpatient pharmacies to obtain the needed pain medication to keep Connie comfortable until the pharmacy in the little town to which she was traveling reopened the following Monday.

On Saturday morning, Connie left for Tennessee. She had her pillowcases and her video with her. Little did we know that shortly after she arrived in Tennessee, Connie's mother had a massive heart attack and mother and daughter both shared the same funeral. We were able to take comfort in the fact that we did the best we could to make Connie's final days comfortable and peaceful.

—Submitted by Jane G. Mason, Our Lady of Peace Hospital, South Bend, IN

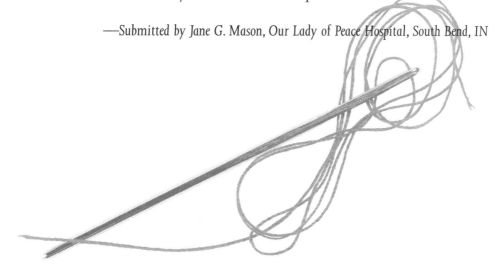

"Never underestimate the difference you can make."

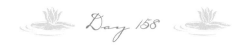

Going the Extra Mile

At Columbus Regional Hospital, our employees often go beyond expectations to show compassion and concern for others. On a recent, hot summer day, a mother and her young child came to the Breast Health Center looking for directions to a physician's office. One of our employees, J., called to find out the office location, which was across town.

The mother explained that they had walked from their home to get this far and there was no way they could make it any further. Because J. knew how important it was for the child to get to his doctor's appointment, she offered to take them there since she was getting ready to leave work for the day.

Before leaving the physician's office, J. told the staff that the mother and child had no transportation and would need assistance to get back home due to the hot weather and the child's age. She gave the staff her home telephone number and instructed them to call her when the mother and child were ready to leave. An hour later, J. returned to the physician's office and gave the mother and child a ride home.

J.'s actions demonstrate how our staff members provide an extraordinary level of caring and compassion for those we serve. We salute the exceptional example they set for all of us.

—Submitted by Columbus Regional Hospital

"Never underestimate the difference you can make."

A Last Goodbye

One cold November morning, my father woke up feeling very weak and unwell. We weren't sure what was wrong with him so we immediately called 911 and he was rushed to the hospital, which was about a mile away. The next several moments were a frenzied blur, as my father was rushed through a series of procedures, questions, and tests.

As it turned out, my father had had an abdominal aortic aneurysm, and being a nurse myself, I knew this was a life-threatening condition. The doctor working that evening was Mary Valvano. Just before Dr. Valvano took my dad up to the OR, she ran over and grabbed my mother and me to take us over to my dad.

It all happened so quickly. Thinking back, it is almost as if Dr. Valvano knew this could be the last time we got to see my dad awake. She rushed us to the elevator. My father's stretcher was already halfway in. There, she gave us just a few moments with him before he was rushed into surgery. We were able to kiss Dad goodbye and tell him how much we loved him. It was the last time we saw him alive. He passed away nine days after his surgery, from which he never awoke.

As I look back, the last day my father was awake remains a haze. The only part I remember well was being able to look at him one last time, kiss him, and tell him that I loved him. That moment is one of my most cherished memories, and I am so grateful that Dr. Valvano had the insight to give us this beautiful gift. She showed us with this one act, how valuable the human side of health care can be.

—Submitted by Mary Beth Miller, Southern NH Medical Center

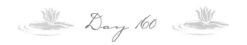

THE PERFECT DATE NIGHT

*B*ack in July, Trauma Services did something really cool for one of our patients. A trauma patient came in with a bad head injury and multiple other injuries. We found out that she was on leave from the Army and was in town with her two kids to visit her mother. They were in a bad accident and she was brought to Deaconess. Her husband was deployed in Iraq at the time. The Army sent a Red Cross message to her husband so that he could join her at the hospital.

Close to her discharge, Trauma Services wanted to try to have a "special night" for her and her husband, because we knew that after her discharge, he would be sent back to Iraq. We created a special table for them with a centerpiece and everything, and brought them food from Biaggi's. This was the patient's first solid food dinner, and she loved it (especially the Tiramisu). To top the night off, we brought them in some movies to watch, one of which was her favorite, *Shrek*. They enjoyed the night immensely. She was so appreciative of all the care that she received here. I was so honored that I got to be a part of it.

—Submitted by *Arvie Webster, Deaconess Hospital, Evansville, IN*

"Never underestimate the difference you can make."

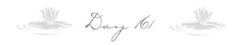

Inspired by Great Care

I was in a terrible accident in October 1991. One night while riding my bike, a drunk driver lost control of his vehicle and hit me. I was thrown backwards and landed on my back. The ambulance arrived and I was taken to Homestead Hospital. Once in the ER, I learned that both of my legs had been broken and that I had a hairline fracture on my right arm. Naturally I was in a lot of pain, I am so grateful to Andrew, my nurse in the ER, who was so incredibly comforting to me during this terrible time. He kept me informed about everything that was going on, telling me that I was going to be fine and not to worry, apologizing for not giving me any medicine for the pain, and explaining that until they knew everything that was wrong with me, they couldn't give me any medication. Through his words, I knew that I was receiving the best possible care.

After my night in the ER, I was admitted to the hospital. Because one of my legs was in traction and the other was set in a cast, I had very little mobility and needed help with everyday activities. Normally a very independent person, it was very hard for me not being able to do things on my own, particularly when it came to something as simple as taking a bath. Thankfully, the staff members at Homestead were so kind and attentive to me. They helped me do everything I could not do for myself. The first time one technician gave me a bath, I began to cry because I was so distraught about not being able to bathe myself. To comfort

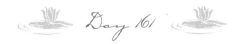

me, she found the perfect words. She told me that God puts people in our lives to help us so we don't ever have to be alone. She said I could ask her for anything I needed or wanted, and she lifted my spirits by telling me that I would heal in no time.

In all, I spent two months at Homestead Hospital. The staff there helped me survive through one of the most difficult times of my life. I was in a strange situation, because my family had just recently moved to Miami and hadn't set up their phone line, so I had no way to contact them. Thankfully, my nurses and doctors took care of me as if they were my family.

When I was completely healed, I made it my goal to work at Homestead Hospital. I knew that any place with a mission to help people in their darkest moments would be a place I could be happy. Unfortunately, at that time there were no positions available. After a great experience working at Baptist Health in Kendall, a position at Homestead Hospital finally opened up several years later. I applied for the job and after being interviewed by my supervisors and peers, I got it!

Now I am a supervisor in our dietary unit, and I oversee our cafeteria staff. Every day, I do my best to make our patients as comfortable and content as the staff made me when I arrived as a patient. I try to brighten their days even if it means just doing something as simple as getting their favorite type of yogurt— as I recently did for one of our patients. It is a great pleasure for me being able to give them the kind of excellent care that I received when I was a patient at Homestead. I work hard everyday to show my fellow coworkers that the compassion they showed me has always stayed with me.

—Submitted by Geraldine Gamboa, Homestead Hospital

"Never underestimate the difference you can make."

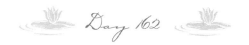

Life Changes

*A*fter 20 years of working as an oncology nurse, it became clear to me how much a person trying to beat cancer needs to regain a sense of normalcy in their lives. Their desire for normalcy prompted me to form Life Changes, a non-traditional cancer support group at Robert Wood Johnson University Hospital Hamilton.

At Life Changes, we as health care providers acknowledge the seriousness of patients' conditions and then move on, focusing on life rather than disease. We teach our patients that it is not the actual illness that influences us, but rather the way in which we interpret and react to the illness. By taking charge of thoughts and actions, we help patients in our group gain control of the way they respond to illness, thus preserving precious energy for living and recovery!

Patients who come to Life Changes often express how they have benefited from the meetings. One young man who started attending after he was diagnosed with cancer came to the meetings with his wife, and for the most part, was a listener more than a talker. At his first meeting, he said he wanted to be a part of Life Changes because he saw that the meetings promoted a sense of normalcy for patients. At the last meeting, he shared that he had recently had a PET scan, and the scan showed that his tumors were shrinking. He attributed his progress to the lessons he had learned as a member of the group about leading a normal, happy, productive life.

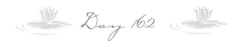

Another group member recently expressed that she very much preferred the way Life Changes operated versus other cancer support groups. She said she didn't like talking about cancer all of the time in the other kinds of groups—something we try to avoid at Life Changes.

Our meetings are not just for current cancer patients. Many former patients continue to come to the meetings after they are cured because their lives are still

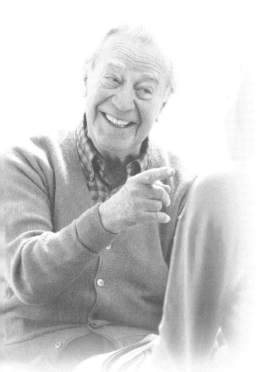

different. After a cure, they must learn to deal with the feelings they have about finishing treatment. Often family and friends of cancer patients also come to the meetings to offer and receive support.

The main goal at Life Changes is to provide our members with a place for healing by experiencing the fullness of life through programs, activities, and companionship. Our goal is to provide patients with a sense of hope in one of the darkest times of their lives. We teach them to just "let go" because that is the only thing that can bring peace.

—Submitted by Jane Finn-Hollenback,
RWJ Hamilton Center for Health & Wellness

"Never underestimate the difference you can make."

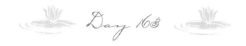

Cultures and Crutches

I work with an extremely diverse group of people as the educational instructor for the Diversity and Language Department at Charlotte AHEC through the Carolina Healthcare System. I train health care professionals in cultural diversity and languages. It is very rewarding to be able to help these people deal with and learn about other cultures so that they can give the absolute best health care possible.

One particular experience was very rewarding for me because I was able to directly help change a foreign doctor's life. I was coordinating the visits of a Ukrainian medical delegation. They were visiting our facilities in Charlotte to see how we did things there. We were touring the facilities with a local delegation of doctors and the two groups were working together to provide one another with a clear view of how hospitals in the United States differ from those in the Ukraine.

Because the Ukrainian doctors specialized in physical rehabilitation, we wanted that to be the main focus of their visit. The Ukrainian doctors were very interested in seeing the tools and procedures we were using for our patients. During the visit, I noticed that one doctor was looking very intensely at the wall.

I asked the doctor what had caught her attention and she said it was a pair of crutches hanging on the wall. She explained that what she found so unusual about the crutches was that they were adjustable. At her facility, there were no

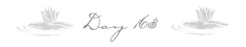

adjustable crutches. her patients were forced to use standard crutches making their physical rehabilitation more difficult than it needed to be.

The prospect of adjustable crutches was even more special for this doctor because her daughter had a medical condition that required her to use crutches every day. From our brief conversation, I learned what an important tool these crutches could be for her daughter and her patients. I felt compelled to help in some way so I set the wheels in motion to make this a very special visit for this doctor.

I told her story to one of the assistants to the vice president of the local delegation. After the story I asked him, "Do you know what I'm thinking?" He was equally moved by this doctor's story and certainly knew what I was thinking. He left to go make arrangements to give this doctor the adjustable crutches she so desperately wanted for her daughter. Not long after he departed, the assistant to the VP returned and nodded to me that our plan had worked. We had received the approval we needed to give this doctor her crutches.

So when both delegations had sat down to eat lunch, I called the doctor up to the podium and asked her to tell her story. She was taken aback at first, but she did share her story and the doctors from the Charlotte facility couldn't believe what they were hearing! In the United States, we take something as simple as adjustable crutches for granted. It was great for them to hear that other medical cultures are still struggling with the simple things while in our culture, we work to master the latest in medical technology.

When she finished her story, I nodded to my colleague who had helped arrange getting her the crutches, and he walked up to the podium and presented her with the set of crutches. When he placed them in her hands, I could see that they meant more to her than I had initially guessed. There were tears not only in

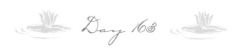

her eyes but also in the eyes of many of the other health care workers in the room. She was so appreciative and happy. She didn't let the crutches leave her sight for the rest of the trip. I think it was the best gift we could have given her to take back to her home.

While this is a simple story, it shows the importance of going the extra mile in health care, whether you are helping patients or doctors themselves. Not only did it make this doctor feel special, but it helped lift the spirits of every doctor in the room. I hope they carried that feeling back with them as they were treating their patients. I still carry it with me as I help other health care professionals understand the importance of learning the ins and outs of other cultures.

—Submitted by Jorge Rudko, Carolinas Healthcare System, Charlotte, NC

"Never underestimate the difference you can make."

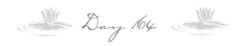
Mary's Roses

During her stay in the department, the Gateway Emergency staff cared for an 89-year-old elderly woman named Mary. While she was with us, we developed a very special relationship with Mary. The staff and her doctor, Dr. Ted Troyer, decided to send her some lovely red roses the day after her admission.

At 5:30 a.m., Dr. Troyer went to check on her and give her the flowers. When he saw how well she was sleeping, he couldn't find it in his heart to wake her up,

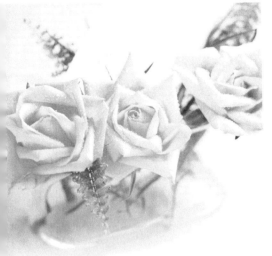

so he left the flowers on her bedside table with a short note so she would see them when she woke up. Dr. Troyer asked me to check in on her later in the morning and let her know he was sorry he missed speaking with her. When I went to check on her, she was so pleased with the flowers and was taken aback by the kindness shown to her by the emergency room staff. This small act really made Mary's day, and I was so proud to see such an act of kindness. It's the spirit of compassion and generosity that truly makes Deaconess an exceptional health care facility.

—Submitted by Diana McDaniel, Deaconess Hospital, Evansville, IN

"Never underestimate the difference you can make."

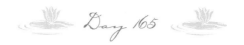

Going Far to Save a Life

My husband Lance had just gone through two major surgeries at Baptist Health Medical Center in North Little Rock, where I am the vice president for patient care. Following his second surgery, Lance was not doing well. He was hooked up to several machines. In fact, I have never seen so many machines used on one person before. Because of the trauma his body had been through, he went into Acute Respiratory Distress Syndrome, a serious condition that can lead to organ failure and even death. He wasn't breathing and wasn't responding to being bagged. I knew if someone didn't act quickly, my husband would not make it.

Thankfully, the hospital had a Jet Vent, which is a machine that could help Lance breathe. We were lucky, because there are actually very few Jet Vents in the state. Still, we weren't out of the woods yet. The Jet Vent had been discontinued by the manufacturer, so we were missing a necessary component we needed to keep the ventilator running. James Lisenbey, the supervisor of the Respiratory Care Unit just happened to know a sales representative who had once worked for the Jet Vent company. He quickly called the rep who just happened to have a box of the very part we needed in his garage!

If James hadn't made such an effort to find the discontinued part, I am sure that Lance would not be here with me today. It just shows you how far people in health care will go to save a life.

—Submitted by *Cara Wade, Baptist Health, Little Rock, AR*

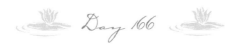

More Than a Coincidence

One rainy afternoon, Julie Phillips was driving to work the evening shift at her job. As a registered nurse, she normally worked in the intensive care unit, but on this particular night, Julie had agreed to work in MICU for the first time. During her hour-long drive, the weather was so bad that people were pulling off the road. As Julie crossed a bridge, she saw that a car accident had just occurred. A man had hydroplaned and rolled down a steep embankment into a flooding creek. She stopped her car and ran down the hill where a group of men were trying to pull the driver from his water-filled truck. Julie could see that the passenger, an older gentleman, was turning purple and she discovered that he didn't have a pulse. Another person at the scene helped her give the unconscious man CPR, and together, they were able to revive the man.

That night Julie worked with a nurse she had never met. Her name was Roelie Ryerson. Shortly after the shift began, Ryerson's sister-in-law called and told Ryerson that her father had been in an accident. When Julie heard what was going on with Roelie's father, she couldn't believe what she was hearing. Julie said, "Oh my gosh, I did CPR on your dad!"

"The likelihood that these two women were on the same shift in the same hospital unit this one night has to be more than a coincidence," says Debbie Bell, MICU supervisor.

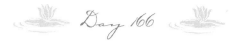

The first time Bill Ryerson, Roelie's father saw Julie after the accident he said to her, "There's my guardian angel." Julie says that things like this really do make you believe in miracles!

—Submitted by Cara Wade, Baptist Health, Little Rock, AR

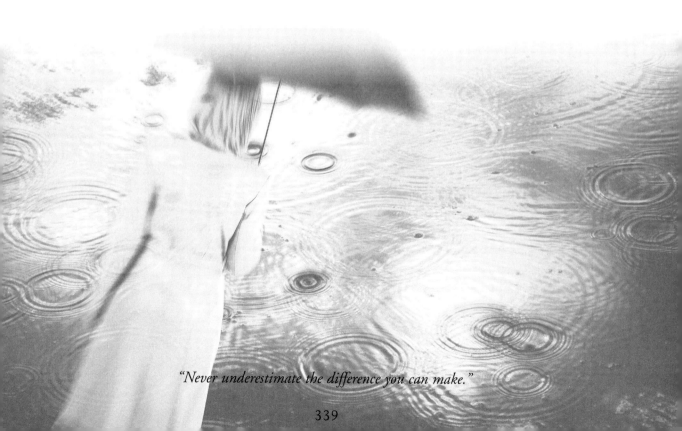

"Never underestimate the difference you can make."

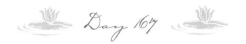

Genuine Compassion

*A*t Columbus Regional Hospital, our employees often go beyond expectations to show compassion and concern for others. Jodi Owen, an Operating Room Technician was on her way to the cafeteria for her break when she noticed an elderly man with a cane in the lobby. Jodi could tell the gentleman couldn't see very well, so she asked if she could help him. He told Jodi that he had just completed a test that required fasting and he was trying to find his way to the cafeteria.

She offered the gentleman her arm and accompanied him to the cafeteria. She gathered his food order and assisted him to a table where she helped him remove his jacket and put it on his chair, all the while encouraging him. Then she cut up his food, salt and peppered it, added sugar to his coffee, and explained where each item of food was located on the tray. The gentleman told Jodi he was 95 years old and apologized for being such a burden. Jodi reassured him that it was no trouble and she hoped that she would be fortunate enough to live that long. Many employees and visitors witnessed Jodi's act of kindness that day and were touched by her genuine compassion.

Jodi's actions demonstrate how our staff members provide an extraordinary level of caring and compassion for those we serve. We salute the exceptional example they set for all of us.

—*Anonymous Contributor, Columbus Regional Hospital*

"Never underestimate the difference you can make."

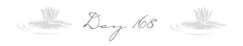

Hero Wall

During one of his appointments, a patient receiving radiation therapy treatments at the Cancer Center asked a therapist if he could possibly obtain a gown to take home with him.

The therapist was quick to reply with a "yes," but then asked the patient why he wanted a gown.

The patient replied that he would like to ask the staff who had administered his treatments to sign his gown. He explained that he and his son have a room in their home where they display jerseys of their favorite sports idols and Nascar drivers. He said some of them are signed and now he would like to hang this gown in tribute to his heroes at SOMC Cancer Center.

"There is no better idol or hero to me than the ones who have saved my life," he said.

On his last day of treatment, the patient was given a gown signed by all those who contributed to his care. We all feel honored to be hanging on his wall!

—*Written by Wendi Waugh, Submitted by Mary Kate Dilts-Skaggs,*
Southern Ohio Medical Center, Portsmouth, OH

"Never underestimate the difference you can make."

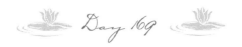
A Special Anniversary

*I*n 2005 in the Oncology Unit, a married couple in their late 40s came in. The husband, Mr. L, was diagnosed with a terminal cancer of the omentum. We found out that Mr. and Mrs. L were high school sweethearts and were coming up on their 20th anniversary. We hoped that Mr. L would be discharged in time for the special day, but unfortunately, due to Mr. L's rapidly decreasing health, he was not discharged.

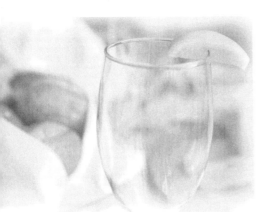

The nurse manager and several of the RNs from the Unit, decided that the Ls deserved a special anniversary dinner. They arranged for a little table with two chairs to be delivered to Mr. L's room. Special linen napkins and place settings were brought in, the nurse manager cooked up a special homemade meal and delivered it in a beautiful basket, and we supplied wine glasses with apple cider and candle light as well as a CD with Mr. L's favorite music.

The Ls had a lovely anniversary dinner and could not thank the staff enough for their kindness. Mr. L was discharged several days later and passed away within two months. After his death, Mrs. L called the nurses station to tell his former nurses about the funeral arrangements and, at the funeral, acknowledged the staff of 5C for their caring and kindness during a difficult yet special time for them as a couple.

—Submitted by Fortuna Borrego, Memorial Healthcare System

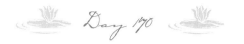
Thank You Notes for Christmas

I was taught from an early age to send thank you notes after receiving gifts. What I did not understand, until reading *Hardwiring Excellence*, was just how powerful thank you notes can be. I have a wonderful team of nurses who deserve a world of thanks. Last year two of my nurses had had a particularly difficult year and had worked very hard to make up for our staffing shortages. At Christmas, I decided I had to do something important for them. I didn't know it at the time, but what I was about to do would impact them for several months.

I found their parents' addresses and sent a Christmas card with an enclosed thank you note, thanking them for the wonderful nurses they had raised. One of the moms read the note at Christmas dinner. When the nurse approached me the following week, we both cried. She said I had impacted her mother more than I would ever know. What she didn't realize was how I had also impacted her. She had been having a rough time with all the extra hours and the increased activity of the floor, but after the thank you note, she was so re-energized that she spread her energy throughout the unit.

The second nurse was having a particularly difficult time during the holidays. Her father's health was failing, and the family was coping with his illness. Her card was also read at Christmas dinner, and again, the impact was very powerful. She called me at home to thank me and tell me what I had done for her family holiday. She, too, was re-energized at work. After doing this, I realized the true power of saying, "Thank you!"

—Submitted by Sally Remington, Canton-Potsdam Hospital, Potsdam, NY

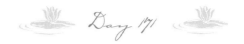
A Powerful Presentation

In the summer of 2005, I was asked to speak to a group of businessmen, civic leaders, and elected officials who were participating in a six-month "Leadership Broward" program. More specifically, these individuals were at Memorial Regional Hospital as part of their "health care day" session, which is designed to expose these influential community leaders to excellence in the health care industry.

I was very proud to have an opportunity to tell the Memorial Regional Hospital story to this group of about 200 of the "who's who" in Broward County. I had prepared a Microsoft PowerPoint presentation in advance, which included information about the many clinical programs of excellence offered at Memorial Regional Hospital. I had prepared slides on financial performance; volume growth and market share; operational efficiency; clinical outcomes; employee, physician and patient satisfaction; staff turnover and vacancy rates; and Memorial's organizational commitment to quality and safety. I shared some of the plans for expansion of the Memorial Regional Hospital campus and in particular, focused on new freestanding facilities for the Comprehensive Cancer Center and the Joe DiMaggio Children's Hospital Pavilion.

I presented information about the many community outreach programs available to those we serve, including our Primary Care Program which sees over 100,000 adults and children annually at three different locations. I spent a good

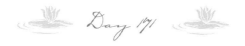

deal of time making sure that the group understood that the reputation for health care excellence enjoyed by Memorial Regional Hospital was not based solely in the bricks and mortar of buildings, the state-of-the-art technology available to patients, or even the wide range of clinical services offered. I told them that Memorial's reputation for health care excellence was earned through the dedication and commitment of our staff to the safety and welfare of our patients, as well as our culture of respect and dignity for staff, patients, and visitors alike.

The prior day, I had received a letter from the family of a patient in our facility who had been hospitalized for more than 45 days. During this time, the patient was in and out of the ICU and had undergone multiple surgeries. The family had been prepared for what seemed like the inevitable. In their letter, the Ashley family wrote about ordinary members of our staff, who never acted as if their "David" was a lost cause. People who had "raised their spirits with hope through their compassion, patience, and concern…offering anything to the family in the way of comfort as they had been camping out for weeks in the waiting room."

They talked about specific people who they described as "Angels of Mercy," and even recognized Dottie from Environmental Services who "always came by with a smile and a cheerful word." The Ashley family wanted me to know how grateful they were for the wonderful difference Memorial's health care team made in their lives and in the life of their loved one, David.

David went home and has fully recovered. I decided that I would read this letter to this group of leaders, hoping that they would understand the powerful difference that engaged people make in great organizations. Much to my surprise, the room broke out in thunderous applause when I finished reading the letter. I felt that they understood the power of people.

This might have been the end of the story, except for the elderly gentleman at the back of the room who quietly asked me if I could speak to him as I was leaving. We went into a corner in the back of the large auditorium where he

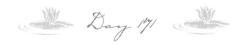

proceeded to tell me that he had listened with great interest as I read the letter from the Ashley family. He went on to tell me that he and his wife had been coming to Memorial Regional Hospital every week for the last two years, and he really knew what went on in my facility. I prepared for the worst!

He then said in a very quiet voice, "My wife was diagnosed with ovarian cancer two years ago by one of your oncologists. For the last two years, she and I have been in here every week for one test or another." He went on to say, "It seems there were always blood transfusions, chemotherapy visits, radiation oncology treatments, doctor's appointments, unplanned admissions, blood tests, if it wasn't one thing, it was another." "Throughout the past two years," he continued, "we were here every week." He then said, "As I heard you read this letter from the Ashley family, I sat here feeling ashamed and embarrassed because I never took the time to write a letter of thanks to your staff."

He went on, "Never once, throughout those two years, did we encounter anyone in your facility who made us feel that caring for us was anything less than the most important thing that they had to do at that moment. They made a difference for me and for my wife, through the most difficult time in our lives." The gentleman then said, "My wife lost her battle with cancer last winter. I am sorry that I never took the time to write a letter to thank your staff for making a difference."

I promised him that I would share his story with our staff. Every two weeks during new employee orientation, I have the opportunity to welcome new employees to the Memorial Regional Hospital health care team. I always tell them this story. I try to impress upon them that at Memorial, even a housekeeper can make a difference in the lives of those we have the privilege of serving.

—Submitted by J.E. Piriz, Memorial Regional Hospital

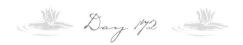

A Moment to Cherish

After our father suffered a hemorrhagic stroke, the physician told us he would not survive. In fact, he had already slipped into a coma. While sitting in the lounge, my youngest brother said he wished he could have had his son christened before Dad became sick. My nephew wondered out loud whether the baby could be christened in Dad's hospital room. I talked to his nurse, Tara Ford, and she said it wouldn't be a problem. We called our minister and arranged all of the details.

After the christening, we realized Dad was holding a package in his hand. Tara had gone down to the gift shop and purchased a present for our father to give to his grandson at his christening.

What a special nurse Tara is. She was so thoughtful and caring. We will always remember her.

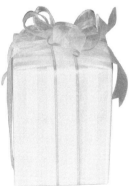

—Submitted by Shannon Johnson,
Deaconess Hospital, Evansville, IN

"Never underestimate the difference you can make."

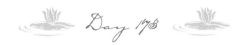

A Golden Anniversary

As quality and risk manager at my hospital, I frequently get calls about customer service issues. I am always pleased when a call comes from a patient or family member for whom we have "made a difference!" A social worker, whom I admire a great deal, called me one morning and said we had admitted a patient that was terminally ill and who wasn't expected to live through his hospitalization. She told me he and his wife would be having their 50th wedding anniversary the day following his admission, and she asked if there was anything we could do to make this anniversary "special."

We decided a very nice meal might be good. I contacted the dietary department and they quickly got to work. The social worker contacted the daughter to ask if she could come to the hospital for their special event!

The next day, at about 11:30 a.m., our dietary department rolled into the patient's room with a linen covered table, fresh flowers, and a special anniversary meal for the couple. The daughter was able to be there as was a large group of staff and the social worker who helped make everything happen.

Many tears were shed on that day since this patient would likely not live to see another wedding anniversary! The daughter called me later and told me how much this meant to her and her parents. While only a small gesture on our part, this would surely be treasured by this family! Just one more day did make a difference! I am privileged to work with these very caring employees!

—Submitted by Karen Harris, Columbia Regional Hospital

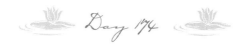

Dedication to Patient Care

uthie had been an ICU nurse for 30 years, but recently she received certification in gastroenterology. Now she works with me in the Gastrointestinal (GI) Unit.

In our department, we often see GI bleeders, and one day the Emergency Room received a man, accompanied by his wife and daughter, who was a GI bleeder. On this particular day, the hospital was completely full and there were no beds open in our unit. It looked as though the only option would be to send the man back down the ER, which wouldn't have been the best case scenario for his medical care.

But then, Ruthie stepped up.

Ruthie came to me, explained the situation, and because of her background in ICU nursing, said she could take care of the man until a bed opened up.

It created a lot of extra work for Ruthie. In fact, I even pitched in to help. But Ruthie understood that this patient and his family were coming from the ER, which is always a hectic place, and she recognized that they probably needed a little extra compassion at this stage of his care.

Ruthie ended up spending the whole day with the family, from 7:30 a.m. until the patient was moved at 6:30 p.m.

About two weeks later, the patient's wife mailed a note to Ruthie at her home address, thanking her for taking the time to take such good care of her husband.

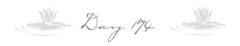

She said she could see how much Ruthie cared for each and every one of her patients and how much she loved her job. It meant so much to Ruthie to receive such a special note from her patient.

—Submitted by Tillie Balliet, Roper St. Francis Healthcare

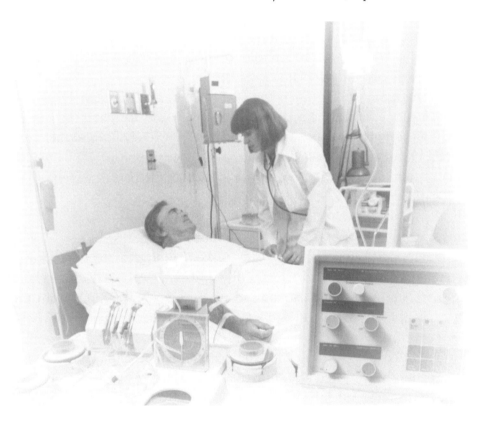

"Never underestimate the difference you can make."

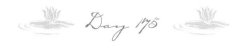

WAITING FOR BABY

Mr. L, who had been a patient in our hospital, stopped by Patient Relations to relay his appreciation for the treatment and care he received under trying circumstances.

Mr. L's daughter was pregnant with his first grandson. During the pregnancy, one of the ultrasounds showed that the baby had what appeared to be a hole in the top of his head with fluid build up. Mr. L said that during the last part of her pregnancy, his daughter had come to the hospital twice a week to have ultrasounds performed to monitor the baby. He said the ultrasound technicians "were awesome" to his daughter.

It had been pre-arranged for his daughter to deliver her baby at Children's Hospital in Columbus so that the baby could receive specialized care. Mr. L explained that on the day they were to take his daughter to Columbus to have her baby, he became ill with a large kidney stone. He came to our hospital's Emergency Department for treatment.

While in the ED, Mr. L said staff quickly got his pain under control and he wanted to be on his way for the birth of his grandson. However, Dr. Schmidt had to admit him for surgery. After the surgery, Mr. L remained in the hospital for the night, due to a history of heart problems.

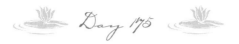

Since Mr. L had not come to the ED prepared to be admitted as a patient, he had not packed anything for an overnight stay. He relayed that his nurse, Dave Knox, was very understanding and went out of his way to assist.

Anxious to be on his way to see his daughter and his new grandson, Mr. L was released from the hospital and headed to Columbus. When he arrived in Columbus, Mr. L discovered his grandson had not yet been born. His grandson soon arrived, with no physical problems, which made for an even more joyous occasion.

Mr. L wanted to make sure that the various caregivers who had helped his family were thanked. He wanted to express his appreciation to everyone in the hospital, from the ultrasound techs who took care of his daughter, to the ED staff, Dr. Schmidt, and his nurse, Dave Knox. Mr. L said the hospital was an asset to the community.

—Submitted by Lori Adams, Southern Ohio Medical Center, Portsmouth, OH

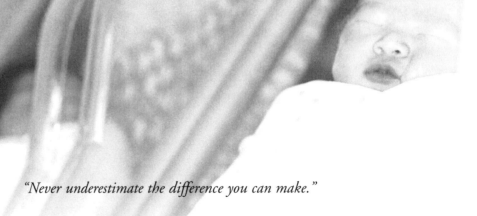

"Never underestimate the difference you can make."

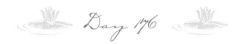

Angels Unaware

Seventeen years ago, my mother became very ill with systemic lupus. She was hospitalized at St. Mary Medical Center Long Beach, for a total of 11 months before she passed away. That year was one of the most difficult and gut-wrenching times of my life. What I noticed most during that time was that because I worked at the hospital, some of the very people I worked with on a regular basis suddenly kept their professional distance. My guess was that they were nervous about another clinician being the "family member."

Mom would get so frustrated sometimes and just cry. She went into a major depression. Sometimes all she asked for was to be able to sit up at the edge of the bed and look out the window in ICU.

One afternoon, I walked in after my shift to see her. Her ICU nurse was a traveler. I so wish that I could remember her name. I can remember her being tall, very pretty, and blond with a sweet southern drawl. She was in the room talking softly to my mom and asking her what she needed. My mom started to cry and told her that she wanted to sit up and look out the window. I stood back watching and listening. I heard her nurse say, "Well then let's go." She helped Mom sit up and dangle her legs over the side of the bed, ventilator tubing and dialysis tubing went too. She had Mom looking out the window, then she herself sat down next to Mom on the bed. She put her arm around Mom's shoulders and let Mom rest her head on her. She rested her head softly on Mom's head too.

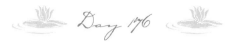

Wow, it is such a vivid memory for me. I can still see it so clearly to this day as I write down this story. My mom passed away not too long after that day. My thoughts go to that verse in the Bible about angels: "Be not forgetful to entertain strangers: for thereby some have entertained angels unaware." (Hebrews 13:2)

I think that an angel came that day to take care of my mom. The touch, the care, and the compassion made the difference that day for both the patient and her daughter. Thank you for allowing me to share my story.

—Submitted by Sharon Sauser, CHW-St. Mary Medical Center, Long Beach, CA

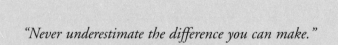

"Never underestimate the difference you can make."

TREATING THE WHOLE FAMILY

After being misdiagnosed by several doctors, my 15-year-old daughter was recently diagnosed with nasal pharangeal carcinoma. Her doctor told us that there was a mass in her nasal area that was starting to mold the skull bone that protected her brain. She was sent to Utah Cancer Specialists, where she not only received great care, but our entire family did as well.

Her radiation doctor, Dr. Aviazonis set her up with seven weeks of radiation Monday through Friday, and Dr. Whisenant set her up for six rounds of chemotherapy. She struggled through the treatments and had to be admitted to the hospital on a few occasions.

At the time of Amanda's diagnosis, I had recently had a baby and was planning on returning to work. But in order to give Amanda the best care, I needed to stay out of work so that I could take her to her treatments. Because they knew about our situation, the kind people at the cancer center had given us help with our bills.

And as if that weren't enough, when Christmas rolled around and I had been out of work for six months, they again asked us what they could do for the whole family. It was such a relief.

There are such wonderful people over there. Although we were happy with Amanda's progress, we cried and cried when we were done with treatment because we loved seeing them so much. They have very big hearts and helped make a very difficult situation for us a lot easier to manage.

—Submitted by Natalie Cervantes, University of Utah Hospital

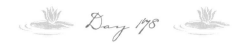

Nail Polish, Crayons, and Mountain Dew

It is a common occurrence to observe our staff giving kind and considerate care to our patients. But the staff of Unit 2100 gave such excellent care to one of our special needs patients that they deserve to be commended.

The patient was a Down syndrome adult with the mental capacity of a child. Unfortunately, she encountered many serious health issues that were difficult for her to understand and that often caused her great fear.

To ease her anxiety, the 2100 staff showered her with items such as crayons, books, a princess crown, nail polish, and her favorite treat of all, Mountain Dew.

With delight, I watched the staff incorporate, as part of her daily care, such activities as coloring, nail painting, positioning her crown, reading out loud to her, and pleasingly responding to her smile and giggles when she was enjoying her Mountain Dew. Even though her condition was serious, her personality positively affected all who came in contact with her.

I know the staff of 2100 will always cherish taking care of this patient, because it was an experience that had such a big impact on their lives.

—Submitted by Belle McCool, Deaconess Hospital, Evansville, IN

"Never underestimate the difference you can make."

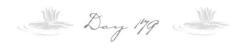

Letter of Praise

I am a director at Glendale Memorial Hospital & Health Center and I received a letter dated Oct. 16, 2006, from a patient regarding one of our lactation educators. It read:

Dear Mrs. R,

I have been wanting to write this letter to you for some time now, but with a newborn, it's been a little difficult to find the time. However, I did think it was very important to bring to your attention that I was so impressed with one of your employees, namely Roza, who was my breastfeeding instructor when I was pregnant and also helped me after my baby was born. She was an amazing teacher and had the whole class captivated with her passion and incredible knowledge. My husband and I learned so much! When my baby was born, she was so patient helping me learn my baby's cues. It is because of her my baby is so healthy and I enjoy breastfeeding him. Roza is a phenomenal educator. I am emotional writing this letter because I have come to understand that there are such gentle, caring, and committed professionals who change the lives of mothers. Roza is one of them. Thank you for a great experience at Glendale Memorial.

—Submitted by Glendale Memorial Hospital & Health Center

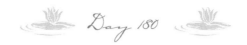

A Special Trip to Disneyland

A month during one winter in the mid-90s, we received several children paralyzed from various traumas. Once these children recovered from the initial injury, we were able to get them into specialized rehabilitation facilities that promote getting the child back into their home environment.

Of the four paralyzed children, three were able to go to a rehabilitation unit, but one child was so severely injured she didn't qualify for rehab. This young girl came to us when she was eight years old. She was paralyzed from her lower lip downward and could only communicate with us by blinking her eyes and clicking her tongue against the roof of her mouth. In addition to her many physical deficits, there were social issues that complicated her care and getting resources for her.

Her family members were frequently picked up and deported from the U.S., sometimes making it weeks, even months, that she had no visitors. Our Pediatric ICU (PICU), which was designed to provide life-saving care to injured or sick children, became a home for two years to this young patient.

She was a physical burden to the staff in her care requirements of lifting and constant suctioning, and she frequently had severe infections despite the best of care. Some of us even had terrible dreams about how it must feel to be trapped in a body with no way to move, breathe, or communicate. Several of us even

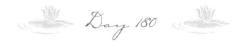
researched trying to take her into our homes to give her a different life, but to no avail.

Driving to work just prior to her second Christmas with us, I heard an advertisement that Target was opening their stores early one morning just for disabled persons to be able to shop easily. Fascinated with this story, I decided we should take this child shopping. Another nurse and I spent the better part of 12 hours getting legal and medical approval as well as making arrangements for transportation.

The event went so well, that the two of us decided that our next outing with her was to go to Disneyland. After weeks of fighting the nay-sayers, issues about volunteer versus work time, transportation arrangements, and those in administration who thought we had lost our minds, we were off.

This child required constant care, including suctioning every 15-30 minutes on good days and more often on bad days. That meant we needed to take a large quantity of equipment with us to Disneyland. I arrived at the park with an entire wagon full of equipment and Disney was gracious enough to give us a room for her care in their first aid area.

By 8 a.m., our patient arrived in tow with two other nurses, a respiratory therapist, her mother, and brother. We as staff even had to pay our own way, but we were committed to doing something positive for this child.

Within five minutes of being in the park, this young girl forgot about her ventilator, wheelchair, and limitations. She acted like any other child enthralled with all that Disneyland had to offer. I will never forget how wonderful the characters were with her. They would make all the visitors stand back while they focused their complete attention on our patient. They would stroke her face and sign her book and we got it all on tape.

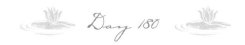

We didn't stop just there. After all, we needed to take her on rides. In order to take her on It's a Small World, we had to disconnect her ventilator, do a total body lift into the boat and hand bag her for the entire ride. The Disney staff was wonderful about letting us take her through several of the rides two or three times in a row. I will never forget the brightness of her eyes, the joy and fascination on her face, and the half smile that her muscles would allow her to make.

We watched shows and parades and, much to the chagrin of our director, decided to keep her at Disneyland until the park closed at 1 a.m. (The PICU had staff present in the unit from 8 p.m. expecting her to return.)

This young girl was so involved with the entire goings on that she refused to let us take her to the first aid station for basic care. Between 8 a.m. and 1 a.m., we only took her to the station three times for bowel, Foley care, and suctioning. She forgot she couldn't swallow and her need for suctioning was significantly decreased.

We also didn't want to destroy her enjoyment, so we figured out how to suction her on the go. Her enjoyment was palpable to all of us, but the day finally had to end and we got her safely back to the PICU.

For the rest of her life, this child watched the video of her day at Disneyland every shift and more often when someone would put it on. The staff grew to hate the music from the electric light parade, but when we saw her face and her enjoyment in reliving the day, we knew it was worth it.

When this child was almost 11, she died in our unit from overwhelming sepsis. The videotape was one of the last things she wanted to see, and she died with a peaceful expression.

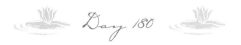
The four of us who took her to Disneyland worked many years before and after her death in the PICU. Despite the many good things we accomplished and the many lives we helped save, each one of us still feels as if for one time in our lives we were able to overcome all barriers and make a difference for a child. We all carry the thought of this young girl and her experiences as our patient and her day at Disneyland in our hearts. We have all identified that that day at Disneyland made us even better health care providers and patient advocates. This child, despite all her limitations, made a difference in our lives that we will never forget.

—Submitted by Anne Wicks, CHW-St. Mary Medical Center, Long Beach, CA

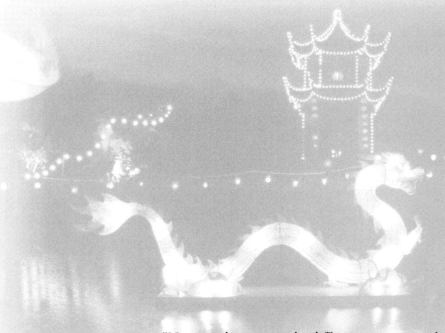

"Never underestimate the difference you can make."

Share Your Own Story

Please share an experience that connected you back to purpose, worthwhile work, and making a difference. You are a big part of what's right in health care!

BRING IT ON!!!

*N*ursing is an extremely demanding profession, and in my opinion, the most rewarding career choice anyone could make. We are tested on a daily basis, and just when we think we have no more left to give, something happens that reminds us why we chose this path in life, and offers us hope for the future, giving us the much needed strength to go on.

I had been working as a staff nurse for a busy Neurosurgery Unit at a large teaching hospital for three years, and I was beginning to feel the first pangs of nurse burn-out. It seemed like each day was worse than the one before. Our patient population's surgeries encompassed brain tumors, cerebral aneurysms, and back and neck problems. Patients were sicker and families were more stressed out. The best I could do was never enough, and I went home remembering things I had either forgotten to do, or simply ran out of time to complete. I felt more like a high paid waitress than a nurse.

One day, I felt particularly low. I had a full patient load, and although several of my patients were to be discharged that day, I knew that more would come in their place, and I would be knee deep in admissions. However, despite all my internal drama, I never allowed the patients or families to see it and had slipped into Nancy Nurse mode.

In the blink of an eye, my faith in nursing was restored, and the Nancy Nurse personality was retired. Tammy was a young woman of 24, who had experienced seizures since she was a child. Due to the severity of her condition and the amounts of anti-convulsant medications she had to take, surgery to remove the

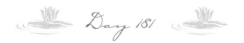

portion of her brain responsible for causing the seizures was performed. During her post-op period, Tammy had a mustard seed pin that she kept on her gown at all times. She would panic if she couldn't feel that pin and would often be observed reaching for it to make sure it was securely pinned to her gown. There was even a note on her chart to alert the staff not to remove her pin. It had become her security blanket.

That day, I was preparing to discharge her for home with her family, when I was called to her room. I walked in and found her sitting up in the bed, with her family standing around, smiling at me. Tammy's husband nodded at her and handed her an envelope, and she in turn handed the envelope to me, and told me she wanted me to have something. I opened the envelope and found a beautiful card thanking me for all the love and care I had given Tammy during her hospitalization, with her cherished mustard seed pin inside the card.

Through tears, Tammy explained that she had been so afraid of the surgery and had prayed to God to get her through it safely, and she held onto hope with that mustard seed pin and shared the story from the Bible of parable of the mustard seed.

By the time she finished talking, there wasn't a dry eye in the room. I placed the mustard seed pin on my name badge and wore it proudly. I learned that when things were unusually rough or stressful, I needed only to remember Tammy and look down at the pin on my badge (which I would often rub for good luck), and whatever dramas were being played out around me, suddenly didn't seem so overwhelming, and I knew I could handle whatever life threw at me.

Bring on the worried families and overwhelmed patients! I can do anything, and I will do it proudly. I am exactly where I am meant to be. I am a nurse.

—Submitted by Rebecca Campbell, Wake Forest University Baptist Medical Center, Winston-Salem, NC

Rosa's Story

*T*his story is a great example of how a health care community can come together to make a difference in the life of one young woman. Rosa is a 15-year-old Mexican immigrant who came to this country last year with her family. As a young girl, she had an eye injury that left her right eye deformed and opaque. She entered the school system here and was having a difficult time with the classes because of the language barrier and a different culture.

One day her mother brought her to us at Southwest Community Medical Center for a check-up. The reason for the check-up was that she had gotten beaten up by a group of girls at the school. It seems that this group of girls had been taunting her for some time, calling her "rotten eye" and other unsavory names, as only adolescents can do. Eventually a fight ensued and the girls beat Rosa up.

Her physical injuries were slight, only bumps and bruises, but between her language barrier and her unsightly eye, her self-esteem was very low. She didn't ever want to go back to school.

That night, I went home wondering what we could do for Rosa to make her life better. I knew there was no money for cosmetic surgery or a prosthesis. Eventually, it dawned on me that a cosmetic contact lens might do the trick. But how could they afford something like that?

The next day I was scheduled to volunteer at San Jose so I stopped by to talk to one of the doctors in the eye clinic. I told him Rosa's story and about the idea

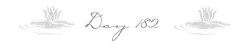

I had to help her. He agreed to see her, but also wanted to have her examined by the ophthalmologist to be sure that her eye could not be repaired.

He said the cosmetic contact lens would cost about $400. That was less than I expected, but more than Rosa's family could pay. I knew there had to be a way to accomplish this for Rosa. I talked to Soccoro Rouse, the nurse in charge of the eye clinic, and she gave Rosa an appointment to see both the optometrist and the ophthalmologist during the same visit.

When we told the family, they were elated. We stressed to them how important it was to be there on time for these appointments. The day of the appointment, Rosa's mother appeared at our clinic a half hour before the appointment time without her daughter. She was afraid to take her daughter out of school after the fighting incident and wasn't sure if she had a ride downtown.

We sent Rosa's mom to collect her daughter right away while I called the school and obtained permission for her to leave. Rosa and her mother took a cab downtown but because of the language barrier they ended up at St. Joseph's Hospital instead of San Jose Clinic.

After wandering around there for a while, an unknown employee took the time to find out what was wrong. When this person realized that they were in the wrong place, he took it upon himself to find a ride for Rosa and her mom so that they could get to San Jose as quickly as possible.

They arrived at San Jose about three hours late for their appointment, but when Socorro heard their story and their misadventures, she made sure that Rosa was examined that day and not rescheduled for another visit.

After several ophthalmologic examinations, it was determined that a cosmetic contact lens would be the best thing for her and that she also needed glasses. The doctor from the eye clinic just happened to know people on the board of the

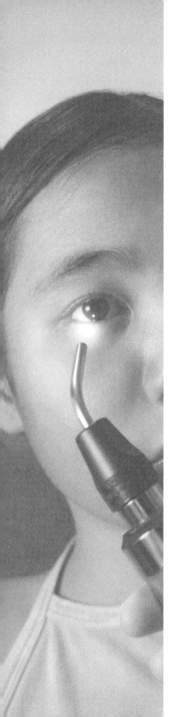

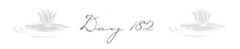

Lyons Club Eye Foundation. He consulted them, and they agreed to pay for Rosa's cosmetic contact lens and for her new glasses.

Rosa has come back to visit the clinic since she has gotten her "new look," and it has given her a new outlook on life. She is smiling now, she's more confident, her hair is styled differently (before she had it in her face to cover her eye), and she is doing much better in school. This is a great example of how people coming together can change the life of a child and make their quality of life so much better. Her smile is the only payment that we need for our efforts.

—Submitted by CHRISTUS Southwest Community Health Center, Houston, TX

"Never underestimate the difference you can make."

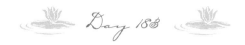

Making Connections

As director of the Living History Program at my hospital, one of my daily assignments is to find appropriate patients to interview for a life story. I look first for the very elderly, the chronically ill or sometimes people I like to call "our loyal apostles"—patients who always come to us for care, who love and support us and who always tell others about their experiences.

On this particular day, I found an elderly lady with a sharp mind and an even sharper wit. She was perfect for my storywriter, Mandy—one of the nurses working in a non-clinical role. Mandy is a great person, with a big heart and someone who needs a little variety in her role as a case manager. She enjoys her time interviewing patients and always comes away with a smile. She considers a Living History assignment a gift!

Mandy interviewed Lila and was able to gather some touching details of her life. She found a very sweet lady who had never married but considered family her most precious possession in life. Lila explained that her cousin, a gentleman about her age, was not only a prized family member, but her "best friend."

The next day, following the interview, Mandy stopped in to visit with Lila. As she was leaving the room, a gentleman came through the door. Lila beckoned Mandy back and did a quick introduction. She said, "Charley, this is the lady who wrote my life story."

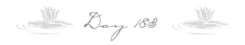

As the gentleman shook Mandy's hand, he noted her name tag and asked about her last name. He said, "I knew a Lynch once. Who is your husband?" Mandy replied with her husband's name. The gentleman said, "Well, I'll be darned…I think I knew your father-in-law," and proceeded to explain that he was the employer Mr. Lynch was working for at the time he was killed in a work-related accident.

He told Mandy about the day Mr. Lynch died and how he chose to go to the home and tell Mrs. Lynch. "It was the hardest thing I ever did." She had five small children. She asked if Charles would go down to the river and "fetch the kids home" so she could tell them the horrible news. As he walked back from the river, little John, age four, cut his foot on a pop bottle and had to be carried.

He sat Mandy down and told her all she wanted to know about the father-in-law she never met. She showed him pictures of her son and he proclaimed how proud grandpa would be. She asked him if she could tell her husband that she had met him.

Excitedly, she called John at work and explained who she had met and the stories she had heard. There was a pause on the other end of the line. Then John said, "I remember that man. I remember the feel of him." Little John had never forgotten the gentle man who carried him to his home on the day his father died.

John, Mandy, and their son were able to establish a relationship with this man who was so kind and gentle to a little boy so many years ago. They were able to spend time with him and hear stories they longed for. It enriched their lives and gave meaning to memories.

Many times, Mandy would thank me for the opportunity to "connect" with this family. It was always my hope when I created the Living History Program that lives would be changed. I wanted people to make real, emotional, compassionate

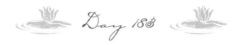

connections that would impact their lives in a positive way and give them a renewed reason to come to work, and love the work we are so privileged to do. That day, I knew I made a difference.

—Submitted by Sheila Brune, Memorial Hospital, Carthage, IL

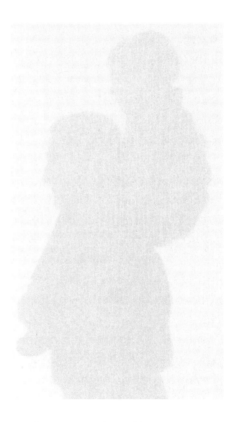

"Never underestimate the difference you can make."

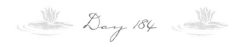

Bedside Marriage Blessing

uth and Gabriel had been dating for two years when they decided to set a date for their wedding. One of their biggest concerns was being sure that her mother would be able to attend. Diagnosed with cancer three years ago, Ruth's mother, Karen, had recovered and gone back to work. She seemed to be doing fine.

Shortly after they made their plans, however, Karen's mother's health began to decline and they learned that the cancer had spread to her lymph nodes. Ruth met with a hospice representative in Kentucky before coming to visit her mother. She also read the book *Final Gifts*, which had been suggested by one of her mother's friends. The book influenced her greatly and provided valuable insight.

"There's a way of listening to those who are dying and hearing what they're saying," she said. "I talked with my mother and I clearly knew what she wanted. She had everything set up as she wanted it. One of the most important things to her was knowing that certain people would look after me."

Her mother was admitted to Hospice of Frederick County. It soon became clear that she was not going to be alive at the time of the wedding. "We decided to have a marriage blessing to give her closure," Ruth said. "My aunt and uncle committed to being my godparents, which was very reassuring to her. She held on and waited until Gabe got here from Kentucky. She loved him. They were so much alike they were like two peas in a pod."

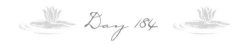

The hospice chaplain, Gary, conducted a sacred ceremony at her bedside at the Kline Hospice House. The service was planned with help from chaplain Gary and members of the hospice staff and included readings of scripture and poetry.

"It was a brief but beautiful ceremony of blessing," Gary recalled. "It was all about life. It was recognition, affirmation, and promise—recognition that we are bound by the limits of our physical beings, affirmation that there is no limit to love, and that relationships last forever, and promise that the life of a loved one will never be forgotten. "The ceremony marked a moment of holding on to her presence," he continues, "but also letting go and knowing she would be kept in the hearts of those who love her." The ritual, he adds, was consistent with the philosophy of hospice that every life is important and continues until the moment of death. In that room, joy and sadness existed in a very sacred way," he recalled. "Happiness and tears have a place in the soul—sometimes at the same time, with joy being an uplifting companion to grief."

Karen was surrounded by family, and her hand was cradled in her daughter's, as her brother and future son-in-law promised to love and watch over Ruth.

Being present was an honor and a privilege for Gary who says creative liturgy is something he embraces as having the potential to fulfill unusual needs.

"The role of a chaplain is to walk with the patient or client in their faith journey," he said, "rather than imposing any specific theology or religious belief on others."

Karen died the day after the ceremony, letting go of life while holding on to the sacred moment she witnessed with her daughter's marriage blessing.

—Submitted by Laurel Cucchi, Hospice of Frederick County,
Frederick Memorial Hospital, Frederick, MD

"Never underestimate the difference you can make."

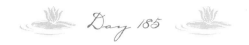

A Celebration to Remember

A critical patient was transferred to our ICU. She was only 43-years-old and needed major surgery, which she was refusing. She was alert, on a ventilator, and in the event of cardiac arrest, had agreed to a "Do Not Resuscitate Order." She was in guarded condition and survival without surgery was not expected.

The patient was told that her daughter from Louisiana was coming to see her and bringing her two grandchildren. The patient had never seen one child and had not seen the other in four years. She desperately wanted to make this visit special. She wrote a note asking her nurse to call her husband and asked him to bring cups and Kool-Aid for the children. When called, the husband refused to bring anything.

Later, when the patient's sister arrived, she asked her if she would get some items for the children. Her sister refused, stating that it was inappropriate. One of our RNs was distressed. She knew her patient was asking for a minimal request, and evidently the patient's family did not recognize how important it was for her. Our nurse was determined and told other staff if the patient wanted a party for her grandkids, then she would make it happen.

With her own money, she asked another staff member to go with her to the gift shop. She made "goodie bags" that contained coloring books, crayons, candy

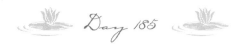
and a stuffed animal for each child. She also purchased two balloons, which the patient signed and gave to her grandchildren.

The visit, and her ability to give the children something, made a tremendous impact on the patient. The next day, the children were still talking about what they got from their grandma and the patient was continually smiling. This act of kindness and caring did so much for all of them. When the attending physician checked on the patient the next day, he asked her how her visit with her grandchildren had gone. Her face lit up like he had never seen before and she indicated it was wonderful. She said her grandchildren loved the presents our nurse bought for them.

—Anonymous Contributor, Conemaugh Memorial Medical Center, Johnstown, PA

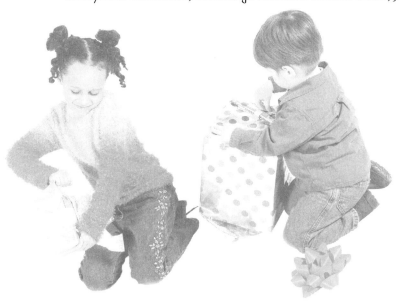

"Never underestimate the difference you can make."

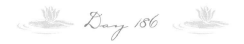

Compassion and Caring from a Hospital Family

This grateful letter was written to the administrator of the hospital where the writer worked:

As you are aware, my mother was recently a patient at North and was very ill. I received a call that she was in respiratory distress and would be taken to the ER. I immediately informed the nurse to take her to North. I truly believe in North and North is my extended family.

My only concern in writing is that I will leave someone out and I do not want that to happen. If I have done so, please charge it to my remembrance and not my heart.

I beat my mother to the ER. Jess was working and reassured me she would let me know when my mother arrived, although I would have to wait to visit. Patricia came out with paperwork and as I started to get up, she told me she would come to where I was. They both were so kind and compassionate.

Jane was her nurse. She listened to me and consoled me. She made me feel so good when she mentioned how my mom's blood pressure had gone down when she heard my voice. My mom doesn't talk or move too much anymore.

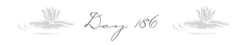

Dr. McMillan had excellent bedside manners, and he explained everything to me.

Gabriel took my mom to 4 North and was so very nice.

From this point, I can only mention a few names because I truly do not want to leave anyone out. The care my mom received was excellent, not only medically, but also spiritually. She had a really bad start and I didn't think she would still be alive. Everyone was so kind to my family and me. My seven-year-old was taken to the office to keep her from being afraid, and she was treated like a princess. 4 North doesn't have one associate that is not caring, compassionate, and kind. Their clinical expertise is life-changing. Respiratory therapy, the nurses, and Dr. Long were all around the bed working on my mom.

There were so many prayers for my mom and me, which gave me the strength I needed. The chaplains came to visit and kept checking on me. Chaplain Chris left from his class on lunch, visited, and prayed with us. Rhonda came with a hug and encouragement. Erin, a dietician, was so sweet and explained my mother's tube feeding to me. She was very caring and made me laugh.

Bruce Wilson and Tanya, RT, were so kind and showed so much love. My office buddy, Debra Savage, was right there with me and even checked on mama after I left the room in the evenings. Monie, a case manager, gave me a hug, which meant so much to me.

Everyone from EVS who entered my mother's room was kind and nice and had smiles on their faces. Mama was transferred to 3 North and discharged back to the North Hospital within a few hours. Cindy Mashburn talked with me and was so encouraging, kind, compassionate,

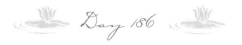
and caring. Brandy, RN, and Mandy, GN, were absolutely wonderful.

I will never forget the care, love, compassion, kindness, and expert skills my mom received from North. It is very different being on the receiving side of the fence. I thank God for North, and I am honored to be a part of the North family.

—Submitted by Diane Anderson,
Methodist Lebonheur North Hospital, Germantown, TN

"Never underestimate the difference you can make."

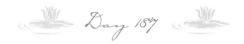
Extraordinary Emergency Care

The following letter was sent to the hospital by an officer in the Coast Guard, who needed emergency medical attention. It is a perfect example of the difference we can make in health care:

I am the Officer in Charge of the Coast Guard Cutter Obion. We patrol the Ohio River from Smithland, Kentucky, to Portsmouth, Ohio. On April 1, while underway in the vicinity of Portsmouth, I needed medical attention. I moored the cutter just below the river wall. Being away from our homeport, the nearest facility that could care for me was your emergency room. I want to take this opportunity to tell you about the excellent care I received from your staff.

From the minute I walked into the emergency waiting room, I was greeted with care and concern. The triage nurse, as well as administrative personnel, ensured I was processed and treated as quickly as possible. Once I entered into the "fast-track" area, I received quick and professional care. My condition was diagnosed immediately, and the proper prescription was issued. At this point, your staff met their obligation in caring for my immediate needs. However, the care did not stop there.

When your staff learned that I had come to the hospital in a taxi cab, they became concerned about my ability to get my prescription. They called two pharmacies that had a courier service, but neither of them

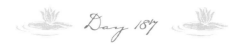

would accept my military insurance. Undeterred, nurse practitioner Warner called Wal-Mart to see if they would help. The pharmacist at Wal-Mart, Ms. Maryanne Osborne, came through and filled my prescription immediately. Your staff, still concerned about transportation, arranged for someone from the hospital to drive to Wal-Mart, pick up the medicine, and deliver it to me. While waiting for the medicine, another nurse brought me coffee and made sure I was comfortable. I had planned to try to get a cab to take me back to my cutter on the river. However, your staff had already arranged a ride for me with one of the local ambulance services.

I cannot adequately put into words the gratitude I have for everyone who was involved in helping me. As an active duty serviceman, even just a few hundred miles from home, I was treated like I was very special. I received the best care I have ever experienced from a medical facility. Any visit to the emergency room is stressful, especially when out of town, and in my case, leaving my crew stranded on the bank of the river. The outstanding care I received allowed me to get back to my crew quickly and back underway on our mission.

Those involved with my care included Susan Warner, NP; Cathy Clark, RN; Doris, ERT; and Maryanne Osborne, Wal-Mart Pharmacy.

Sincerely, Brian Williams, United States Coast Guard

—Submitted by Mary Kate Dilts-Skaggs, Southern Ohio Medical Center, Portsmouth, OH

"Never underestimate the difference you can make."

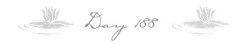

A Baby's Touch

There was a car accident involving several victims from the same family. They were all brought to Regions Hospital, a level one trauma center. As happens in the ER, the patients were placed in separate rooms while the teams of providers began caring for the patients.

One of the ER nurses noted that the mother seemed particularly upset, but without having the interpreter immediately present, the nurse couldn't figure out the source of her distress. Then, the nurse put herself in the mother's place, and realized that her anxiousness was resulting from being away from her baby.

The nurse found the baby in another room, and once the baby was stable, brought the baby's bed into the room. She placed the mother's bed and baby's bed next to each other, and put the baby's hand in the mother's. The interpreter arrived at about this time, and noticed the actions of the nurse, and the immediate calming effects they had on the mother. It was one of those special human moments worth remembering.

—Anonymous Contributor, Health Partners, Minnetonka, MN

"Never underestimate the difference you can make."

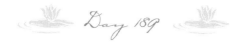
Helping Charlie

Early this June, my family and I were thrown a curve. It happened when Charlie, my 12-year-old son, was diagnosed with diabetes. It happened during the middle of May. Charlie had baseball almost every night, the weather was warm, and he was running all the time. I noticed that he was drinking Gatorade as fast as I could get it for him, and his appetite was increasing day by day.

I thought this was normal for a growing child until I noticed that he was urinating constantly, four to five times an hour. He also developed a skeletal look in his face as he was losing weight rapidly. In February, he weighed 112 lbs. By May, he was down to 99 lbs. We decided to take Charlie in for a blood test, which confirmed our suspicions that he was diabetic. In fact, his glucose level was over 600, and he was admitted immediately.

Upon arriving on the pediatric unit at Mary Greeley, Charlie was hooked up to his IV. Dr. Richard Carano explained to my wife and I what was going on and what they would be doing for Charlie. I found Dr. Carano to be compassionate and was always a true professional.

Tara, Charlie's nurse on the unit, was exceptional. She inserted his IV with ease, was friendly to us, and kept us all informed of what was going on. She made a scary time easier for us to handle.

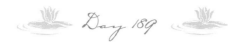

The day after Charlie was admitted, Dr. Carano was at Charlie's bedside following up from the previous day. Things were progressing nicely and Charlie's blood sugar was lowering to safer levels. That morning, we also met with Jolene Wolf, the dietitian assigned to the pediatric unit and a certified diabetic educator. She began by asking him what he might eat in a normal week and used those food choices to come up with a meal plan. She showed a great amount of compassion and professionalism to us all.

As the day progressed, Tara was there giving Charlie his insulin and teaching him how to give himself his own shots. Later in the day, we were notified that Charlie would be discharged that evening. My wife and I were concerned because we weren't yet comfortable with treating Charlie on our own. Again, Dr. Carano, Tara, and Jolene came to the rescue ready to answer our questions.

Before our discharge, we met with the diabetic educator, Barb Fatka. Her focus was entirely on Charlie. She taught him everything from how to read his glucose monitor to how to give himself his own shots. She was a great teacher.

That weekend I had to go out of town. My wife, Beth, was a little nervous about being home alone with Charlie and not knowing what to do in the event of an emergency. Barb immediately offered her cell phone number to us in case Beth needed help. Sure enough, that Saturday evening, Beth called Barb on her cell phone for some advice. Barb was there and helped her through it. She was truly an angel to us during our time of need.

I realized early this summer that we can't do things on our own. We need other people we work with. We need them for their knowledge, their professionalism, and their compassion.

—*Submitted by Matt Hart, Mary Greeley Medical Center, Ames, IA*

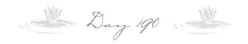

A Last Goodbye

Karen is a very tall, lanky nurse that has worked in Banner Baywood Medical Center's pre-op holding area for many years and has been a nurse for more than 30 years, dedicating most of that time to our organization and our Arizona community. Naturally, over the years, she has experienced many changes in health care. Karen's heart is truly as large as she is tall. One story, in particular, shows the heart of gold that Karen possesses.

One day, an elderly woman presented in pre-op holding with her family. She was scheduled to undergo joint replacement surgery. Upon arrival, the patient's family members informed Karen that the woman's husband of 50 years had undergone a cardiac arrest the evening before and was currently a patient in our Intensive Care Unit (ICU). He was gravely ill and his condition was deteriorating rapidly, but he was still lucid.

The family had chosen not to tell the woman of her husband's critical condition for a few more days so that she could concentrate on her own surgical recovery. Instinctively, Karen checked the status of our patient's husband in the ICU and discovered that his was deteriorating. Karen then visited with the family and suggested that it might be in the patient's best interest if she was told of her husband's condition and was allowed to visit with him before her surgery.

The family talked about her suggestion and ultimately decided to tell our patient. That is when Karen leaped into action. Our patient did indeed want to

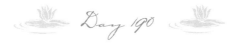

spend those few precious minutes with her beloved husband before her surgery. Karen arranged the visit with the physicians and ICU nurses and took the patient to see her husband. It was touching to see them holding hands and saying goodbye.

Our patient then made the decision to proceed with her surgery. Her husband passed away that afternoon before our patient was discharged from the PACU. Those few precious minutes were very important and special to our patient, as they were the last time that she saw him alive.

Karen provided this loving couple who had had a long-lasting relationship with one last opportunity to say goodbye. This is truly a great example of Banner's service excellence standards and exceeding expectations.

—*Submitted by Christine C. Halowell,*
Banner Baywood Medical Center, Mesa, AZ

Intensive Care
Unit

"Never underestimate the difference you can make."

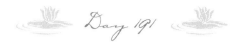

Thanks for an Angel

The following is excerpted from a letter of thanks expressing the gratitude of a patient and his family for Faby, a great financial counselor:

We have worked so hard to recover from a complete loss of personal possessions following a fire. Married for 16 years, this has been a painful challenge. No complaints—just find it difficult to write this letter and share our financial situation, especially at our age.

We have NEVER found ourselves in such a position of despair, and we have never asked for assistance before. Health problems and job loss combined can change one's life in a short period of time. I am able to ask for your consideration because I don't know what else to do.

Tragically, my husband has delayed/refused to get radiation/chemo treatment because he has been waiting for approval. The day my husband had surgery at your wonderful hospital, I remember looking at a sign that said, "Provena Mercy Medical Center."

I truly understood the word "mercy" when Faby reviewed our circumstances and informed us we were pre-qualified for 100 percent financial aid. Faby is a wonderful representative of your hospital. She treated us with a sense of dignity, kindness, and caring. We refer to her as

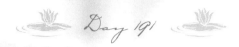

our "Little Angel." She even called us after discharge to see how we were doing. She is so kind and gentle.

When you are in our position, the world feels a little hard and a bit crusty, and when someone takes the extra time to be gentle with you, it is unexpected and much appreciated. Our experience at your hospital has been a very positive one, and we will always be thankful and feel blessed for finding our way to your facility, the staff, and physicians. We appreciate you. Thank you.

—Submitted by Barbara Novak, Provena Mercy Medical Center, Aurora, IL

"Never underestimate the difference you can make."

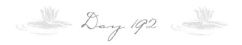

Christmas Angels

We would like to share the story of a true guardian angel in our Nutrition/Food Service Department. Her name is Linda Rabe, Nutritional Representative. Her tenderness and kindness toward all patients makes them feel like they are the only ones in the hospital. One year, starting in the fall, Linda began making Christmas Angel ornaments to place on our patients' Christmas meal lunch trays. The angels were made with the same love and compassion that she gives to her patients each day.

Our administration received a note from the daughter of a patient who had been given an angel. The daughter wrote that her mother had passed away, and she wanted Linda to know how much her mother cherished the hand-made angel. The letter said that her mother had requested that if she passed away, the angel be buried with her in the casket. Her daughter wrote that she had granted the wish. She was grateful that from the time her mother had entered the hospital Linda had shown her great amounts of care and compassion. We are so lucky to have a guardian angel walking our floors!

—Submitted by Nancy Stephens, Banner Baywood Medical Center & Banner Baywood Heart Hospital, Mesa, AZ

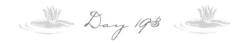

From Behind the Scenes

*T*he first time I publicly shared this story was at a Leadership Development Institute meeting on finance. My hospital's management team was quite surprised to see how much a medical incident from many years ago could shape the career path of just about anyone—including one of their own leaders.

When I was 16, I was watching television one day after school. I had an itch on my leg, but when I scratched it, I felt something very strange. I ran right upstairs and told my mother that I thought I needed to go to the doctor right away. She was worried and she wanted to know what was wrong. But I was reluctant to tell her exactly what the problem was. I just explained that I really needed to get to a doctor. She kept asking why, and grew very concerned so I told her that I had found a lump and it was not right. She asked to see it because she wanted to help. I finally had to tell her that she couldn't see it—it was on my testicle.

Our HMO at the time had an urgent care clinic, and that is where we went. The female doctor that came in looked barely older than me, and the exam was terribly uncomfortable. All she said was that I needed to see a urologist right away, and she made an appointment for me the next day. After my exam with the urologist, he told my mother and I that it could be a few different things and one was cancer. That didn't sit well with me at all, and my mother was angry that he would scare me by saying such a thing that just couldn't be possible.

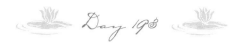

Tests at the time showed a mass, and the doctor said it had to be removed. A short time later, it was, and as I feared, the result came back positive for cancer. The next step was a lymph node biopsy, where many lymph glands would be removed to determine if the cancer had spread. Well, after a long hospital stay of six weeks, it was done. The cancer had never spread, and everything was back to normal. Everything, that is, except me.

At 16, a six-week hospital stay can change your life. What is most amazing, however, is how 10 minutes of that stay can define one's life. It was late one day, and I was waiting for a CT scan to find out why my bowels were not functioning. I was alone in the waiting room when another patient was wheeled in on a stretcher. Clearly, this person was fresh out of brain surgery as there were three enormous incisions across the person's head. The patient was hooked up to more machines than I had ever seen before and no one attended to them. I sat alone, in a small waiting room with this person and could not even tell if it was a man or a woman. That wait seemed like forever.

When I finally left the hospital, I swore to myself that I would never ever set foot in a hospital again, but things change. I have now worked in a hospital for many years, and could never ever imagine doing anything else. What I learned in that waiting room was that there are things in this world a lot bigger than me. I work hard every day, in a hospital, behind the scenes, to give back all that I can to those who helped me: my doctors, nurses, techs, food service people, everyone. And I dedicate every day to that person in the waiting room. People need help in their lives at times. I know I did. People were there for me, and I want to thank them all by being there for others—even behind the scenes.

—*Anonymous Contributor, Blue Hill Memorial Hospital, Blue Hill, ME*

"Never underestimate the difference you can make."

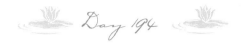

Living the Standards Every Day

Like most Phoenix Baptist Hospital staff members, I'm pretty familiar with the "standard of the month" posted by the elevators. And honestly, I really do try to live by the standards, though I have to admit that when rushing off late to a meeting, it could be tempting to just point to the lab or radiology rather than walking the visitor there in person. While I believe that all the standards are worthwhile in delivering excellent customer service, something happened recently that showed me that our standards are not only good for our patients and visitors—they are also good for our families.

Two weeks ago, I was working well into the evening to meet a deadline. As I wrapped up the day, I grabbed my belongings and hurried toward the door thinking about dinner for my kids and wondering what homework monsters were lurking in their backpacks. As I swung through the main lobby, I came upon a petite woman slowly shuffling with a cane and a bag marked "patient belongings." Visions of the "Five and Ten" rule poster flashed before me as I slowed to make eye contact and say "hello." Her response was so heartfelt, I stopped to complete the next step—I asked, "Is there anything I can do for you?" As we passed through the door into the night, it was obvious that her ride was not yet there. Hesitating to leave her alone outside, I asked if I could call anyone for her. The cab driver she was expecting had a ride that had taken him far across the Valley making him at least 30 minutes late in rush hour traffic. At that point,

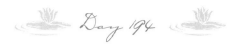
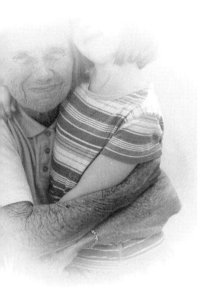

I knew I was hooked. This charming grandmotherly figure looked up to me for help. There seemed no other choice than to take her home myself—dinner and homework would have to be late that night.

On the way to her home, I learned that both she and her husband were holocaust survivors. She rolled up her sleeve to display the ID tattoo she received in a concentration camp. She met her husband of 61 years when American soldiers liberated their concentration camp. Both had lost their families in the camp. He now lay in our hospital as a patient. Hearing her survival story suddenly put my petty concerns in stark perspective.

When I finally arrived home, my kids were hungry but anxious to know why I was so late. I shared with them about the very special lady I had befriended. Later that night, still full of questions, my fifth grader and I visited several holocaust websites to learn more. My daughter asked if she could ever meet my new friend. Over the next few days, I checked in on her and her husband each day as I got to know them better. She was more than willing to meet my young daughter and we set a date for the coming weekend. During their visit, my daughter was able to hear first-person history about one of the 20th Century's most horrifying events. It impacted her like no website or textbook ever could. As I watched their visit unfold, I realized it was all because of our Five and Ten Rule. In my effort to serve our visitors, I received a reward I would have never known otherwise, and my daughter received a history lesson she will never forget.

—Submitted by Richard Holland, Phoenix Baptist Hospital, Phoenix, AZ

"Never underestimate the difference you can make."

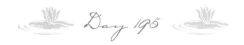

Message of Thanks

The following is a voicemail message that was left from a Deaconess patient's family member. He was genuinely thankful for the compassionate care that his family received from one Deaconess employee in particular:

"My name is Mark S. I was in your hospital last night, and too many times people complain about things that people do wrong. I wanted to let you know you have an employee who went above and beyond her call of duty. Joyce was her name.

We had a very bad case going into surgery last night. She took time out of her schedule to spend time with my family, pray with them, talk with them, and I just want her to be commended for the great job she does."

She's a great example of what an employee should be. I just wanted you to know; Thank you very much."

—Submitted by Kathy Clodfelter, Deaconess Hospital, Evansville, IN

"Never underestimate the difference you can make."

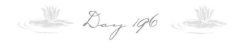

It Takes a Lot of Heart

As far as Mr. C is concerned, every day is a great day. Minister of Music, Senior Adults, and Administration at a Baptist church, Mr. C began Thursday, April 6, 2006, the way he begins almost every Thursday. First, he met two friends at a local restaurant for a 6 a.m. prayer breakfast, then ran home for a quick change of clothes before reporting to work at his church.

While at the prayer breakfast, Mr. C noticed that he was having chest pains, but chalked it up simply to catching a cold. He found that the pain came and went, and at times he was able to cough and get some relief.

He went about his regular course of business Thursday morning—making preparations for the church's upcoming Easter services. This included preparing the church's order of worship for Sunday, burning a CD for the choir's anthem, checking on a microphone for the services, preparing for that night's praise team practice, and running out to make a few purchases associated with the Easter services.

While taking care of all of these tasks, he noticed that the pain that had been confined to his chest began to move to both sides of his jaw. He went into the church's main office, and upon bumping into one of his buddies from the earlier prayer breakfast, asked him if he knew the symptoms of a heart attack.

Naturally, the question worried his friend and within minutes they were in a vehicle, headed the six blocks to the Emergency Care Center (ECC) of Self

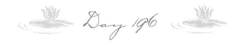

Regional Healthcare. Mr. C was immediately wheeled inside and hooked up to an EKG machine. Shortly after his doctor, Dr. Bruce Cook, medical director of the ECC, informed him he was experiencing a heart attack and that the hospital staff would do everything in their power to help him.

He was given four aspirins and was being prepared for a heart catheterization. Just as his wife, Bonnie, arrived on the scene, he coded. Mr. C said, "The room just closed in around me—very similar to passing out. In fact, when I regained consciousness, I thought I had been asleep, even though I was being bagged and there was a lot of activity around me. I could hear my nurse telling what medications to give me, but I still did not connect with what was going on."

Flat on his back, breathing with the help of the bag and about to code again, Mr. C realized the seriousness of his situation. He became aware of health providers using defibrillators on his chest, and how the burning of the shocks differed from the other chest pain he was experiencing. Before leaving the ECC, he coded a total of three times.

As he regained consciousness, Mr. C became aware of Dr. Cook standing over him and offering reassurance, "We are just trying to keep you with us," Dr. Cook told him.

Mr. C recalls, "I replied for him to do his magic, and I knew that either way I would win. There was still a lot of activity around me as more medication was being administered and they were pushing me out of the cubicle to the cath lab."

Following what Mr. C described as "the fastest stretcher ride I've ever taken," he was in the Self Regional Heart Center being prepped for a diagnostic catheterization to determine the exact severity of his problem. Dr. Tom Pritchard, a cardiologist, performed the procedure. Mr. C had to be shocked again in the cath lab to restore his heart rhythm.

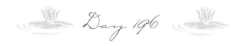

Mr. C had drifted out of consciousness when Dr. Pritchard made the diagnosis. One vein of his heart was 100 percent occluded. One of the other three veins pumping blood through his heart was also totally closed. The doctors concluded it had been that way for seven or eight years as evidenced by the secondary branching that had occurred to bypass the clot.

Dr. Paul Kim, an interventional cardiologist, was called in to insert a stent into one of the blockages. After the procedure, Dr. Kim accompanied him to the Cardiac Intensive Care Unit (CICU) and remained with him an hour to make certain his heart rhythm stayed normal.

When he awoke in his CICU room, Mr. C saw his faithful wife and his CICU nurse by his side. Outside his room, in the unit's visitor waiting area, a number of his family members, friends, church members, and even people he did not know were praying for his recovery.

Later, after talking to some of the health professionals, he began to understand what a close call he had had. Had he been 10 minutes later getting to the ECC or had it happened two years earlier—in the days before the Self Regional Heart Center had interventional capability, he probably would not have made it.

Nearly a year later, Mr. C is back in the routine of daily life both at home and at church. He completed the cardiac rehabilitation program at Self Regional

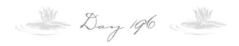

Healthcare's Optimum Life Center recommended by his doctor, but elected to continue at least through this spring.

"Dr. Kim and the staff at cardiac rehab have been very helpful in establishing a program that allows me to achieve maximum benefit," he said. "I am feeling great."

Not only does he feel great, he also looks forward to the opportunities of each day more fully now than ever and knows that nothing should be taken for granted.

—Submitted by Dan Branyon, *Self Regional Healthcare, Greenwood, SC*

"Never underestimate the difference you can make."

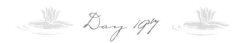

Ramping It UP!

W oody Tatman and Al Kozlowski may be occupational therapists, but their commitment to their profession reaches much further into the community.

One of their patients, a man with multiple sclerosis who was recovering from a broken hip, bought an electric wheelchair to increase his mobility. However, this solved only part of the man's mobility challenges. After discussing the situation, Al and Woody realized this gentleman needed a sidewalk to cover a distance of nearly 60 feet which stretched from his driveway to his front porch ramp.

Woody and Al devised a plan. They were soon at the patient's home, measuring and breaking up the ground with Woody's hand tiller. When that was finished, they were off to the local handyman store to buy boards for framing the sidewalk. Next, they arranged for a concrete mixing truck to arrive and pour cement, which Al and Woody leveled and smoothed. After several days of work on their own personal time, Al and Woody stepped back to gaze at a perfect sidewalk. Of course, no one was more elated than the patient! Now, with a sidewalk that allows him to navigate from his wheelchair ramp to his car, he is able to get to work at a local high school, where he helps handicapped kids prepare for future employment. What a great story he has to share with his students, thanks to two occupational therapists who made a difference for a grateful patient.

—Submitted by Linda Pledge, West Tennessee Healthcare, Jackson, TN

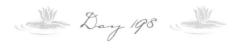

I Have Time

As a health care attorney for longer than I care to tell, I've learned more about clinical care in the last few months than in all my prior years combined. The reason? My organization began daily administrative rounding.

On a recent rounding experience, I was in a room with a patient who was describing her pain to the nurse as a nine on a 10-point scale. Her demeanor made it obvious that she was in a great deal of pain. There was also a housekeeper in the room with us, working quietly as the nurse and patient interacted.

However, when she was finished, she approached the patient, put her hand on the patient's arm, and said, "I've finished cleaning your room, is there anything else I can do for you, I have time." For the first time since I entered the room, this patient, who had a nine on the pain scale, actually smiled, said "no," and thanked the housekeeper. I was grateful to witness quality health care in action.

—Anonymous Contributor

"Never underestimate the difference you can make."

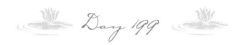

Making Change

*I*n the late summer of last year, I was attending a hospital-sponsored conference on customer service featuring an internal speaker. The speaker happened to mention during his talk that his secretary had a problem with an infusion service. My ears perked up, as I am the director of clinical operations at the Cancer Center, where many of the infusion services are provided. After the conference, I approached this leader and asked if he would give me the details so I could follow up on the situation. He did, and I called his secretary that afternoon. She told me that she had breast cancer and was receiving chemotherapy in our infusion area. She told me that she was frustrated because her wait times for infusion were often several hours in duration. Infusion is an area that is amazingly complex and difficult to keep running on time because of the synchronicity required in the components of the service. At that time, we were often running at greater than 90 percent capacity, which leaves little wiggle room for anything unexpected and can result in lengthened wait times. I explained all of this to her in detail and explained what we were doing to fix some of the issues.

On the last day before Christmas break, I received a phone call from her. Again, she told me that she was frustrated with the wait times in infusion. I explained to her the progress that we had made since we spoke last—that we had a multi-million dollar expansion project approved, that we had design plans already developed, and that there was light at the end of the tunnel.

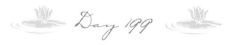

Day 199

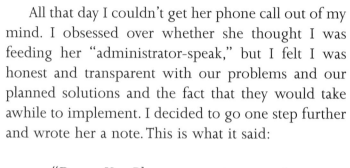

All that day I couldn't get her phone call out of my mind. I obsessed over whether she thought I was feeding her "administrator-speak," but I felt I was honest and transparent with our problems and our planned solutions and the fact that they would take awhile to implement. I decided to go one step further and wrote her a note. This is what it said:

> "Dear X, Please accept my sincere apologies for your recent problems in our infusion area. Unfortunately, I can't restore the time you wasted, but I can try to make sure you have a nice dinner (on us!). Please enjoy. I hope your holidays are bright and restful. Remember to call me if you have any further issues or if I can help you in any way."

I enclosed a gift certificate for a local restaurant and sent it to her via internal mail.

I came back from the holidays to the news (from a colleague) that this secretary had died. I was stunned. I couldn't believe the courage and sincere desire for improving service that this employee demonstrated by spending what was, in essence, her dying hours telling me how to improve our service.

At that moment, I dedicated myself, in her honor, to insuring that I came up with some expedient fix that would positively impact infusion wait times for everyone. Within 90 days of the day I received the call

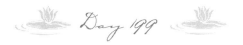

that she had passed, we had opened (on a shoestring budget) a seven-chair infusion expansion in temporary space. To do so, we fought all levels of organizational mulishness and were even able to figure out a way to avoid the dreaded capital budgeting process.

I was on a mission—I understood my role in impacting the issue, and I understood that nothing would happen quickly unless I personally made it happen.

It was a seminal time for me as a leader—I was able to bring together a sense of purpose and worthwhile work to contribute toward making a real difference for our patients.

—Submitted by C. Jane Martin,
University of Michigan Comprehensive Cancer Center, Ann Arbor, MI

"Never underestimate the difference you can make."

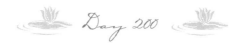

Very Good Care

A nurse sent the following letter to Mike Murphy at Mary Birch Hospital regarding her experience as a patient.

My husband and I just arrived home from Mary Birch Hospital after a most tragic event. Despite our enormous grief, we felt compelled to write to you so we could recognize those that truly made a difference in our lives these past few days.

I was eight months pregnant with our first child, a baby boy to be named Evan Flannery Murano. We had just had our baby shower and the baby's room was ready for his arrival. I had begun preparations for my maternity leave from Sharp Rees-Stealy and was busy planning this new stage of our lives. I went into SRS San Diego Main to see nurse practitioner Janet Bargabus for my routine appointment and expressed my concerns that the baby's movements seemed to have slowed down. I was worried that things were not okay. I told her that on Monday, I had heard the baby's heartbeat and that all was well, but that I was still concerned about his movements.

Janet was unable to find his heartbeat and put me on the ultrasound machine. After a few minutes, she told me that she could not see his heart beating and she went to get a doctor. Dr. O'Hara is my OB, but he was not in the office, so Dr. Barmeyer came in. He advised me that there was no heartbeat, and that Evan was gone.

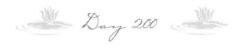

I don't think there is anything in life that can prepare anyone for such devastating news. I am a seasoned ICU/ER nurse, and I have seen the worst possible tragedies happen to families with absolutely no warning, but we never think that one day those things will happen to us.

I was alone and hysterical, trying to reach my husband to tell him to come to the doctor's office, so that we could figure out the next step. Janet was wonderful and so supportive.

My husband is a nurse for Sharp Rees-Stealy as well, and we assumed that I would need to go to the hospital and deliver the baby. I couldn't believe that I would have to go through the long and arduous labor process, knowing that at the end of it, my husband and I would bury our son. It seemed unimaginable and the pain and sadness were overwhelming.

We arrived at Mary Birch on February 2, at 8:30 a.m. All the arrangements had been made ahead of time and the staff was well aware that they were dealing with a fetal demise. We were escorted personally to our room and introduced to our nurse, Polly Martin.

Needless to say, I was not doing well. I was trying to maintain a sense of calm, but was so overcome with grief that I was crying the minute we walked into our room. Polly was absolutely wonderful from the very beginning. She welcomed us with open arms and sincere condolences. She explained everything that was going to happen initially, and assisted in getting me settled to wait for Dr. O'Hara.

This was my first real experience as a patient in a hospital setting, and I have to admit that being on the receiving end as a patient, I discovered that I was rather terrified. I have a huge fear of needles and was dreading the thought of having an epidural. Polly was so kind to me through all of this. She arranged for the

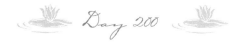

anesthesiologist on duty to talk me through the epidural process and answer all of my questions.

Meanwhile, Polly was at our bedside constantly, tending to not only my needs, but the needs of my husband and our two friends who were with us. She cried with us, laughed with us, shared stories with us, and respected us as colleagues. She seemed to sense when we needed some company and when we needed to be alone. When it was time for her lunch break, she brought the nurse that covered for her into the room and introduced her to us. I was starting to have labor pains by then, and she made sure before she left that I was given pain medication to make me comfortable.

Polly answered all of my questions and explained to me how my pain would progress and that eventually the pain medication would cease to be as effective and then it would be time for the epidural. I had strong labor pains that progressed to severe labor pains. Despite copious amounts of narcotics over the course of three hours, I eventually arrived at the conclusion that I had to have the epidural.

As luck would have it, the timing of all of this was adding to my anxiety. Polly's shift was coming to an end which meant I would have a new nurse. Dr. O'Hara had gone home for the night and I would have to deal with a new OB doctor that I had never met. In addition, the anesthesiologist would be replaced by another.

This is where Polly truly went above and beyond. She assured us that Jocelyn, the night shift nurse, would take excellent care of us. She then introduced us to Jocelyn and told us that the OB, Dr. Bolch, was kind and patient and that I had nothing to fear. She even stayed a few minutes late to be there for me as I was getting the epidural.

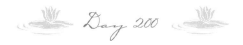

My husband and I were able to get some sleep as we waited for my labor to progress. I was given more medication to progress my labor, but it would be more than seven more hours before we saw our son's face.

Jocelyn made sure she understood our wishes for how things were to be handled on Evan's arrival. She explained various choices. We could spend time with him or not, we could hold him or not, we could have pictures or not. We could choose what was best for us without fear of judgment from her or anyone else. It was truly up to us.

At 2:19 a.m. on February 3, Evan Flannery Murano came into this world, even though his spirit had already moved on. This was such a bittersweet and heartbreaking time for my husband and me as we got to see our little baby's face but realized that we were also saying goodbye. He was a roadmap of us both. He had my husband's wild curly black hair and beautiful brown eyes. He had my little nose, lips, and chin. He had my husband's torso and long piano man fingers. His legs were all my husband's, but his feet were definitely mine, right down to the funny third toe that is infamous in my Flannery clan. We held him, we took pictures, Jocelyn made impressions of his feet and hands, and we created other memories to cherish. We were given time and privacy and treated with the utmost respect and tenderness by all the staff that entered the room.

So Mr. Murphy, I just wanted to tell you our story and let you know about the wonderful people working at Sharp Mary Birch. My husband and I lost our child, but the incredible people that took care of us made a huge difference and brought us some comfort during a tragic time.

I have been an employee of Sharp going on 13 years and my husband has been going on nine years. We have both witnessed the changes that have taken place with the Sharp Experience and have taken part in creating that change. We have never been more grateful or more appreciative of Sharp's commitment than we were this week, experiencing the Sharp Experience first hand as patients. Additionally, our friends and coworkers within Sharp Rees-Stealy have also rallied around us to give comfort and be there for us in our time of need.

Thank you for all that you have done and all that you do to make sure that every patient has the same very good care that we received.

Sincerely,
Maureen Flannery, RN

—Submitted by Maureen Flannery, Sharp Rees-Stealy, San Diego, CA

"Never underestimate the difference you can make."

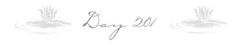

Last Wish

My wife, Laura, is a paramedic. While on a call to transport a woman from an Emergency Department to hospice care, Laura encountered an elderly man who was near death. His daughter begged Laura to transport him to the family home, which was about 10 miles away. It was this man's fervent wish to die at home, surrounded by his large family.

Laura put the man and his daughter in the ambulance and took off towards the family residence. Along the way, the gentleman became very ill and appeared to be near death any moment. His daughter begged Laura to do something—and not allow her father to die in the back of an ambulance.

At that moment, Laura took a risk. She had the driver turn on the lights and siren in order to quickly get the man to his bed so his last wish could be fulfilled.

They arrived at the man's home safely, and his family was able to say goodbye at his bedside, as he had wanted.

Laura escaped disciplinary action and was instead complimented when the ambulance company found out about her diligent action on behalf of a dying man. They agreed—she had done the right thing in fulfilling the man's last wish.

—Submitted by Bob Murphy, Studer Group, Gulf Breeze, FL

"Never underestimate the difference you can make."

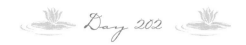

Helping Others Walk

J erry Segal is an amazing person. In 1988, he underwent surgery on the West Coast that was supposed to be relatively routine. In the recovery room, however, Jerry Segal discovered that he could not raise his arm to scratch an itch on his forehead. Following the unsuccessful surgery, Jerry returned to Philadelphia and was admitted to Magee Rehabilitation Hospital in December 1988. At that time he had no movement below his shoulders. Before coming to Magee, the prognosis was that he would spend the rest of his life in a wheelchair. But Segal vowed to walk again, and after much hard work, he did. At his discharge, he walked out of Magee Rehabilitation—despite his quadriplegia and having no feeling below his neck.

On re-entering the community on the day following his discharge, he went to a restaurant in center city Philadelphia. When he got out of his car, he discovered that basic steps such as leaving the car, going up a slanted curb, climbing steps, and getting through the doorways of the restaurant were extraordinary challenges. He quickly realized that the hospital setting, with its tile floors and smooth walkways, was not representative of what he faced in the community. He approached Magee about building a community skills center, complete with uneven walkways, varying terrains and curb heights, cobblestones, and much more. He not only put forth the concept, he also

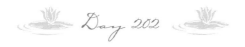

contributed and raised much of the money to complete what is now the Jerry and Carolyn Segal Center for Community Skills.

The Center, on the rooftop of Magee Rehabilitation Hospital, allows people with disabilities to practice skills that will help them meet the challenges they will face in the real world. Jerry's dream was funded by the Jerry Segal Classic, an annual one-day golf charity event he founded in 1990. The first Segal Classic raised $56,000 for Magee. Since then, the Classic has enlisted the support of over 1,000 individuals and corporate contributors and has become the Philadelphia region's most successful one-day golf fundraiser.

Unparalleled in its success, in 2006 the Segal Classic raised an event-record $1 million, bringing the 17-year total of funds raised for Magee's patients to more than $6.2 million. "Through the dollars we raise at this outing, maybe other Magee spinal cord injury patients can be where I am today, walking, working, living independently," says Jerry. "Maybe, with the extra support, they can accomplish what I have accomplished."

The event is directed and organized by Jerry Segal and The Friends of Jerry Segal, all of whom volunteer their services for the benefit of Magee Rehabilitation. An executive committee of dedicated volunteers provides hands-on leadership for the event. Edward G. Rendell, governor of Pennsylvania, has served as honorary chairman of the event since 1992. Jerry's wife, Carolyn, also volunteers her energy and expertise, and serves as executive director of the Jerry Segal Classic. This special brand of volunteerism assures that all proceeds go directly to patient programs and services at Magee.

Jerry Segal, now a member of Magee's Board of Trustees, is steadfast in his determination to help Magee's patients. He also makes numerous visits to patients, offering them his personal support and encouragement. He advises

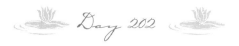

them to stay positive and to work diligently both to overcome personal challenges and to achieve their goals for independence. Through his own courage and heroic recovery, he has become an inspiration and a role model for patients with physical disabilities. And he has personally assured that patients in need are provided with the necessary equipment that improves health and well-being, enhances their quality of life, and allows them to pursue their goals for independence.

Jerry Segal has demonstrated unstinting philanthropy and tireless service on behalf of the patients at Magee Rehabilitation Hospital. He is dedicated to providing people with disabilities every possible opportunity to reenter the mainstream community. "Persons with disabilities should be given the freedom to do until they can't do anymore," he says, adding that the more he tries, the more he is able to do. "Who knows what strengths can come back. I always hope that tomorrow I'll be able to do more than I did today. I go through every day thinking things are going to get better."

—Submitted by John Martino, Magee Rehabilitation Hospital, Philadelphia, PA

"Never underestimate the difference you can make."

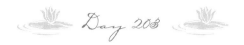

Mom's Final Days

My story begins with the care of my mom. My mom was an awesome individual, one whose smile was contagious to all those she met. She was a very caring individual, and I was blessed to have her as a part of my life for 79 years.

My mom fought a courageous battle with cancer for nine years, going into remission several times before her last bout was too much for her to handle. She lived with me for the last 18 months of her life, until she was admitted to our Covenant Hospice Care Center at West Florida Hospital.

As a non-clinical employee, it is rare that I get see the impact that our caregivers really *do* have on our patients. Visiting the care center several times each day and seeing the relief and sense of comfort on my mom's face from the day she arrived, I began to see the big picture. The RNs, LPNs, home health aides, chaplains, and physicians that visited and cared for my mom on each shift while she was there, were there because they wanted to be, not because it was their job. These individuals truly live the mission of "adding life to days when there aren't many days left to live." So much time was taken to meet my mom's needs, from the food she ate, her bathing, the combing of her hair, and even what she wanted to wear that day! It was truly amazing how happy she was and how thankful she was every day to be in a comfortable home-like setting, knowing that help was only a step away at all times.

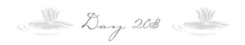

My mom remained at the Care Center for three weeks, until she went to Heaven in late July 2006. Her death truly left a void in my heart, but once again, the staff was there for me, as the caregiver, to comfort and provide emotional support as well as prepare me and my family for what lay ahead in preparation for the funeral and transport of my mom to her home in Cincinnati, Ohio. Even today, I receive cards and phone calls from caring staff from all of our branch offices, checking up on me to see if I need anything at all. This is very rare occurrence in this day and age, and absolutely amazing to me!

From the day I arrived, I have loved my job here at Covenant Hospice, but the reasons I stay have escalated 10-fold since this experience. I have always been an employee advocate, ready to do whatever it takes to recruit and retain those individuals who we *need* to meet the needs of our customers, *their* customers—the patients and families. My customers, our staff, whether clinical or non-clinical, are the best of the best and as such, deserve the best in return.

The Human Resources staff at Covenant Hospice is a team second to none. We serve more than 800 employees organization-wide and do it every day with a smile and a commitment to excellence. Hospice care is so very needed in the lives of so many. When our department works with newly-hired staff members to explain their benefits, help with staffing needs, listen to concerns, or make improvements to policy and procedure, we do it because we really care. I am so very proud to be associated with the members of this HR team, and I know that if ever I need an ear or a shoulder to cry on, someone from Covenant Hospice will be there for me, as I will be for them. The employees at Covenant Hospice are the cream of the crop, they strive for excellence all the time and it makes the job of the leaders of this organization so much easier.

—Submitted by Pat Holtman, Covenant Hospice, Pensacola, FL

"Never underestimate the difference you can make."

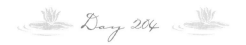

A Song of Comfort

I have had the honor of being a nurse for almost 15 years. During this time, there have been many moments when I know that I have touched someone's heart and even more moments when a patient or family member has touched mine. Recently, I chose to go down the path of nurse educator, and I now work as a faculty member at the same college of nursing from which I graduated years ago.

Being able to share my passion for nursing with students has been a true joy. One bit of wisdom that I try to impart upon my students is that every patient has different needs. As nurses, the challenge we face is finding the best way to identify and care for those needs, whether they need an IV started, pain control, or simply need a reassuring smile or touch.

One of my students was able to witness this as she and I provided daily care for an elderly patient. The elderly woman had a long history of Chronic Obstructive Pulmonary Disease (COPD). This woman had one son, who lived out of town, and as a result, spent much of her time alone. As I assisted with the woman's bath, I was softly humming a tune. It was then that the woman asked from behind her venti-mask if I would sing for her. I asked what she would like me to sing and she replied, "Why 'Amazing Grace' of course." I proceeded to give my best rendition of the beloved hymn and with tearful eyes she thanked me. We finished our work and said goodbye.

The next day, upon returning to the unit we were told that our patient had died the previous evening. Tears came to my eyes as my student said, "Now I see what you mean about giving your patients what they need. I bet you didn't expect that what our patient needed was a song of comfort for her dying day." I can only hope that that simple act of compassion brought a sense of peace to our patient, and that she knew, in her last hours, that someone cared.

—*Anonymous Contributor*

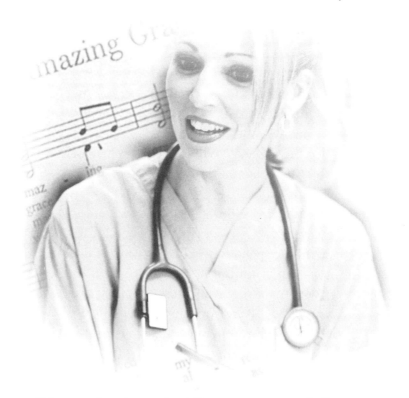

"Never underestimate the difference you can make."

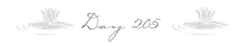
Caring for Your Own

*I*am a laboratory assistant at Alameda County Medical Center in Oakland, California. My job is to perform phlebotomy venipunctures on a daily basis for Fairmont Hospital and the John George Psychiatric Pavilion.

It is safe to say that I am used to traumas as I often have to draw blood from critically ill patients, but nothing could have prepared me for what I experienced in September 2006.

Never in my wildest dreams did I ever expect one of my family members would receive care from one of my coworkers. On Sept. 20, 2006, a neighborhood friend came to my home and told me that my youngest son, Bobby, had been shot and that he was at the fire station.

My husband and I jumped in our car and rushed towards the fire station. When we arrived, the paramedics had finished loading him into the ambulance and were headed towards Alameda County Medical Center. I was thankful because I knew that if my son was going to have a chance at survival he would find it through the care provided there.

When we arrived at the hospital, the deputy sheriff saw the state of panic I was in, and immediately began to help. He helped us find parking and escorted us into the trauma area where the surgeon on duty informed us of my son's condition. The bullet had entered his back area, through his kidney, and had gone into and out of his lower intestine. At the time they did not know if his spleen

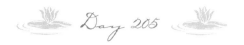

was damaged, and he told us that they may have to remove it once they went in for surgery.

My son's surgery took six to seven hours. While he was in surgery, the deputy sheriff was kind enough to check on my family and me. We also received a lot of support from my coworkers in the laboratory.

In recovery, my son's nurse was very attentive and actively helped him with his pain, tending to both his mental and physical state. When he was stable, he was transferred to Kaiser Hospital where he continued to recover.

My hat goes off to all of my coworkers at Alameda County Medical Center. If not for the skills of the surgeons, lab assistants, the quick diagnosis of the lab, the one-on-one care given in recovery, and the mental support provided by the deputy sheriff, my son, my family, and I would not have made it through this difficult situation.

I am proud to be a part of an organization that has the skills to perform nothing short of miracles. Thank you again to Alameda County Medical Center for giving my son back to me. He is mending just fine!

—Submitted by Mona Hall, Alameda County Medical Center, Oakland, CA

"Never underestimate the difference you can make."

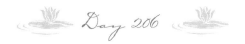

Gathered Belongings

At Columbus Regional Hospital (CRH), our employees often go beyond expectations to show compassion and concern for their patients. Recently, Jennifer Everroad, RN, of Tower 4, admitted a patient who had been involved in a motor vehicle accident.

All six of the patient's family members were brought to the hospital by ambulance with nothing but the torn, bloody clothes they were wearing. Their vehicle was towed to a local junkyard with all their belongings still inside. Jennifer realized that she could help this family by finding their belongings before they were dismissed. So, after work, she went to the junk yard, crawled into the mangled car and brought back all the personal items she could find. The family was very appreciative of Jennifer's efforts. Jennifer says, "That's what we're all about at CRH."

Jennifer's actions demonstrate how our health care workers can provide an extraordinary level of caring and compassion for those we serve.

—*Anonymous Contributor, Columbus Regional Hospital, Columbus, IN*

"Never underestimate the difference you can make."

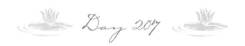

Because She Cared

Debbie Seals deals with many different customers in her role as a Cardinal Access financial services representative, but one instance of a reluctant patient stands out.

Debbie was called to the Cardiology Department to talk with an upset patient. The man was scheduled for surgery on an infected gallbladder, but had become upset because he could not pay for the procedure. He insisted on canceling the surgery and leaving the hospital.

After talking with her supervisors, Debbie contacted the patient at home and convinced him to come in to fill out an application for Cardinal Access. He reluctantly agreed and qualified for assistance from the program for uninsured patients.

Debbie successfully arranged emergency surgery for the man, but she had to chase him down in the parking lot to convince him he could be treated for his condition in the Emergency Department right away.

Two days later, she visited the man in recovery. He thanked her for her care and attention, and confessed that he would have died painfully of gallbladder failure had she not insisted on helping him. He told Debbie he considered her a friend and still keeps her updated on his condition.

"Deb is a dedicated CHS employee who personifies the CHS Customer Service Standards and Core Values," says Debbie Mace, director, Patient Financial Services. "She is very compassionate and cares for her patients and their needs. She goes above and beyond to meet their needs."

—Submitted by Debbie Mace, Ball Memorial Hospital, Inc., Muncie, IN

Going Home

In mid-November 2005, we admitted a 33-year-old male patient who was an undocumented worker. He had suffered a trauma that left him paralyzed from the neck down. He required mechanical ventilation and eventual placement of a tracheotomy and feeding tube. He had many invasive procedures and was in the ICU for a prolonged time due to the complications his condition had caused.

Eventually, he was weaned from the ventilator and transferred to 4NE. He slowly began an extended recovery period. He was able to eat small meals with some assistance, and he was able to be lifted into a wheelchair. Most importantly however, he was awake and alert.

He had been so very sick and now he was getting well enough to be able to go home. What incredible progress! This was the point when our real teamwork at the hospital began. Imagine trying to meet all the needs this patient had, but to meet them in an at-home setting, away from our modern equipment and around the clock nursing care. He would require tracheotomy care and suctioning, skin care, and turning each hour, plus bowel and bladder management. Furthermore he would require medications, plus a special bed, wheelchair, oxygen concentrator, and suctioning machine.

We had our work cut out for us since we had no resources to pay for his care. Well, we did it anyway! We were able to secure donations of $1,605 for

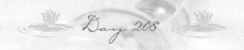

equipment needs. This was an amazing feat in itself. There were few detours along the way, but with diligent planning, great teamwork, and pure persistence this patient was discharged on February 10, just three months after arriving. Our patient certainly was grateful. He was so excited to be going home.

—Submitted by Sherry Petrillo, Methodist Dallas Medical Center, Dallas, TX

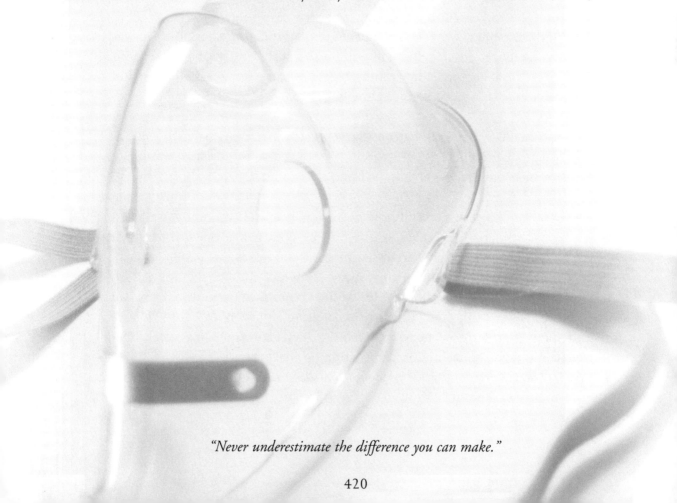

"Never underestimate the difference you can make."

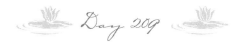

TAKING THE TIME

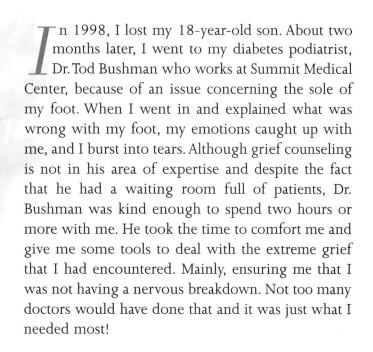

In 1998, I lost my 18-year-old son. About two months later, I went to my diabetes podiatrist, Dr. Tod Bushman who works at Summit Medical Center, because of an issue concerning the sole of my foot. When I went in and explained what was wrong with my foot, my emotions caught up with me, and I burst into tears. Although grief counseling is not in his area of expertise and despite the fact that he had a waiting room full of patients, Dr. Bushman was kind enough to spend two hours or more with me. He took the time to comfort me and give me some tools to deal with the extreme grief that I had encountered. Mainly, ensuring me that I was not having a nervous breakdown. Not too many doctors would have done that and it was just what I needed most!

—Submitted by Diana Neely,
Skyline Madison Campus HCA Tristar, Madison, TN

"Never underestimate the difference you can make."

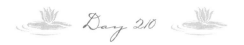

THE DRIVE

An ICU nurse came to work one day and saw an elderly woman sitting alone and crying. She learned that this woman had been on a bus trip for senior citizens bound for Branson, Missouri, with her husband of 50 years. They stopped in Valparaiso to have dinner when her husband had a heart attack. Despite the efforts of the ICU staff, he passed away.

She was still in the ICU because she had nowhere else to go. The hospital was making arrangements to get her back to Ohio on a bus, because the seniors' trip had gone on without her the previous night.

After learning this, the nurse immediately told her supervisor that she needed emergency time off. Then she introduced herself to the woman and asked if she would like a ride to Ohio. She called her husband and asked him for directions, because she had never been to Ohio.

On the drive the nurse kept the woman's mind off her husband's death by chatting with her about their families, careers, and lives. The time flew by for both women.

The nurse was surprised when she received thank you cards from the woman and her loved ones. The nurse had only been doing what she would like someone to do if her mother went through something like this.

—Submitted by Donna McHenry, Porter Hospital, Valparaiso, IN

"Never underestimate the difference you can make."

Share Your Own Story

Please share an experience that connected you back to purpose, worthwhile work, and making a difference. You are a big part of what's right in health care!

BY HER SIDE

Working as a social worker on the oncology floor is not always easy. There are times that I feel so impotent that I wish I had divine powers to cure people from the terrible diseases that consume their lives. I was constantly wishing for those powers in the case of one of our patients who I'll call A.G.

For more than two years, I regularly interacted with A.G. at both the Spanish cancer support group that I facilitate, and during her multiple admissions to the hospital. Throughout her illness I provided ongoing support to her and to her young adult children.

I felt a special kinship with A.G. because we had many things in common: we were born in the same country, had the same birthday, and we both shared the goal of achieving the American dream. I knew of A.G.'s struggle to prolong her life; to remain active; to continue being a loving mother and grandmother and a good friend; and above all, to keep a positive attitude so she could encourage other cancer patients to go on and not to lose faith.

Unfortunately, the time that we all feared had come—the time that the disease would win the battle. During her last weeks, A.G. was in pain and confused most of the time. She was bed-bound, cachectic, and her beautiful eyes were like two deep precipices. I dreaded going to see her—it was just too painful. I had no idea what to tell her. How could I tell her that she lost the battle she incessantly

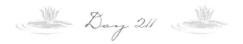

fought, and that her end was close? However, I tried to overcome my emotions, and I continued visiting her almost every day. Even when A.G. was very confused, she would recognize me, call my name, and reach out for my hand. Then I would sit by her side, hold her hand, play some music from our country, talk about foods that she liked so much but was no longer able to eat, and finally we would talk about the "old times." A.G. would always fall asleep with a peaceful smile. It was then when I learned that those moments were more powerful than any morphine or Ativan.

One night, A.G. died in her sleep, and I spent long hours with her family as we all worked on accepting the fact that she was gone. It was hard for everybody, including myself. We all cried and worked hard on understanding that when our bodies give up, our spirit takes a long journey. A journey to a better place, a place in which suffering no longer exists.

—Submitted by Noemi Vidal, St. Joseph Hospital, Orange, CA

"Never underestimate the difference you can make."

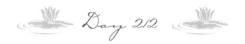

Keeping Time

Recently, one of our Emergency Department nurses, Donna Dellinger, RN, was triaging a patient. The patient, a female, related that she was homeless. Donna proceeded to talk with the patient and asked her if she had any valuables, like a watch, etc.

The lady said to Donna, "No, I don't have a watch, but I'd love to. It's almost impossible to know the correct time, given the way I have to live. Do you know where I could get a watch?"

Donna is a very compassionate person. She left work that day, purchased the patient a watch and had another staff member take it to the patient (who was admitted after her ED visit). Donna did all of this anonymously. She is indeed a very special person and one whom we are so fortunate to have on our staff.

—Submitted by Elaine Haynes,
Carolinas Medical Center-Lincoln, Lincolnton, NC

"Never underestimate the difference you can make."

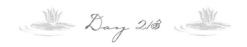
Persistent Care

One day, an elderly patient of mine missed his appointment so I called him to ask if maybe he had forgotten. He explained that he thought the appointment was tomorrow, so I rescheduled him for the next day. Early the next morning the patient called our receptionist and stated that the pharmacist had given him the wrong medication. He asked if we could come over and pick it up and return it to the pharmacist.

I called him when I arrived to work that day. He told me that he had fallen, and he had been up all night because a woman had broken into his apartment. He proceeded to tell me that the woman had then come back and was now sitting on his couch and would not leave. I asked him if he had called the police and he said that he had, but they would not come because they were too busy. I instructed him to tell the woman to leave and the patient did, but he said she refused to go.

It occurred to me then that the woman could have been a home health aide, so I asked to speak with her. The patient said she would not come to the phone. I called the patient's emergency contact person to report the interaction between myself and the patient. Because I still felt uncomfortable with the situation, I also called the landlord to see if she could check on the patient to make sure he wasn't being harmed. The landlord agreed and said she would call after she checked on him.

After arriving at his apartment, the landlord called me back to report. She stated that the patient was still in his pajamas, had toilet paper unrolled all over his house and was introducing her to an imaginary woman. The landlord, together with the patient's relative, assisted in getting him the proper medical attention. He was admitted to the hospital later that day, found to be hallucinating and received a medical work-up to determine the cause. As a result of knowing the patient and persistence in determining what was responsible for his sudden personality changes, I helped him get the proper care he needed.

—Submitted by Theresa Strassberger, Faxton St. Luke's Healthcare, Utica, NY

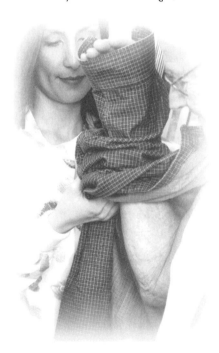

"Never underestimate the difference you can make."

Angel On Your Shoulder

Laurel is an LPN at Southwest Washington Medical Center and is a member of the IV therapy department. One morning during her rounds on the oncology unit she entered a patient's room intending on restarting an outdated IV site. As she introduced herself to the patient she noticed the patient seemed very distressed. Knowing it wasn't the best time to change the IV site, Laurel explained to the patient that she would leave and return at a later time to change the site.

Seeing her patient in such a stressful state, Laurel wanted to do something to brighten her day. She went to the hospital gift shop and purchased a small angel pin. When she returned to the patient's room, she restarted the IV site and then pinned the angel to the patient's gown. Before she left the room, she said to the patient, "You need a little angel on your shoulder today. She will help you get through the day."

Several months later, Laurel was assigned again to the oncology department and entered a patient's room to place an IV site. She was greeted by this patient, who was on a return admission. The patient was excited and happy to see Laurel. She said, "I was hoping to see you during this admission! I want you to know how much your kindness meant to me during my last visit here." She then opened her purse and gave the angel back to Laurel. She asked her to pass it on to the next patient who needed some support. Laurel has been giving angel pins to patients for years now and still does so today.

—Submitted by Debbie Mahoney, Southwest Washington Medical Center, Vancouver, WA

When I Close My Eyes

At Columbus Regional Hospital, our employees often go beyond expectations to show compassion and concern for patients and their families. Bonnie Plummer, Unit-Based Case Manager on Tower 3, became a source of comfort for the family of a man battling cancer.

To help the family have lasting memories, Bonnie took pictures and video of her patient interacting with his family during his last days. She then asked an employee of Holdaway Medical Services (a supplier of oxygen for the hospital) to write a song for the family to go with the pictures and video. This man has been writing poetry for several years and recently began writing music, and he used his talent to compose a song called "When I Close My Eyes" for the family.

Bonnie then created a CD combining the photos, video, and song. She presented a CD to the patient's wife, son, and daughter. The family said the CD was a gift and very uplifting during this difficult time. Due to Bonnie's love and caring, they will always remember their husband and father more dearly. Bonnie's actions demonstrate how our staff members provide an extraordinary level of caring and compassion for those we serve. We salute the exceptional example they set for all of us.

—Submitted by Columbus Regional Hospital, Columbus, IN

Out of the Darkness, Into the Light

A.J. felt life had no meaning until Magee's wheelchair rugby team led him to happiness and a gold medal. His story is one of triumph and of the powerful influence great health care can have in a patient's life. In his case, Magee helped A.J. get back in the game of life in his darkest time.

Following a devastating karate injury in 1994 that caused the then 21-year-old to become a quadriplegic and rely on a wheelchair, A.J. felt as if he had lost everything, from his athletic prowess to his dreams and aspirations. He was the epitome of despair, spending more time in his bedroom than outdoors and not caring about life in general.

The darkness threatened to engulf him for good until an unexpected glimmer of hope appeared. While at Magee, for an outpatient visit a few years ago, he saw a flyer for the hospital's wheelchair rugby program. He decided to try the sport, and the decision changed his life forever. A.J. joined the Magee Eagles in 2002, and the team has given him new confidence, direction, and, most of all, instilled in him a sense of purpose.

His passion for wheelchair rugby also earned him local and national honors. In August, Philadelphia Mayor John Street presented him with a city proclamation for being named to the developmental USA Olympic wheelchair rugby squad. The following month, A.J.'s dream year turned golden when he and his Olympic

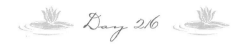

teammates captured the gold medal in Rio de Janeiro, Brazil. A.J. never thought he would be happy again after seven long years. Now it is hard to wipe the smile off this young man's face.

"Wheelchair rugby turned my whole life around and improved my outlook on life," says A.J. "I was excited to be a part of a team, and it opened so many doors for me. I was able to pick myself up off the floor for the first time and do everything on my own. I have so much more confidence. Now, I'm back in school, and I just bought a house."

His happy-go-lucky attitude seemed improbable a decade ago before wheelchair rugby came into his life. When he was admitted into Magee, he thought his best days were behind him. He became a bitter person who did not want to associate with anyone or the outside world.

"My impression of everything was pretty dark," he recalls. "I did not want to be in a wheelchair, I didn't want to talk to others who were in a wheelchair, and I did not want to be seen in a wheelchair. I was very depressed and I didn't feel like an important part of society. I just felt like a burden for others. Being in a wheelchair, I felt like I couldn't do anything."

His perspective soon changed when he witnessed his first rugby practice. He realized that wheelchair athletes were just that—athletes. "It was great to see the team practice," says A.J. "It was a bunch of people in armored chairs banging into each other. It looked like a lot of fun."

A.J.'s excitement about the squad influenced him to drive a month later to watch the players compete in a sectional championship in Warm Springs, Georgia. Soon thereafter, he was on the court himself as part of the Magee Eagles. He experienced some growing pains during his rookie season. He was the slowest player and didn't see much action, but he challenged himself to do better.

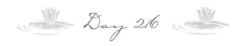

His efforts paid off during his second season as he cracked the starting lineup. His dramatic improvement raised eyebrows among his coaches.

"When one of our speedy guys makes a great play, you can look back to where the play developed and see it all started from an A.J. pick," says Magee Eagles head coach Thomas Hamill, who guided the Eagles to a second-place finish in the 2005 U.S. Quad Rugby Association (USQRA) Division II National Championships in April. "One of our goals as a team this year is to play smarter, to do the little things that can swing two or three extra goals our way. A.J. is one of the best athletes we have for understanding those nuances of the game and making them happen. You can see with A.J. that he's not all about the glory, he's a great team player."

With his confidence soaring, A.J. chose to test his athletic skills against the nation's top wheelchair rugby athletes. Though he didn't qualify for the USA Olympic team, he was invited to try out for Team USA's developmental squad. Competing against players who have been participating in the sport two to three times longer than him, A.J. held his own and was named to the 16-member squad.

"It was an awesome feeling to be selected," he says. "I trained so hard to get to that point. I trained everyday in the off season, pushing five to seven miles a day on Kelly Drive three times a week. It was gratifying to know that I accomplished my goal."

A.J. and the rest of the USA team members headed to South America to realize the rewards of their efforts. Team USA was split into two evenly matched teams, USA Stars and USA Stripes. Both squads battled the world's best, but ultimately squared off against each other in the finals. When the dust settled, A.J.'s USA Stripes team took home the gold medal after defeating the USA Stars, 42-39.

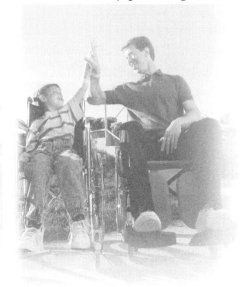

"The trip to Brazil was a blast," says A.J. "I was very proud and honored to represent my country at the World Wheelchair Games. It was a cool feeling when they put the gold medal around my neck. My parents were there watching, and they were very proud. To be considered one of the best in the world at what you do is a great feeling."

A.J. also gets a great feeling helping other wheelchair users. As a member of Magee's volunteer Spinal Cord Injury (SCI) Peer Mentoring Program, he helps lead inpatient groups and conducts one-on-one peer counseling. He listens to patients and empathizes with them as well as educates them on practical tips for performing activities related to daily living and staying healthy.

"It makes me feel good to talk to patients at Magee because I can relate to them," he says. "If I can help incoming patients adjust better, then that makes me proud." Looking back at his darkest hours, A.J. says he is thrilled that he was able to escape and be in the place he is in today. He adds that he couldn't have done it without the support of Magee. "I realize now that I made myself miserable," he says. "My injury had nothing to do with how unhappy I was. I was making myself unhappy and that is what I try to explain to patients at Magee.

"Magee is a special place, but what makes it more special is all the programs and the activities and sports, like wheelchair rugby, that it offers," he adds. "I just feel so lucky to be allowed to do what I'm doing. I am really blessed."

—*Submitted by John Martino, Magee Rehabilitation Hospital, Philadelphia, PA*

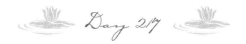

A Walk for Life

When I first started working at Regency of Northwest Indiana, I encountered a moment when a patient's physician wanted him up and walking around the unit. However, the patient was ventilator dependent and no one had taken a ventilator patient out of his or her hospital room before. Luckily, I had had experience with this at a pediatric facility where I had worked previously.

First, I confirmed that the ventilator had a half-hour back-up battery. Then, I found a connection that would work to bleed in oxygen so we could disconnect from wall oxygen, and I let the rehabilitation staff know that the respiratory staff was ready. The patient got up and dressed for his stroll around the halls. Rehab and respiratory worked side by side every day to take this patient for walks and help build up his strength. After a few weeks, he was off the ventilator and continuing his rehab with a trach collar and oxygen tank, then with a cannula and oxygen tank, until the day he was able to walk out of the hospital without oxygen and without assistance.

—Anonymous Contributor, Regency Hospital of Northwest Indiana, East Chicago, IN

"Never underestimate the difference you can make."

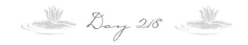

SHIRLEY'S PASSING

One son was very quiet and the other showed every emotion he had ever felt for his mother. He shared her birthday because, being a C-section, she chose to have him on that date. Her husband complemented the daughters in law, one of whom was ready to have a baby any minute. Her son, Steve, apologized for crying and I stood toe-to-toe and cried with him. Again and again, I told them what a wonderful job they were doing and that they would always remember and be proud, as well as forever changed, for the incredible gift of compassion they gave their mother and wife.

The next day, at 8:30 p.m., Shirley died. Her husband called quickly as her respiration slowed. I reassured him that he just needed to sit and hold her hand. He wanted me to come over but she died before I arrived. They were very calm. They told stories and they thanked all the nurses by name, from Katie and Pam, to all the nurses at the infusion center. She called the nurses her angels. He thanked Dr. M., and even tried to comfort him. Then he shared a touching story.

He told how Shirley hoped she would live to see this latest baby born. She didn't know the sex of the baby because they wanted to be surprised. But in the end, the last day, the only person that knew, whispered the sex of the baby into her ear. Her glazed eyes brightened and her final smile appeared. I know that baby will forever know how Grandma loved him or her and how he or she pleased her

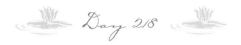

in the last moments of her life. Life goes on and the loved one goes on without them. They give and guide even in their weakest moment and darkest hour.

As I left the family that night, Shirley's son was crying and he gave me that hug that doesn't want to let go. I feel so blessed that they would share these deep, personal feelings so openly. They told me they were certain it wasn't a coincidence that my name was Shirley also.

—*Submitted by Shirley Irby, St. Joseph Health System, Home Health Network, Orange, CA*

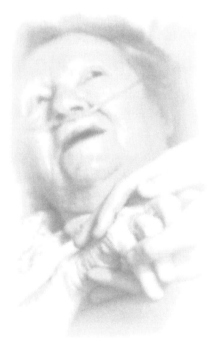

"Never underestimate the difference you can make."

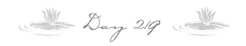

DAY AND NIGHT COMPASSION

*T*here was an outpatient on the Oncology Unit scheduled to receive a chemotherapy infusion after several units of blood overnight. At 2 a.m. the staff on the unit determined that the medication had expired, due to a short stability once mixed, before the patient could complete the transfusions. The BMH Pharmacy did not have enough additional units of the drug available so the nursing staff paged Brian.

Brian responded to the page in the middle of the night, located, and picked up the needed drug that was available at a facility in Indianapolis, then drove to BMH to prepare the infusion, and delivered it to the nursing staff responsible for the outpatient.

"This particular event was just one example of how Brian displays the true heart of an oncology pharmacist," says Dani Williams, RN, manager, Oncology. "The staff greatly appreciates Brian for his sense of compassion towards oncology patients and for his enthusiasm to help provide great care every day."

—Submitted by Dani Williams, Tina Love, and Ellen Keyes,
Ball Memorial Hospital, Inc., Muncie, IN

"Never underestimate the difference you can make."

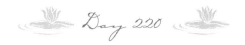

Hold Her Hand

A beautiful nine-year-old little girl was pushing her bike near her house on the crest of a hill. She stepped in front of an oncoming motorcycle, and although the driver tried to swerve and miss her, he hit her straight on.

We received her at 6 p.m. The Code Team on standby that evening was falling apart around me in the chaos that occurred as we tried to stabilize her. She was in full cardiac arrest with massive internal injuries. We worked on her frantically for 10 minutes, at which point I alerted the physicians to bring in her parents to see her.

We weren't sure how her parents, the staff, and administration would react to this. The child did not look good, as her face was extensively injured along with the rest of her body. We prepared her for viewing the best we could, all the while applying compressions and monitoring her status.

Her mother slid down the wall and sat on the floor in complete shock and her father was very distraught. He was immediately drawn to her even in his horror. I encouraged him to speak to her and to hold her hand. Soon both parents were stroking their daughter's hands and talking to her. Our Code Team mourned along with the parents, cried with them and stayed with them as she left this world.

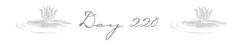

For weeks afterward, I struggled with the decision to bring the parents in for fear that they would only remember how their daughter looked at the end. Three weeks later, the father told a nurse on another floor, "They let me hold her hand."

It is so important for us to let families and friends hold the patients' hands. The power of touch is an unspoken language of love that can make painful transitions more meaningful and special.

—Submitted by Jeanie Flanagan, Claxton-Hepburn Medical Center, Ogdensburg, NY

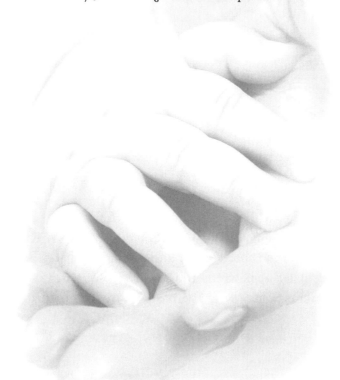

"Never underestimate the difference you can make."

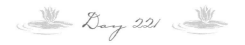

Birthday Brownies

My hat goes off to a great team of people who gave one of our patients a very special, very happy birthday. This team of individuals clearly exhibits our values of teamwork, spirit of serving, and compassionate care.

One morning, I walked into a patient's room, and she just raved about the wonderful surprise she had received for her birthday the day before.

Carrie Urista and Lessie Givens found out from a family member that one of their patients had a birthday that day. They told Chris Fowler, who came to me and asked if we could get a cake from our food service area. I knew the patient was on a gluten-free diet, which meant that he could not have any wheat products such as bread, cake, or any of the usual desserts that a person would normally have on her birthday.

I contacted Kathleen Lipko in food services. Kathleen left the hospital and went to several grocery stores until she found a gluten-free brownie mix. She took the mix to our cook Jose Gonzales who, even though he was very busy, stopped what he was doing and made the brownies.

When they were done, they took the brownies upstairs to 4BT where the nursing staff joined them in singing "Happy Birthday" to our patient. She was thrilled, but none of this could have happened if everyone had not been persistent and followed up. In just one day, these workers were able to achieve what seemed to be an impossible task for a hospital that feeds so many patients and staff. Their efforts really made this day very special for our patient.

—Submitted by Pat Travis, Methodist Health System, Dallas, TX

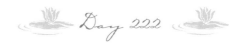

PATRICK AND THE PIANO

I began my career as a physical therapist in New Orleans. There, I spent three years working in a burn unit where I watched patients who had burns covering up to 90 percent of their bodies recover and walk out of the hospital. Needless to say it was extremely rewarding to participate in their rehabilitation.

Then I moved back to my home state of Connecticut where I started working in a sports medicine facility. The change in patient population was quite dramatic and I found myself struggling with whether or not I was truly making a difference in my patients' lives. Sure, I improved a tennis swing or returned an athlete to his respective sport, but I couldn't forget my days in New Orleans and the impact I knew I had been making before.

Enter Patrick, a concert pianist who had sustained a devastating shoulder and arm injury that really jeopardized his career. I worked with him three days a week and continuously encouraged him. I wanted him to believe that he would one day be able to play the piano again. He would remind me often that he needed to have a complete return of shoulder function in order to return to his profession. His physician told him that he would probably never get full motion back.

Every session we would work in a crowded treatment room. I remember him yelling at the top of his lungs to "push harder." I could sense that other patients

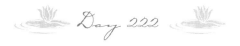

were uncomfortable with his mannerisms. He was definitely a little odd, but the fear in his eyes kept me on a determined path to getting him back to his livelihood and passion—if it was the last thing I ever did. Six months later I discharged him with a 100 percent return in function.

I thought about Patrick a lot. About three months later, I received an invitation to a concert and silent film showing. Here I saw Patrick's extraordinary talent at work. He finished the concert to a standing ovation. I remember how proud I was of the effort he put into getting back to this level.

He invited me backstage after the event. I stayed in the background and watched as so many of his friends and supporters crowded around him. Our eyes met and he waved me over to his side. In the flamboyant manner he did most things in his life, Patrick went on to recognize my efforts in his recovery in a way that touched my heart, even though it embarrassed me a little! Patrick had such a profound effect on my career. He showed me that every day I really do influence the patients that I help.

—Submitted by *Annie Torza Fortnam, Paradise Valley Hospital, Phoenix, AZ*

"Never underestimate the difference you can make."

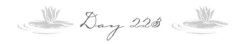

Patrick's Story

The following letter was sent to us by James and Kathleen B., parents of Patrick:

My wife and I are from New York City and we were on vacation at the Lago Mar resort in Fort Lauderdale when my son Patrick became ill. We decided to seek medical attention when Patrick's lethargy and vomiting worsened.

Before leaving the hotel, I asked the doorman where I should take my son. He unequivocally stated that I should go to Joe DiMaggio Children's Hospital even though the drive was a bit longer than the closest hospital.

I drove Patrick to the emergency room at Joe DiMaggio Children's Hospital on April 27. He was judged to be constipated and was released from the E.R. in several hours. The next day, Patrick looked even worse and I took him back to JDCH for re-evaluation. This time, the triage team noticed that Patrick's heart rate was slower than expected. Dr. Stephen Mathew led the E.R. team and we are grateful for his thoroughness. Among the other tests, he ordered a CT scan of the head, which revealed a very large (nearly 8 cm) brain tumor. By the next morning Patrick decompensated clinically, requiring intubation. He also had a seizure. During a long operation by Dr. Ian Heger, the tumor was removed that same day. We are so thankful for his considerable skill.

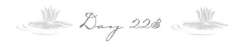

Not only was the surgery a success, but the post-operative care Patrick received was nothing short of outstanding. Patrick was unable to walk or talk for the entire time we were in the hospital. The pediatric ICU team not only provided excellent medical care, but also provided tremendous emotional support to me, my wife, and our other son, James, who was three years old at the time. The Child Life program was of particular help to James. Dr. Theresa Duncan was the team leader for much of our time in the ICU and did an absolutely incredible job. She also displayed tremendous compassion and made us feel at home in South Florida. Dr. Iftikahar Hanif led the oncology team and pointed us in the right direction to pursue chemotherapy back home in New York. His insight, intelligence, and tremendous knowledge of brain tumors were a great help. The nursing staff was uniformly excellent. We had so many incredible nurses over the week we were in the ICU that we regret we can't thank all of them individually. The physical, occupational, and speech therapists were also amazing.

I think that one of the reasons I was so impressed by the quality of care at your hospital is because I am a physician. I have worked in several "Centers of Excellence" in the New York area, but I have honestly not encountered the high level of customer service and attention to detail that seems to pervade JDCH. My experience as a parent at JDCH has made me a better physician.

Patrick has now completed a six-month chemotherapy protocol in New York, including an autologous stem cell transplant, and is doing quite well. His tumor has not relapsed to this point and we remain hopeful for a cure.

—*Submitted by Cindy Friedewald, Joe DiMaggio Children's Hospital, Hollywood, FL*

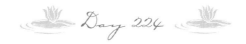

The Letter

A hospital operator received a phone call from a woman who was nearly frantic. Her mother was dying in our hospital. They lived in another state and she could not afford to come to Porter Hospital to see her. The dying woman's granddaughter had written and mailed a letter and the woman expressed concern that there was no one to read the letter to her mother.

The operator assured the caller that the letter would be read because she would go read it herself when she got off her shift.

After her shift was over, the operator went to the patient's room and introduced herself. She told the patient that she understood she had a letter waiting to be read. The patient, who was nearly blind, began to cry. The operator asked if she would like her to read it. The patient said "yes" and asked if she could hold her hand. The operator said, "Of course."

In the letter, the granddaughter told her that she was so sorry she could not be there. She said there was no place she would rather be, but she could not afford to come to Indiana. She said that no matter what happened, she wanted her to know that she was the woman she is today because of the values her grandmother taught her. The letter said that her legacy would live on with her children and that she would never be forgotten. By the end of the letter, both ladies were crying. The patient asked if she could hug the operator, and they held each other and cried. What a gift.

—Submitted by Donna McHenry, Porter Hospital, Valparaiso, IN

Heather the Feather

They called her "Heather the Feather." Weighing in at 15 3/4 ounces on August 29, 1981, Heather was the smallest premature baby to survive at OSF Saint Francis Medical Center in Peoria, Illinois.

She was a challenge for the team of caregivers in neonatal intensive care, to say the least. Dr. Tim Miller headed the unit at the time and back then there was simply no technology available to support such a tiny life. Due to the fact that data on such small babies did not exist, even calculating her chance of survival was difficult.

But Heather proved that she was no lightweight when it came to fighting for her life. Her mother, Cheryl, was told that Heather had zero chance to live. In fact, the doctors didn't know why she lived two hours. She was a fighter.

Recently, Heather's family and caregivers shared many memories with each other and with Heather at a birthday party in honor of her 22nd birthday, which was hosted by Deb Weseloh, a respiratory therapist who became a close friend of Cheryl's after caring for Heather.

Deb vividly remembers the day Heather was born. At the party she recalled how she was there when Heather was carried into the unit and how Dr. Miller brought her over wrapped in blue sterile towels. He told Lois Schleuter, who has since retired but was the charge nurse that day, to just put her in a room and keep an eye on her. Deb went on to say how she was surprised when she saw that

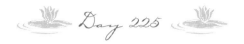

Heather was still there the next day. Then it was two days…and three days…and two weeks. The staff was just so shocked that she lived.

At the reunion, Cheryl Colgan, NICU's clinical educator, also shared her recollections of caring for Heather and talked about how they had Heather on a warmer and how they didn't expect her to live. They had never seen a baby that small—Heather's weight actually dropped as low as 12 ounces and stayed under one pound for a month. They were all fascinated with her.

What the staff lacked in technology they made up for in ingenuity as they came up with innovative ways to care for such a small baby. Everything they did was new.

They had never had one so small, so they just played it by ear. The staff waited to see what would work, and she responded more than they imagined. The nurses started thinking up ways to keep her warm and fix it so they could even weigh her.

Knowing that Heather would need more than the resources they had at their disposal, the people in Heather's corner turned to another source for help. They had prayer chains all over the place.

Throughout Heather's hospitalization, her parents, Cheryl and Walt, had faith in God and the staff caring for their tiny daughter. Cheryl and Walt just lived day by day and did a lot of praying, and it all worked out. Dr. Miller was always two steps ahead of everything. He always anticipated what might happen and got his plan of action ready. He gives most of the credit for Heather's survival to Heather herself.

If love is a factor in the healing process, Heather certainly had that going for her.

Her mother was always so loving toward Heather. The staff spent a lot of time with her mother and noted at the reunion how she was there all the time. She loved baby Heather so dearly. Everybody was rooting this little baby on.

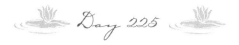

In addition to reminiscences, the partygoers exchanged hugs with the guest of honor and presented her with birthday gifts. They also caught up with what had been happening in the life of this young woman, whose lifelong love for animals had led to a job as an assistant in a veterinarian's office.

The guests also viewed memorabilia related to Heather's hospitalization that her parents had saved and viewed a videotaped segment about Heather that appeared on a television show called *PM Magazine*.

The gathering at Deb's home proves that the expression "out of sight, out of mind" certainly does not apply to the attitude NICU staff have toward a patient. They are concerned about outcomes, not only when a patient is in their care, but even decades later.

—Submitted by Theresa Schieffer, OSF Saint Francis Medical Center, Peoria, IL

"Never underestimate the difference you can make."

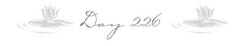

Mr. H

Debbie Buzzard met Mr. H about 34 years ago when she was a new respiratory therapist. He was a frail, elderly Hispanic man in his mid-eighties who suffered from a severe pulmonary disease. He would always request that Debbie be the one to perform his outpatient breathing treatments when he came into the hospital.

One day Mr. H tried to place something in Debbie's pocket during his treatment. Debbie politely informed him she could not accept any gifts from patients. During another visit Mr. H again tried to place an object into her pocket and again Debbie explained to him that she could not accept any gifts from her patients. Finally, one day Mr. H placed his index finger over his lips to shush Debbie's rejection of his gift. He looked up and pointed towards heaven and then he pointed to his heart. "This is between me, God, and you, Debbie," he explained. "I want you to have this gift from me." As he slipped a very old silver dollar into her pocket, he said, "Each time you look at this, you will think of Mr. H."

That was the last time Debbie saw Mr. H. She still has that silver dollar, and Mr. H was right: every time she looks at that gift given to her so many years ago, she remembers the frail, kind gentleman, Mr. H.

—Submitted by Debbie Buzzard and Pat Lucken, St. Mary Medical Center, Long Beach, CA

"Never underestimate the difference you can make."

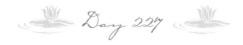

Key Words

A few years ago, when I was working as the clinical manager of the emergency department on our Scottish Rite Campus, I had come in to help supplement a nursing shortage on a particularly busy winter night. We received word that we were getting a very sick six-year-old girl named Taylor from an outlying county. She had suspected bacterial meningicoccemia and was being flown in by a helicopter.

When she arrived, we rushed her into the trauma room and began to treat her. Purpura was blossoming all over her body as we worked. She had lost IV access during the flight and it was critical that we get antibiotics administered as soon as possible. She was going to need to be intubated and rushed to the ICU. In our haste to try and stabilize her, we didn't think about the fact that she was still awake and aware of what was going on. As I was cutting off her clothes, I looked up and our eyes met and she said, "Am I going to die?"

My heart ached. We had been practicing using key words for years. If anyone ever needed an explanation of what was happening to her, it was this little girl, right now. I said, "Taylor, I'm one of your nurses and my name is Marianne. This is your doctor, Dr. Sharna and P.K. is your respiratory therapist who is going to make sure you can breathe. You are very sick right now, but we are going to do everything we can to try to help you get better."

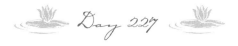

A good deal of the terror left her eyes and she actually said, "Okay." Both Dr. Sharna and P.K. then explained everything they were going to do to this child. We had to sedate and intubate her; then we moved her to the ICU.

Within the hour, the entire family arrived, consisting of seven adults and two more children. We called Infectious Disease and they said that all of them should get a Rocephin shot since they'd been exposed. We were all pediatric nurses but we gowned and administered shots of antibiotics to all seven adults. It was some night for customer service. Even more importantly, Taylor survived and is now a healthy, happy eight-year-old. It's one of those patient stories that I'll never forget and I'll never regret going to help my staff that night.

—Submitted by *Marianne Hatfield, Children's Healthcare of Atlanta, Atlanta, GA*

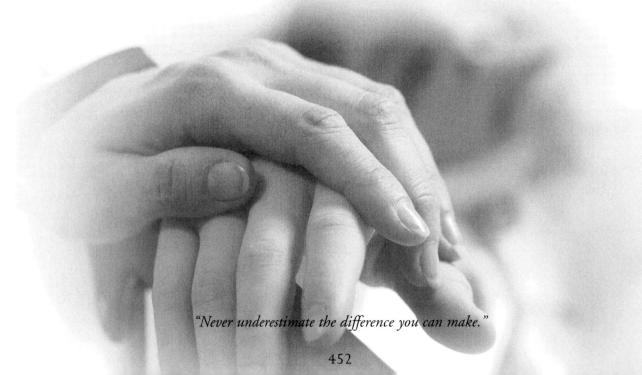

"Never underestimate the difference you can make."

Someone Special

I am a member of the dietary staff at Clark Regional Medical Center, and I met Ms. H in outpatient services when I was a patient myself. She was sitting in a wheelchair waiting for someone to come and pick her up. She was smiling, talking to the nurses, and then she noticed me. She said, "Hi, honey, what are you here for today?" I explained that I was there for a procedure, but I wasn't worried about it.

At this time, Ms. H told me that she was there for her cancer treatment. She did not go into any details but she assured me that I would be fine.

At the time I met Ms. H, I did not realize she was a resident on our transitional care unit. From looking at her, she appeared to be in her 50s, very attractive, and had a faithful heart and hopeful eyes.

One day while doing menu rounds, I was on the TCU. I walked into a resident's room and said, "Good morning." I heard a familiar voice say, "Well, it's good to see you again." From that day forward we became friends. We shared family stories and current events, and she shared with me her strong faith. Ms. H was like sunshine on a rainy day for all of us who knew her.

She often had difficulty with food after her chemo treatments, and food odors made matters worse. Nutritional services tried to go the extra mile for her on good days and by grilling her favorite steaks on Fridays. They made taco salads at her request and even took a trip to Wendy's for an outside hamburger.

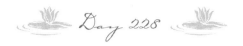

This extra "TLC"—and special attention to Ms. H's meals on the days she could eat—made a huge difference in her care. It really brightened her outlook.

One day I walked into her room and saw her sitting in bed crying, so I sat down beside her, took hold of her hand, and asked her what was wrong. I had never seen her so upset, and it broke my heart when she told me that the cancer had gone to her brain and she didn't know how much longer she would be here. I really didn't know what to say, but I hugged her and told her that it would be okay. She had fought this battle for a long time and could overcome anything. I told her that I would pray for her as she had prayed for me.

A few months later, as the cancer got worse, Ms. H had difficulty recognizing anyone who came into her room. One day I walked into her room and said, "Ms. H, how are you doing today?" She replied, "Hi, honey, I'm doing okay." Then she looked up at me and asked, "Who are you?" I said, "Ms. H, it's Barbara." She told me that she was sorry, that she didn't remember me. I kissed her on the cheek and told her that she was okay.

A few days later, Ms. H passed away. She will always be in my memory. She will always be my friend. I have other friends here at the hospital that I may have to give up sometime. This one was special.

—Submitted by Barbara Hisle, Clark Regional Medical Center, Winchester, KY

"Never underestimate the difference you can make."

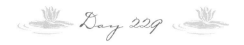

Molly

As a diabetes educator, I deal with all ages…from the very young to the elderly. In dealing with different attitudes and various degrees of compliance, it is suggested that each patient with diabetes attending class have a support person accompany them.

One morning on my daily rounds, I received a call from our pediatrics floor to see Molly, a newly diagnosed patient with type 1 (insulin dependent) diabetes. Upon arrival at the bedside, I faced a very thin, pale, seven-year-old attached to an IV. When I met her, Molly had a very difficult time keeping her eyes open. Her extremely anxious father was sitting beside her, holding her hand. After a few minutes of conversation, he looked at me with tears in his eyes and asked, "Is there something we should have done? Will this diabetes go away?"

Probably the most difficult concept parents of diabetic children must realize is that there is nothing they could have done to prevent the diabetes from occurring. As the child's primary support system, they are forced to quickly accept the situation and be educated in all aspects of the daily intervention required for their child. During the next four days, every available moment was spent teaching Molly's parents insulin technique, glucose monitoring, and food exchanges. We also encouraged them to come to the diabetes class sessions we offer.

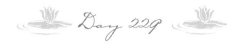

Over the next few days, Molly's condition improved as she became hydrated, was regulated on insulin, and began to regain her weight. During this time, Molly's parents were able to work through some of their fear and anxiety, but seeing these improvements made it all the more difficult for them to accept the fact that she would never be "cured." My constant suggestions for them to attend classes usually resulted in a swift change in conversation. On Friday afternoon I spoke with Molly by herself explaining how very important it was for either or both of her parents to come to class with her. When I left work that day I felt that I had failed Molly.

On Monday morning before breakfast, I went to visit Molly. She looked much better and her eyes seemed to light up as she said, "Someone is going to come to class with me today!" Upon questioning her she responded, "You will be happy."

Monday's class was about to start when Molly charged into the room, tugged at my arm, and pointed toward the door. "Look!" she said. "They are going to help me!" There stood Molly's parents, her sister, her two brothers, and even grandma and grandpa (who has type 2 diabetes). Classes were particularly rewarding that week, as the various family members became actively involved in Molly's health. Molly's sister helped her through an insulin reaction, her mother helped her choose an appropriate lunch, and Molly instructed and demonstrated the use of her glucose meter on her grandpa.

On Thursday afternoon Molly's father stayed after class to speak with me. "We can never thank you enough for being so kind and patient and not giving up on us," he said. "Molly will not be alone; we can all benefit from this improved lifestyle."

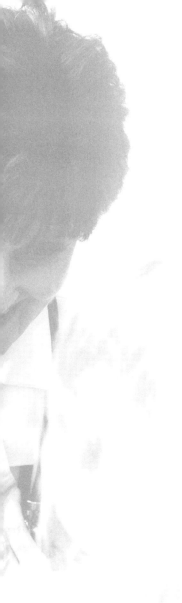

Molly was right…they were all going to help her! We often do not realize how we have touched the lives of another person. The time we spend encouraging and educating our patients and their families may result in some of our most rewarding memories.

—Submitted by Kay Leonhart,
Humility of Mary Health Partners/St. Elizabeth Health Center,
Youngstown, OH

"Never underestimate the difference you can make."

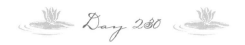

A Good Lesson

As nurses, more often than not, we forget that we are caring for not only our patients, but for their families as well. It is easy to get caught up in the "hustle and bustle" of the day with all of the different situations, issues, and problems that unexpectedly arise. In a perfect world, every nurse would have time to sit with each of his or her patients and spend quality time getting to know them and their families. Unfortunately, we don't live in a perfect world, but this does not mean that we can't try and include the families when discussing the plan of care and help them to understand what is going on with their loved one.

Several months ago, I was at the nurses' station getting a report from a nurse. A visitor came to the desk with a frantic, wide-eyed look on her face and said to the secretary, "Excuse me, but I think my mom's nurse needs to come to her room right now." The secretary proceeded to tell her that the nurse was not around, but that she would page her and send her in. The woman exclaimed, "But I need a nurse now! She was supposed to go home, but I don't think she's ready because she's not doing well." The secretary looked as if she didn't know how to handle the situation and began to mumble something about paging the nurse again.

At this point, the woman's frantic state began to escalate and I overheard her trying to bargain with the secretary while pacing in front of the nursing unit. I came to her and said, "Hi, I am the charge nurse. It sounds like you need some

458

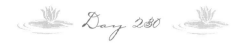

help. Let me go with you to check on your mom." As I stepped in the doorway of the room, I already knew that something was wrong. I could hear the patient breathing in a rapid and struggling manner. I walked in and put her oxygen tubing back in place. Then I cranked it up as high as I could and got on the phone to call the nurses' station. The tele-tech answered, and I immediately told him to send a nurse in STAT. Within seconds about three RNs were there and I told them to grab a non-re-breather oxygen mask and a pulse oximeter. We checked the patient's pulse-ox and it was in the low 80s. I did not need a stethoscope to know that the patient was in distress and was filling up with fluid. I could hear her gasping from where I was standing across the room. I called the operator and paged respiratory therapy to come to the room. I then told the patient's nurse to call the attending doctor and get an order for I.V. Lasix and a Foley catheter and asked if we could transfer her to the unit. She told me the doctor who was seeing her was not on call anymore and had already discharged the patient. I looked at the patient's daughter and I told her, "Look, your mom is in respiratory distress and we have her on as much oxygen as she can possibly be on. We are going to do whatever we can to make sure she is okay. I am going to leave the room for a few minutes and find a doctor to give me some orders. If that doesn't work, I will call a 'code blue' and we'll have all of the help we need. Whatever we have to do, we'll do it."

I went out to the nurses' station and grabbed the first doctor I saw. He just so happened to be the doctor who was on call for the patient's normal doctor.

He told me that he didn't know the patient but asked, "What can I do?" On our way to the room, I told him I thought the patient was in distress and it sounded like she could use some extra I.V. Lasix right away. I asked him if we could get her to the ICU.

He stepped into the room and gave me an order for I.V. Lasix, asked me to put a catheter in, told the respiratory therapist to draw ABG's, and told me to transfer

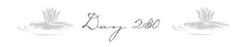

her to the unit. It was exactly what I wanted. I introduced the doctor to the patient's daughter, and she was so relieved at this point that all she could say to the doctor and me was "thank you" over and over again.

Within about five minutes of getting the Lasix on board, her breathing improved and her oxygen saturation level had increased to 93 percent. I went out to speak with the daughter, who was talking to the chaplain and told her that her mom was doing much better and she would be going to the ICU for closer observation. She told me she had mentioned her concerns about her mom to another nurse earlier in the day but that the nurse kind of "brushed her off." She also felt that when she went out to the nurses' station and was having trouble conveying a sense of urgency with the secretary, it was happening all over again. Here she was, having to try and convince someone else that her mother truly was not doing well. She proceeded to tell me that she felt that if I hadn't been there and offered my assistance that her mom might have died. Then she gave me a big hug and kissed my cheek. She said that she believed that God put me in that place at that particular time, because He knew they would need me there. I told her jokingly, "I am not an angel, but I believe that God has a way of knowing what we are going to need and when we will need it." She was so overwhelmed with gratitude that she kept hugging me and even hugged the doctor!

This experience was a wake-up call. It made me remember why I chose to become a nurse, and that, despite the ups and downs, being a nurse really is a rewarding and special part of my life.

—Submitted by Sarah Atchison, St. Joseph Hospital, Orange, CA

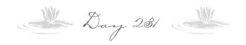

Cookie

ookie Bannon sets an example of Christian love and compassion as she serves people through her role as community representative for Children's Hospital of Illinois and in her personal life.

This talented singer-songwriter uses her gift of music to entertain and comfort hospitalized children and their families and to communicate the message of Children's Hospital to community groups. Cookie's work can best be described as a music ministry. On the surface, it might not seem like *Six Little Ducks, Baby Beluga,* or *Grandma's Featherbed* belong in that category, but they do when performed by Cookie. Before entering a hospital room, she often prays that the Holy Spirit will put the right song in her heart so that she can put a smile on a youngster's face or bring peace to a family.

It is evident that Cookie makes a positive impact on people's lives during trying times, by the fact that they remember her long after that period is over. She is asked to sing at birthdays, weddings, baptisms, and other celebrations. Sadly, she is also called upon to sing at funerals. Despite the fact that she herself grieves when a child dies, she consoles and strengthens families with her comforting words and caring presence to help them find peace.

Whether singing to one patient in a hospital room, or to hundreds of guests in a banquet hall, Cookie connects with her audience. She has a gift for knowing what songs to sing and what anecdotes to tell to touch their lives. In her 23 years

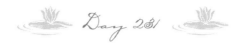
of experience, Cookie has found that music can be an effective form of communication and a powerful tool in the healing process.

Cookie actually began her career as an activity therapy assistant working with adult patients. It was not long, however, before God gave her a "tap on the shoulder," as she puts it, directing her to pediatrics. It immediately became apparent that interacting with pediatric patients was her true calling.

In response to requests from her young patients to record her music so they could continue to listen to it after their discharge from the hospital, Cookie made her first recording, *A Cookie That Sings?*, in 1988. Six other recordings have followed: *A Christmas Cookie, Another Batch from Cookie, Count Your Cookies, Not Your Crumbs, Cookie Live, Always a Child,* and *The Other Side of the Bed.* Proceeds from the recordings benefit Children's Hospital of Illinois.

Cookie's most recent recording, *The Other Side of the Bed,* released in 2003, features 12 of her original compositions and a companion book in which Cookie shares the stories behind the music. (Her first literary effort was a finalist in the 2003 *ForeWord Magazine* Book of the Year Awards. She was inspired to write about experiences from her personal and professional life after her adult son became paralyzed in a car accident in July 2000.)

As she went from her longtime role of caregiver and servant to the unfamiliar role of family member of a critically injured patient, and the person being served, Cookie was overwhelmed by the outpouring of support from everyone—from people whose lives she had somehow touched over the years to strangers moved by her story. *The Other Side of the Bed* is Cookie's thank you to a caring community.

In the following passage from her book, Cookie describes this time in her life, giving the reader insight into the fact that, through the indomitable faith and spirit, she managed to turn adversity into an opportunity for spiritual growth:

"As the days of my life unfolded, never did I believe that I was immune to a catastrophe within my own family. Few escape the devastation on its intrusion, yet through faith, many transform it to triumph. In the blink of an eye, I went from servant to being served. Nothing has humbled me as much. So, with each obstacle balanced by a miracle, the minutes became hours. Surpassing every barricade, we approached a new dawn as the days transformed into months of healing."

Although Cookie has always been empathetic and sympathetic to others' suffering, her experience as the mother of a patient has given her firsthand knowledge of what families she encounters at Children's Hospital are going through. She now realizes more than ever the devastating effect an illness or injury can have on a family.

Cookie's service to others goes beyond music. She genuinely cares that their needs are met in other respects as well. For instance, when a family from out of town had been away from home for an extended period due to a child's hospitalization, Cookie thought that they were probably missing home cooking. So, she prepared a pan of lasagna and a salad and delivered the meal to them at Children's Hospital. Cookie delivered groceries to the home of a family of a dying patient, knowing that their preoccupation with their loved one had kept them from attending to this themselves. Sometime after the young patient's death, Cookie offered to spend the evening with the surviving children so that the parents could have a much-needed "date."

To the countless children and families Cookie has ministered to over the years, she is the embodiment of what's right in health care.

—Submitted by Theresa Schieffer,
Saint Francis Medical Center/Children's Hospital of Illinois, Peoria, IL

"Never underestimate the difference you can make."

CHARLIE'S CHAPLAINS

In 1991, Chaplain Robert Ford approached Pastor Dana "Bubbles" McKim to discuss the possibility of establishing a clown hospital ministry at Frye Regional Medical Center. Chaplain Ford found his inspiration for this idea when he read about a similar ministry that made its visitations on a three-wheeled humor buggy. McKim loved the idea and joined forces with Pastor Danny "Snickers" Leonard to help forge this new adventure. Both Dana and Danny were already involved in clown ministry, and they devised a training program, which trained 45 eager students. Thus was born "Charlie's Chaplains" at Frye Regional Medical Center in Hickory, North Carolina.

"This was a big experiment in creative humor therapy and we had a great time. We didn't have difficulty getting a crowd of people to respond," Danny Leonard explains. "We are just thrilled beyond imagination that something would continue to grow and gain worldwide attention as Charlie's Chaplains has now. The group's mission has always been to do nothing more than to cheer the patients up through a gentle presence as a means of taking the patients' minds off their current health condition or painful situation.

"The goal of Charlie's Chaplains is very simple," Leonard says. "It is about providing a holy interruption, if only for one second. When you enter patients' rooms, if they can forget the situation they're in—it has been a successful experience."

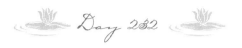
After sixteen years, a new generation of Charlie's Chaplains entertains monthly at FRMC. The group encompasses a number of professional entertainers who donate their services, along with other specially trained community volunteers who offer uplifting performances. The hospital ministry is now a creative ministry, representing several disciplines with the group's talent pool, and was recently featured on the front page of *The Hospital Clown Newsletter*, which is distributed worldwide through paid subscriptions.

Charlie's Chaplains makes rounds to cheer FRMC patients monthly and has a party for the children at the hospital's mental health facility. The group also participates in select community events in tandem with FRMC.

Patients are always our primary focus during visitation. Charlie's Chaplains is comprised of members with varied interests and talents, which adds to the mix when entertaining the patients. We have a well-known professional teen magician, "Magic's Royal Duke Sammy Cortino," who performs simple close-up magic routines. Another seasoned clown juggler, Vince "Zenzel" Ferretti, brings a real air of wonder to our traveling show. Music is an added element to our visits, as one of our professionals is international award-winner: "The Whistling Woman," Phyllis Heil. Several of our members bring along puppets to interact with the patients and their visiting team members.

The rule of the day in rounds is that simple is always best. If the patient is under heavy medication, he or she will not really be able to fully

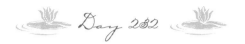

participate or grasp the concept of a long or intricate presentation. We try to notice and consider the patient's condition and alertness.

Analyzing the environment in the room also plays an important role in determining our performance—Are there visitors? What is the mood in the room? Sometimes our gentle presence is enough, with a smile and wave, to brighten a patient's day. Sometimes that is all the energy they may have to take in what we can offer.

We entertain the staff at the nurses' station and in the hallways, as schedule allows. The staff appreciates stress-relieving moments with us. Visitors are often treated to entertainment in the patients' rooms, but sometimes we catch them by surprise in the hallways, waiting rooms, elevators, and lobby.

Over the years, we have had many experiences that have left indelible prints on our collective hearts. The patients, visitors, and staff often tell us how much they enjoy our visits and performances, and sometimes we are even surprised by our patients' reactions to our work. We were all thrilled when a gentleman in his seventies whipped out his harmonica and played us a tune after we sang *Happy Birthday*.

Our clown ministry gives us the opportunity to brighten patients' lives as they experience trying times. We are grateful to be able to collectively heal our community with humor, joy, and love.

—Submitted by Becky Cortino, Frye Regional Medical Center, Hickory, NC

"Never underestimate the difference you can make."

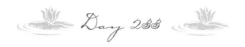

Washing Feet

Being thorough, I remove a holey sock,
to view a diabetic man's filthy feet.
I use the time to complete our talk
of what drove him to live on the street
as I wonder how any of this can help.

While he tells me more of his medical past,
I run warm water into a stainless bowl.
I immerse both his feet, and begin to ask
myself what good it does for this poor soul
to allow himself to undergo this ablution.

Silently I sluice the water between his toes
and soap the crusty callous at his heel.
I marvel at his arch, and notice how closely
it fits my palm. I know he can feel
this proximity too. He shuts his eyes.

Months of useless layers peel away,
revealing layers useless weeks ago.
Removing the tough brown hide of yesterday
yields clean pink skin, but we both know
this ritual will be useless days from now.

Still, this moment may withstand time's test,
teaching us each lessons unknown before.
I learn the medicine of selflessness.
He learns what medicine is really for—
the hope that basin, soap, and touch can bear.

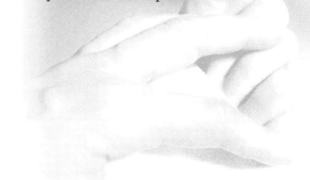

—Submitted by Robert Fawcett M.D., *Associate Director*
York Hospital Family Medicine Residency, York, PA

467

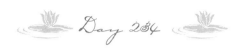

A Tiny Angel

We had a baby who had been a patient for most of his short life. His family was Spanish-speaking and had very limited resources. Near the end of the infant's life, he was transferred to another setting. Unfortunately, soon after, he lost his life. The baby's parents had no resources with which to bury the baby and their religion would not allow cremation.

Our hospital team knew this was the time to do something good for the family. Because I am a social worker, I was able to find a cemetery that would donate a burial plot. Our staff collected enough money to pay for mortuary services and a casket, which was discounted for us.

The main problem we encountered was the issue of transportation. The expense was so high that we could not cover the cost even with donations. So after researching some state laws, two of our nurses volunteered to drive the mother and her baby back in one of their personal cars. The mother held the baby the entire trip and was able to say goodbye with dignity. The way everyone rallied together really made me proud to work in the health care industry, where kindness and compassion really do make a difference!

—Submitted by Dee Mann Aust

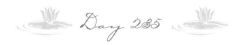

Creative Solutions

*I*n my work, we take care of pediatric dental patients who can't have their dental needs met in a regular office setting. Some have medical issues that put them at a higher health risk, and some have mental challenges such as autism and Down's syndrome that keep them from being treated in an office.

We had one such patient, a 13-year-old girl with autism. She was minimally interactive and was given a "doodle board" to draw on by our child life therapist. She was happiest when someone was next to her, drawing for her. Her father drew for a while but as surgery time approached, the question became, "How do we get our artist into the operating room with the least amount of struggle?"

The anesthesiologist ordered intra-nasal Versed, which required three or four nurses to hold her arms to administer. After ten minutes or so, it became apparent that sedation was not enough to ensure the cooperation needed to have a smooth transition to the OR.

A nurse suggested that we keep drawing with her so she might cooperate more. The nurse climbed into the patient's bed with the "doodle board" and invited the patient to come draw with her. She then put on a hat "like Katie's" and off they went together, both being wheeled in the bed to the operating room.

The anesthesiologist was surprised to see two people instead of just one, but the nurse kept talking and drawing with the patient. The doctor was able to mask

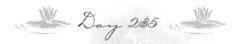

the patient to sleep while she and the nurse next to her continued to draw. The patient was then moved to the OR and the surgery ensued smoothly.

This was a successful process do to the recognition that sometimes we have to be a little flexible and creative in order to ensure a positive outcome.

—Submitted by Cathy Smith, St. Joseph Hospital, Orange, CA

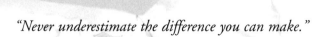

"Never underestimate the difference you can make."

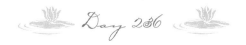

Okay to Let Go

One day I was working in the ICU and we received a report on my patient who was an actively dying and a DNR. I proceeded on with my usual morning routine. I checked my labs, checked my vitals, and completed my a.m. assessment. There was something about this particular patient that made me feel the need to pray. As I gave her a bath, I found myself silently praying. Then I started to talk to her and found her unresponsive. Still, I let her know that I was there and it was okay to relax. I sat in on patient rounds with the charge nurse and found out that this patient had no family.

I went to lunch and when I got back from my break another nurse helped me turn the patient from her right side to her left side. At this point she took a really deep breath. Her heart rate slowed down and her respirations became slower and labored.

I called the chaplain, Frankie, into the room. I didn't want to leave her bedside. Frankie and I held her hand and we reassured her that it was okay to let go. We prayed. It seemed to me like time stood still and there was such a peaceful silence in the room. She passed away within minutes. As I stood there holding one of her hands and caressing her hair, Frankie gently leaned over to me and offered to sit with me if I needed someone to talk to. I felt so full of emotions and so proud to be a nurse. I felt honored to offer myself to the patient at that moment. In what other profession can you offer yourself that fully to another

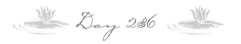

person? I hold all of these emotions in my heart, and I hope that someday when it's my loved one in the bed dying, they will be blessed enough to have a nurse by their side.

—Submitted by Kathryn Cosgrove, St. Joseph Hospital, Orange, CA

"Never underestimate the difference you can make."

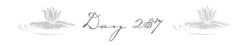

The Reunion

Perhaps one of my most profound experiences as a medical social worker was with Steve and his family. I went to visit Steve soon after his admission to Hospice of Lubbock. In the course of providing information for my psychosocial assessment, Steve related how he had walked away from his family as well as from his "suit and tie" job as a supervisor soon after his divorce 14 years ago. Steve left behind two sons—ages 16 and 18 at the time—never to return.

My thoughts immediately went to his sons. I asked Steve if I could call them to let them know of his current situation. Steve was reluctant and stated, "Maybe in time." I knew that his time was limited. After a few days of thinking about it, Steve allowed me to call his sister, Salese. However, he did not want her to visit because he did not want her telling him what he should do.

Salese was pleased to receive my phone call and later she called one of Steve's sons, Brian. Brian called me to find out more about his dad. Brian, now 30 years old with a daughter of his own, wanted very much to see his dad. Brian explained how he had worked through his anger after his dad left and had come to forgive him. Now, after all these years, he wanted to see his father.

During my next visit with Steve, I told him about my telephone conversation with Salese and Brian. Steve was still not yet ready to see them. However, he was willing to talk to them by telephone.

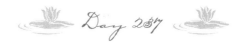

The next time I saw Steve, he appeared very pleased to have talked with Salese and Brian, but was still reluctant to allow them to visit.

Brian called me several times over the course of the next week asking about his dad. Upon my next call from him I was surprised to learn that he was in Lubbock and wanted to meet me at his dad's. I was thrilled! Brian had made the decision to come even without Steve's knowledge. Their reunion was an event that is simply beyond words. They were so happy to see each other!

After catching up on each other's lives, Brian gave his dad three choices. He told Steve that he could either go home with Brian to Houston so Brian could take care of him; he could go with Brian to Houston and stay in a nursing home near Brian; or Brian would stay here in Lubbock and take care of him. Later that day, Steven told Brian that he would go back to Houston with him and stay there.

With a flurry of phone calls, I was able to get Steve transferred to a hospice in Houston and he and Brian were able to leave the next day.

While Steve's other son, Mark, chose not to see his father, he did talk with him by phone.

Steve died ten days after arriving in Houston with Brian and his family at his side. Not long after Steve's death, I received the following notes from Brian and Salese:

Dear Linda,

Thank you for caring and your sincere devotion to our family and Steve. Because of your strength and thoughtfulness, Steven experienced a closure with his boys and me. We were able to say our goodbyes and renew our relationships. I have wonderful memories of our childhood, as

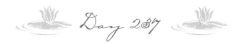
does Steven. You were able to give Steven dignity after he had apparently gone through some bad times in his life. But now that is all behind us and our family has reconnected, thanks to you. You are a very special person!

> Thank you,
> Salese

Linda,

There is no way that I could put in words what a difference you have made on my dad's and my life. A simple phone call and a ton of extra effort from you have made me a better and happier person. My dad was able to pass with someone who truly loved him. How do you repay something like that? And then it hit me…you are an "angel" sent from God to help people and you will be rewarded someday. You gave me the opportunity to mend a deep hole in my heart before it was too late! I do hope that you will stay in touch and I will email you pictures of my family so you can see the lives you've touched!

> Thank you. You are my "Angel!"
> Love,
> Brian

—*Submitted by Linda Cook, Hospice of Lubbock, Lubbock, TX*

"Never underestimate the difference you can make."

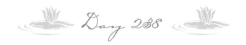

Finding Home

When a patient at OSF Saint Francis Center for Health in Peoria, Illinois, mentioned his poor living conditions to a nurse, he got far more than a sympathetic ear. That casual conversation became the catalyst for a major change in his life, thanks to the concern, compassion, determination, and benevolence of the caregiver.

"I was admitting this patient for cataract surgery, and it takes about 45 to 50 minutes to do that, so we had an opportunity to talk," explained the nurse, Kim Morris, who works in pre-post surgery. "This guy just seemed to kind of have a rough life. He gives a lot to the community as a social worker who counsels troubled teens. He works long hours with them, just giving, giving, giving, and then he had to go home to a rough home environment."

The neighborhood where the middle-aged patient lived was noisy, unsafe, and populated mainly by young people, according to Kim. The patient said that he had been attacked near his home.

"It just wasn't a good situation," Kim said. "But because of his poor vision, he wasn't extremely motivated to get out and look for a new place to live. It bothered me that he had to go home at the end of the day and be concerned for his well-being."

When the patient learned that Kim lives in West Peoria, he expressed that he would like to live there because it is a nice area and it is near his place of

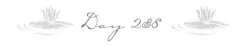

employment. Kim offered to be on the lookout for available rental units while jogging through the area. The patient appreciated the offer and gave her his phone number.

"Sure enough, within a month I found a little house that became available," Kim says. "The previous tenant had lived there 30 years. It was well maintained and in a quiet area. I thought it would just be perfect for him, and that he would fit in well there."

But they weren't home free quite yet. When Kim contacted the landlord and said she was calling on behalf of "a very nice man in desperate need of a new place," the landlord told her that he prefers to rent to older women because it has been his experience that they are the best tenants. Kim said, "What can I do to make this happen?"

Because appealing to the landlord's humanitarianism didn't seem to be working, she decided to try the practical approach. Knowing that the house was in need of painting and cleaning, Kim offered to do this work if the landlord agreed to rent the house to the patient. Deal.

Kim added some other touches, such as window treatments, to help turn the house into a comfortable, attractive home for her patient. Her coworkers also donated some furniture and household items. Kim and her husband also helped the patient move his belongings.

The patient got more than a new place to live; he has formed friendships with the other tenants in the small housing complex.

"They've all become good friends," Kim reports. "It has given him kind of a little family, too. I couldn't be happier about the outcome. It worked out really well. It has been life-changing for him! Just moving a few miles from where he was put him in such a better position."

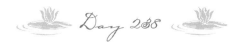
Kim is hesitant to accept praise for her good deed, insisting that anyone in her position would have done the same thing for the patient.

"It's just one of those things," she says. "I was in the right place at the right time, and he spoke to the right person who knows the area. I was surprised at how it all fell into place. It makes you feel good to know you can make such a positive change in someone's life by doing something so simple."

—Submitted by Theresa Schieffer, OSF Saint Francis Medical Center, Peoria, IL

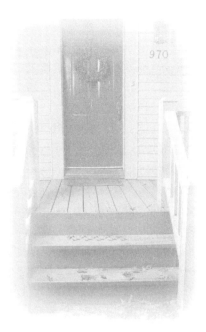

"Never underestimate the difference you can make."

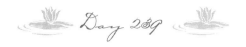

Friends in a Day, Friends Forever

I keep the precious, original, tattered piece of paper laminated on my clipboard as a memoir to my "Friend in a Day, Friend Forever" Lisa. It has my mindless doodles on it, a coffee mug stain, and slurred print, but it also has the treasures from Lisa's last day. That little scrap reminds me of the afternoon before she died when we talked for hours. Feeling something significant happening, I tried hard to scribble as many of her gems down as I could. I felt the need to take in whatever she said and she had an urgent need to talk.

We began our friendship the day she called the hospice's "on call" service and I was the nurse on duty. Though we had not yet admitted her to our service, she wanted advice on making a decision to go to the hospital to be hydrated. She knew this was a temporary fix to help her feel well enough to return home to see her three young children, the youngest of whom was only five. She wanted to be there for their first day of school. I applauded her decision to go. This was a tough choice to make, because I believe she knew in her gut that she would not be returning home, ever again. I tried to imagine the searing agony of a 33-year-old mother leaving home, knowing she may never be able to soothe her babies, tuck them in, feed them, or see them to the bus on the first day of school.

Once admitted to the hospital, Lisa called me many times during my shift. It was hard for her to be alone when her family needed to leave for any amount of time. I happily spent this precious time with her for I knew I was talking with a

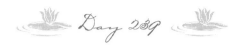

very dear and important person who would soon die. I am so grateful I was "on call" this day.

Our conversation flowed easily, sometimes gaily, only occasionally solemnly, as we spoke of what was most important to us. We laughed about our similarities that included very close birthdays and our love for the color blue. We share an insane love for animals and concern for the environment so we made up a song together about trying to save them. She told me her favorite prayers and I told her mine. I told her of other patients' journeys, their prayers, and what was said at some of their funerals. She spoke of her deep love and concern for her children. She told me that just that morning her youngest was sad having to leave with her dad, so Lisa wrapped her in her own, big sweater to comfort her. She felt an enormous sadness for them.

Something was happening to us while we talked. After some time on the phone, I felt as if it was more than Lisa's voice, but rather some force reminding me of things I had so easily forgotten. The phone call started to transport me and I believe Lisa was feeling this strength as well. We were on fire, feeling so energized by our connection. I started to feel that maybe I was getting more from this conversation than was fair.

I was so curious about how she managed the enormity of her disease. I asked Lisa how she managed the pain of saying goodbye to her children and husband and how she proceeded through years of chemotherapy and being desperately ill. Quoting from my scribble, she said, "Sometimes you have to go ahead like a soldier." I'll never forget that one. She also said, "If I didn't believe in God, I never would have made it this far." Our conversation centered on her faith and how it helped her march on.

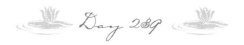

"Dear God, the river is so wide and my boat is so small. Please help me," was another prayer she loved. I asked her about anger. She said, "I was mad. I was upset. Then I began to think about what it is when you have a gift. Do you say, 'It's not good enough'? God gave me this day. How can I complain about His gift?" I hope I won't forget that one either.

I asked her about her fear. She said, "I'm not afraid because I've been so sick." I hear similar feelings from my other patients of having had enough. They are exhausted by illness and sorrow, and they become ready to leave it behind. They begin to believe in something better, and start to surrender to it. Lisa had complete faith in God that she was going somewhere wonderful.

As Lisa and I drifted in her wee boat on the wide river of conversation, we created a friendship. I picked up her oars and rowed awhile. I told her I wanted to write her story down, along with other hospice patients' stories, and she, in the most emphatic tone she could muster, told me to entitle the book, "Friends in a Day, Friends Forever." This became our mantra during the succeeding phone calls. She wanted her story told to others who might find strength in it, so that her story could help them across their own river. I believe Lisa and I connected for this reason. I needed to hear her incredible messages and we both needed to pass them along to as many people as possible. Knowing I would be sharing her story gave her hope that she would not be forgotten so fast. We are all afraid of being erased prematurely from people's memories. Lisa's words would keep her memory alive.

Lisa's last words on the phone were prayers for me, not herself. Her very final words to me were, "God bless you, Peggy," and then she thanked me for being her "Friend in a Day." She was a spigot flowing with good energy and love, and it seemed she was going to keep it open as long as she could.

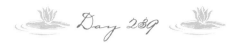

Later that night Lisa began to hemorrhage and flowed in and out of consciousness—her life force becoming a mere trickle. Her family was with her, her oldest daughter wiping her forehead as she died. The next morning her mother called to tell me she died and to say Lisa mentioned me in her last conscious hours. "Mom, tell Peg it's really okay. It's good. I am okay."

I thought *Man, she is still giving.* I wrapped her sweater of warm words around my own shoulders. My friend I never saw is gone from this realm, but she is in my heart forever and I feel her presence. I felt keenly aware of her while I wrote this.

Thank you so much, Lisa, for the power behind your words and your message of love and gratitude despite adversity. Because of you, our boats are a bit bigger and the river not so wide.

—Submitted by Margaret Crawford, Cranberry Hospice, Plymouth, MA

"Never underestimate the difference you can make."

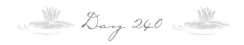

Serving God's People

Each day in the emergency department is different. But from the beginning of the day until the end, a whirlwind of excitement, stress, and contentment are common emotions that I feel. Each day this reminds me of why I wanted to become a nurse. I may move from stress one minute to joy the next. Sometimes just a smile from one of my patients is enough to make me say a little prayer of thanks to God for giving me such a wonderful opportunity to serve His people. There is one particular day that sticks out in my mind.

It was already a busy morning. I was caring for a critical patient in one of the rooms when I looked out and saw that the paramedics were placing a critically ill man into the next monitored room. It was one of those moments when your heart drops. The patient didn't even look alive. I watched for any sort of recognition, eye movement, or sign of breathing…anything, when I finally saw his eyes turn slightly to look at me. It was at that moment that I knew in my heart that everything was going to be okay.

I quickly began to care for this elderly gentleman and initiated treatment. After lab work, intravenous fluids, and a CAT scan of his head, it was determined that he was anemic and suffering internal bleeding. I had cared for people with this diagnosis before, but what struck me as special about this patient was the dynamic held with his family.

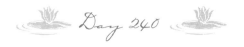

His wife had joined him approximately 15 minutes after he arrived. In apparent distress, she sobbed for her "amour," her love, her husband. She cried out to him over and over, "Don't leave me!" My heart wrenched in pain for this woman, and at this point I realized that my role as a nurse was now to not only care for the emotional and spiritual aspects of the patient, but for this family member as well. After the patient's clinical care, I pulled up a chair for her, prayed with her, and explained everything I could to her, medically, about the situation. I explained the meaning of his vitals, the meaning of the doctor's reports, and did anything else I could to make her understand and calm her down.

Soon after, I began the blood infusion, per the doctor's order. This plus the fluid bolus improved the patient's circulation and vitals. Finally he acquired a more lively level of consciousness. After a short while, the patient was able to verbalize, all of which didn't make sense, but it was still a good sign.

I tried to make his wife see his improved vitals and speech as a good sign, but she was still very distressed by his deteriorated health. She couldn't understand that she wasn't going to lose him at that moment. As she cried, she told me the best day of her life was the day she met him. She proceeded to tell me how they had met and what a wonderful husband he was. She repeatedly told me, "He always honored me and loved me so much." She told me that they would be married for 50 years in December.

Just before this gentleman was transferred from the emergency room to the CCU, he was able to recognize his wife. I proudly transferred this patient and his wife to his new bed on the floor. I only hoped that they would touch the life of another the way that they touched mine.

Although his normal baseline of mental status was yet to return, I still believe that the nursing care I provided, and his wife's love and the spiritual domains that

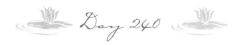

encompassed the entire event, were the reasons that I saw such improvement in this patient.

This story will never leave my mind. The fact that I was able to physically and spiritually care for this patient, so he and his wife could continue on in their love, makes me so proud of the work that I do. This is the type of day that brings me a sense of accomplishment and contentment with my work. I smile to myself and once again say a little prayer of thanks to God for giving me such a wonderful opportunity to serve His people.

—Submitted by Anna Morris, St. Joseph Hospital, Orange, CA

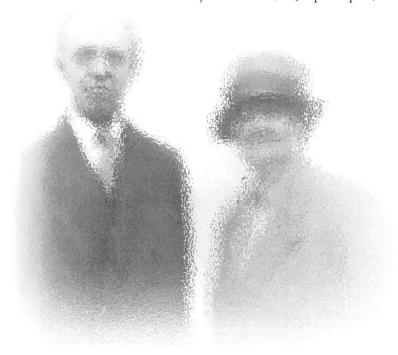

"Never underestimate the difference you can make."

Share Your Own Story

Please share an experience that connected you back to purpose, worthwhile work, and making a difference. You are a big part of what's right in health care!

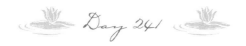

Unexpected Miracle

It was June 14th, 2005. I wasn't teaching my usual childbirth education class that evening, because I was on low census. Still, I was at Sherman working on the computer for Julie Kane, our Nurse Systems Analyst. I finished at about 9:15 p.m. and walked out to the parking garage to leave when I heard someone yelling "There is a woman having a baby in the front of the hospital!" I hurried out, thinking that I would simply escort the woman into the hospital and up to Labor and Delivery, as the main entrance doors were all locked because it was so late at night.

When I walked around the corner from the garage to the front of the hospital, I couldn't believe what was happening. There was a woman lying on the ground in the grass and a couple of people standing by helplessly watching. One woman finally called 911 on her cell phone.

I knelt down by the woman on the ground and recognized the look on her face: she was pushing. I asked her not to push and she looked at me as if to say, "I can't help it."

I thought that I had better see what was going on with her so I lowered her pants enough to see that there was a baby being born. The head of the baby was already out and I had no idea how long the baby had been in this situation.

Now, I am an RN, and I have L&D experience from years ago, but I had never been in a situation like this before. I was outside in the dark with very little light

487

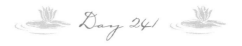

from the garden lamps, with no gloves, no bulb syringe to suction the baby, and no blankets for warmth in the cool June night air. I looked up and silently prayed, *God, it's you and me.* I gently reached around the baby's head to see if the cord was around the neck. It wasn't. I could hear the baby's father saying, "Baby gonna die! Baby gonna die!" I thought to myself, *Not if I can help it.*

There was a new baby blanket in the woman's bag and I slipped it under her hips. I then encouraged the woman to push, and I applied some gentle traction to help ease the shoulders out. A few pushes later, the baby was born. Someone handed me a shirt to wrap around the baby. I dried the baby and stimulated it until I heard a cry. I didn't even know the sex yet. I was just so relieved to hear that tiny cry. It was all I could do to hold the baby and hold pressure on the umbilical cord until help arrived. I finally managed to raise the baby up to see what sex it was. He was a little boy.

The paramedics arrived. Someone had called the L&D unit and it seemed they all arrived at once. I thanked God once again.

We took the baby up to the Special Care Nursery in the warmer the L&D nurses brought down with them. He was fine. I went to see the mom after washing up in the nursery. The doctor was repairing a tear to her perineum that occurred during her pushing. She had leaves and twigs on her head from lying on the ground. She smiled at me and I assured her that her baby was doing well.

Later, I found out that this was this woman's fourth baby. Her husband had dropped her off at the front door so she wouldn't have to walk from the parking lot. He didn't realize that the doors were locked after 8:30 p.m. for security and that the Emergency Room was on the other side of the hospital. I also found out that the mom had some complications with high blood pressure during her pregnancy, which thankfully seemed to be under control. God was certainly with us all that night.

—Submitted by Claudette Wagner, Sherman Hospital, Elgin, IL

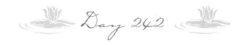

Sincere Care

Our hospital received this heartfelt letter from a patient:

I sit here at home looking out the window, gazing at the new fallen snow, reflecting on my whole experience with the team at Saint Mary's Healthcare before, during, and after the surgery I had on January 9th. I have repeatedly told others with praise about the wonderful care and genuine concern I have felt from all of you at your office…words cannot describe how wonderful and safe I felt in your hands and care. In today's world, it is a rarity.

My past surgery experience back in 1995 had me scared and worried. That was the most horrible hospital experience you could ever imagine.

I have to say *thank you* for all this team has done for me. My doctor was so gentle and kind, and all the while he made me feel secure. Even the doctor's assistant in surgery, Teri, was so concerned for my wellbeing. She bestowed such kind words upon me and was absolutely wonderful. Darla, who spoke to me over the phone was so understanding with my many questions. She was so gentle with me and I could feel her smile even over the telephone.

I realize this is just everyday business for everyone I have mentioned, but what they do daily really impacts people. It has impressed me so much that I have been contemplating a career change. My passion and gifts include the ability to bestow mercy and compassion. Who knows, someday I too may be able to give back what has been so graciously given to me…just honest, sincere care.

A Grateful Patient

—Submitted by John Bremer, Saint Mary's Healthcare, Grand Rapids, MI

"Never underestimate the difference you can make."

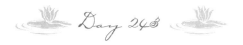

Family First

Social worker Shawna Smith is one of those rare individuals who can look at a total stranger and see him as a brother, worthy of compassionate service and genuine love. That's what happened when she met Jake and Otis.

Jake, a Hurricane Katrina evacuee in his 80s, had lost his two grown children and his bed-bound wife. Otis, another evacuee, was a recent stroke victim in his 30s who couldn't speak or walk. Though she credits her co-workers with so much, Shawna virtually adopted these new residents, going far beyond the call of duty to help them.

For instance, she worked diligently to locate and identify the bodies of Jake's family so that a memorial service could be held at a local church. She and her family drove him to Meridian, Mississippi to live with his niece. Shawna also worked to reunite Otis with his estranged family, flying all night in a cargo plane to accompany him.

"Now I have family there," says Shawna. They will always be a part of me."

—Submitted by Maria Macras, WellStar Paulding Nursing Center, Dallas, GA

"Never underestimate the difference you can make."

MORE LIKE HOME

At Mercy Clermont and Anderson, we have what we call "The Angel Cart." It is stocked with items that are intended to comfort a patient at the end of life. There are CDs of quiet music, tissues, and spiritual readings. And each dying patient is covered with a beautiful quilt or afghan, made by the fingers of "angels," which are a group of our community volunteers. Their quilts and afghans make the hospital room seem more like home, bringing comfort to the family and to the patient.

Recently, one of our chaplains was working with a family at the bedside of a patient as she slipped into the dying process. She placed an afghan on the bed and put a CD of Bluegrass Gospel Music into the CD player. The family remarked, "This is perfect. Mom grew up in Eastern Kentucky and she was always making things for others. The afghan and the music suit her just right."

The family gathered around the bed for prayer. At the very moment she took her final breath, a Bluegrass version of The Lord's Prayer was heard. The family grew silent as the prayer ended. On the "amen," tears began to fall as the prayer brought home the realization that God was calling his child home.

Also present was a neighbor of many years who watched over their mom every day. The family unanimously decided to give the afghan to her. She had spent a great deal of time caring for the patient during her final days, in the same way that their mom had always cared for others.

—Submitted by Marty Hoffman, Mercy Hospital, Clermont, Batavia, OH

"Never underestimate the difference you can make."

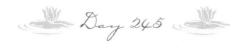

A Flute Was His Only Wish

*B*eing hospitalized during the holidays is tough. It really increases a patient's levels of anxiety, stress and loneliness. That's why our hospital came up with a "Holiday Giving Adopt a Patient Program"—a program that, among other things, allows each patient to create a wish list of gifts that they would be interested in receiving.

One patient in particular benefited from the program. He was a middle-aged man named Jim who told the Patient Access staff who chose him that what he really wanted was a flute. The staffers told him that unfortunately, a flute was pretty expensive, and they did not believe they could fulfill his wish because of the instrument's cost. Instead, they suggested gifts of clothing, pajamas, or toiletries that would be useful while on the unit. They even asked if he would like some candy or fruit as a special treat with his gift.

The patient expressed gratitude for their offer but said that a flute was his only wish. He smiled and said, "Have any of you ever been to a pawn shop? You could probably find a used flute there, really cheap." He went on to tell them how he played the flute many years ago until the debilitating symptoms of his illness kept him from being able to focus on his music. He said that with the care he had received in the hospital he felt he was becoming more stable and was ready to play again.

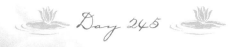

Wanda Cummings, MSW, the Director of Behavioral Health Therapy, reported, "The most heartwarming part of the holiday party was when the Patient Access staff presented Jim with a pair of pajamas, t-shirts, socks, and a beautifully wrapped basket of fruit and candy. He graciously thanked the staff for their gifts, but dropped his head in disappointment because he didn't get the flute he really wanted. Then a staff member left the room and returned to lay a small case on Jim's lap. He looked at the case, raised his head, and began to cry. He stared at the case in amazement and with tears streaming down his face, said, 'I can't believe it, I really got a flute, a real flute.' There wasn't a dry eye in the room."

It seemed as if time stopped; the entire room was silent. Then he got up, hugged everyone in the room and then proceeded to play a beautiful Christmas song. To everyone's amazement, he seemed to be an accomplished musician. To meet his wish the Patient Access Staff had gone out to pawn shops all over the Philadelphia area to find a flute for him. Each contributed money to make his dream come true.

Wanda said, "The feeling of warmth and good will that was palpable throughout the room continues in the hospital today."

She summed up the experience by recalling a comment she overheard from a staff member: "This is a moment I will cherish forever; I have a warm feeling in my heart after seeing how happy we've made the patients today. It has to be the best Christmas gift I have ever received. This is what Christmas is all about."

—Submitted by Doris Quiles, Temple University Hospital/Episcopal Campus, Philadelphia, PA

"Never underestimate the difference you can make."

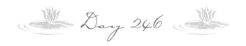

A CINDERELLA STORY

*I*t was afternoon when Hannah arrived in Orlando, Florida. She had flown from her home with her mom, her dad, and her brothers and sisters. Only one thing was on all of their minds: to make her dream come true. With the help of the Make-A-Wish foundation, the little girl, who had been battling cancer, had come to see her heroine…Cinderella.

The family's excitement built as they stayed at Give Kids the World Village, a non-profit resort for children like Hannah who are battling life-threatening diseases. Hannah's brothers and sister went with her dad to Universal Studios for a day of fun, but Hannah wanted to stay in and rest for her upcoming visit with Cinderella at Disney World—a visit scheduled for Friday morning.

Unfortunately, on Thursday afternoon, Hannah took a turn for the worse. An ambulance transported her to the Emergency Department at Orlando Regional Medical Center. No one thought she would make it longer than an hour.

The young, frail girl lay in bed, her parents looking at their unresponsive daughter. They were not prepared for this. *She was supposed to see Cinderella. The cancer was not supposed to win. She was supposed to live to see at least that dream come true.* Tears streamed down their faces as nurses in the ED cared for their daughter.

The ED bustled with activity. Everyone was busy, even more so than normal. Kim Hogan, assistant nurse manager, went to see if she could offer any assistance before going home for the evening. She checked with Hannah's nurse, Emily

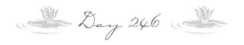

Marcella, who was updating Ann Marie Wood, another nurse, on Hannah's situation. "Hannah had been totally unresponsive, and now she is alert and even asking for chocolate milk," she shared. They were all excited about the young girl's improvement.

"Can you ask the parents if they would like us to try to get Cinderella to come here?" Kim suggested to the nurses. Emily shook her head "No," tears spilling from her eyes even at the thought of asking them. "I will just cry," she admitted. She had already become emotionally connected to the family. Ann Marie offered to pose the question.

"If you can, that would be great," Hannah's mother responded to the offer. Just like the mice in the Cinderella story, the team members of the ED worked to make Hannah's dream come true.

Kim placed a call to a friend asking if he could pull some strings to get Cinderella to ORMC that night. That set the Disney magic into motion. Characters covered for each other, even staying late, to allow Cinderella to leave. Within five minutes, Kim received word that Cinderella was on her way.

The staff scurried around, still caring for all the patients in the hectic ED, making sure they pulled all the curtains and closed all the doors so Cinderella could slip in unnoticed for her special visit with Hannah.

Carrie Lavrich, unit secretary, called Make-A-Wish and arranged for them to bring Hannah's older siblings to join Hannah in seeing her dream come true.

Bryan Draper, advanced clinical tech, raced to the gift shop to purchase a couple disposable cameras to capture the moment. And Tina Hunter, teenage volunteer coordinator, brought over a digital camera with video capabilities.

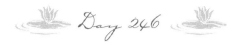

The team members transferred Hannah into a bigger room to better accommodate her family. And just like in the movie, just in time, all the preparations were finished. And in walked Cinderella.

For the next hour, the little girl who barely clung to life lived her dream. Cinderella talked to her. She held her hand and gently rubbed it. She smiled and laughed. It was like a fairytale. "She never missed a beat. She stayed in character the entire time. No matter what Hannah said, she related to it as Cinderella," says Kim with fresh tears.

"Mommy, we can turn the Cinderella movie off now," said Hannah, whose eyes were exceptionally sensitive to the lights. Cinderella left the room with tears brimming in her eyes. "You just don't know what this will be to us. The closure you have provided," her father told the ED staff.

Hannah's battle with cancer ended the following day.

"This is one of those moments you hold onto forever. It really touched us all," says Kim. "We could not save her life, but we helped make her dream come true."

—Submitted by Mary Tomlinson, Orlando Regional Healthcare, Windemere, FL

"Never underestimate the difference you can make."

BEYOND THE CALL OF DUTY

O n January 20, 2007, a man was jogging with a group of people from the YMCA near our hospital, Deaconess. The man, who was trying to complete his jog with friends, began complaining of cramps. Suddenly he stopped, grabbed a street sign, and fell.

Officer Hoover, of Deaconess EPD, was off-duty when he observed a group of people standing around the man. When he reached the group, he saw that Sarah Craft, Deaconess RN on unit 5100, was already on the scene. The man was breathing and 911 had been contacted. However, before an ambulance arrived, the man stopped breathing. Knowing that they needed to act fast in order to save the man's life, Sarah Craft and Officer Hoover gently rolled the man over. They found that he didn't have a pulse. Working together, they began to administer CPR. After performing CPR for several minutes they were able to get a pulse. The man was then transported to Deaconess Hospital.

Sergeant Guenin, of the EPD, spoke with the physician who stated that the man would have died if Officer Hoover and Sarah Craft had not taken action.

Officer Hoover and Sarah Craft saved the life of this man. Their preparation and willingness to act is commendable, and their efforts should be recognized. Officer Hoover has been recommended to receive a Merit Award. And Sarah Craft has been recommended to receive a Citizen's Award.

—Submitted by Kathy Clodfelter, Deaconess Health System, Evansville, IN

"Never underestimate the difference you can make."

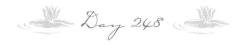

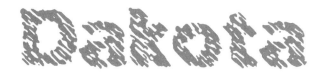

The family member of a patient shared the following story with our hospital:

My boyfriend and I came into the Pediatric ER on Saturday May 13, 2006, with his son, Dakota, who had a broken arm. The staff at the hospital made the situation bearable. From the moment we walked through the doors, the security guards were pleasant and the administrator was all smiles. They made all of us feel so calm.

We went right into the ER. Eddie was our nurse. He was so attentive to all of Dakota's needs and our needs as well. Then we met Dr. Haynes. My goodness, how wonderful to be around a doctor who laughs and smiles when your son is scared! We never felt like we were forgotten. Anything we asked for, they were right there to help with. Even Andrew, who was, I believe in Maintenance, was amazing! He saw me shivering and brought me a warm blanket, then a chair so I could sit down while they were setting Dakota's arm. Thank goodness Dr. Haynes and Eddie were able to set the bone and keep Dakota from needing surgery.

I do not know the names of everyone we came in contact with, but they were all wonderful. I think nowadays when you come across people who are there not just for the job but for the rewards and the people they serve, they should be applauded!

—*Anonymous Contributor, Joe DiMaggio Children's Hospital, Hollywood, FL*

At Home in a Foreign Land

As a young woman entered the front doors of Orlando Regional South Seminole Hospital, guest services representative Isabel Taylor immediately noticed her swollen abdomen. She could tell that it would not be long before this young woman was ready to deliver. The woman looked around nervously, obviously unfamiliar with the hospital. "She's scared," thought Isabel as she began moving toward her to offer her assistance.

"Seeing someone look so scared breaks my heart," she shares. "I just want to say, I'll take care of you. Don't worry."

The young woman, Maryela, began saying in Spanish that she was new from South America and was afraid to deliver her child in a strange country. "I could not help but see myself in her," Isabel shares. "It was not that long ago that I came here from Spain."

It has not been long since Isabel found herself in the Orlando airport, with two small children and her only suitcase stolen. Getting started in America was difficult. "I remember the first Christmas," she recalls. "I hadn't any money to buy presents for my children. However, just before Christmas I received a call from CNL saying they had adopted my family. They brought food for a wonderful meal and presents for my kids. To this day, it is my most cherished Christmas. I thought that day, 'One day, I want to help someone else like everyone has helped me.'"

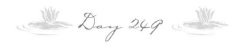

Though Isabel often acts as a translator or helps others navigate South Seminole Hospital, she had an immediate connection with Maryela. She escorted her to Admitting and helped her pre-register for the upcoming birth. Understanding the anxiety of being in a new country, Isabel gave her cell phone and home numbers for Maryela to use to contact her if she was at the hospital or needed help with translation. "I wanted her to enjoy the birth of her child and not feel anxious about being in a new country," Isabel shares.

When the time came to deliver, Maryela called. "Will you please join me?" she asked. Isabel returned to the hospital and stood by her side through the entire process. She acted as a translator and brought confidence to Maryela and the South Seminole Hospital team. "I have been more blessed than anyone in this situation," Isabel shares. "I was there to help that baby be born."

Maryela has since returned to thank Isabel for her help. "She treats me like a celebrity," says Isabel. "She is so appreciative, but really, I did nothing. I could see myself in her eyes. So many strangers helped me out. I just got to repay the favor."

Isabel has worked at South Seminole Hospital since August 2005. "When I saw the title, Guest Services, I knew this job was for me," she says.

Isabel, who used to dream of being a flight attendant, now delivers world-class service to the guests of South Seminole Hospital.

—*Submitted by Mary Tomlinson, Orlando Regional Healthcare, Windemere, FL*

"Never underestimate the difference you can make."

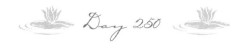

That Was My Duty

I had just left the night shift. It was 6:50 a.m. on a Thursday. The traffic was heavy and my eyes were tired. I soon perked right up as a young man on a black motorcycle sped by my car at lightening speed. I yelled, "Slow down!" Not a second later, the driver lost control and flew into a ditch on the side of the freeway. My heart beating in my throat, I knew I had to pull over. As it turned out, the young man had died on impact. There was nothing I could do. There was nothing the paramedics could do. They thanked me for pulling over and told me to drive safely.

I walked back up the embankment back to my car. Looking at the scene one last time, I felt like I had failed. *What kind of nurse am I?* I wondered. I drove home shaking, and later I was unable to sleep. I kept wondering about his family and how many other people would be affected by his death.

A week later, I had cut out the newspaper article about his death. It was a very small article because not many people knew why or how it had happened. That evening at work, I was taking a small break when a patient came in with chest pains. I asked the woman how she was doing that evening. She proceeded to tell me in detail about a grandmother who had lost her grandson in motorcycle accident last week. My heart jumped back into my throat as I realized instantly that I had seen it happen. I did some research on the name, and sure enough, her

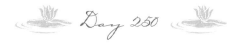

daughter was the mother of the accident victim. I asked her nurse if she thought it would be a good idea to let her know I had been there when it happened.

I began to question my judgment. Why would I want to talk about this tragedy again? A young, 32-year-old man was gone. I didn't know his past or his relatives, but I did know I was there when he died. I did know that he hadn't suffered.

The nurse on duty prepared the grandmother, and I walked into the room, afraid to face it all again. She grabbed my hand and I sat at the side of the bed. I said to her the words I had rehearsed, not giving details. I told her I was there when her grandson passed and that he did not suffer. We shared tears as she told me what a great man he was. Ultimately, I enabled her to rest and feel some peace knowing that her grandson did not die alone.

I did not save his life that misty morning but I was able to bring a family peace in the end. That was my duty.

—Submitted by Teri Fredrick, St. Joseph Hospital, Orange, CA

"Never underestimate the difference you can make."

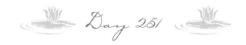

Caring For the Family

My husband Rob was in an accident at work on June 30, 2006. I received a call that he had been sent to the Emergency Department from his work. I work at the hospital as a Rehab nurse, and I immediately ran to the Emergency Department. I was greeted by a nurse who asked me, "Who are you here to see?" I explained that my husband was being brought in by Bedford Park ambulance. She told me he was there in the trauma room and that a nurse would be right with me.

They allowed me to go in and see my husband. He was alert and oriented. He told me he hit a pole while on the forklift. The nurse was constantly monitoring him and told me he had blood in his stomach and would be going to surgery. I did not realize the severity of his injury because he was talking and joking with the staff. (Later I realized he was in shock. He does not remember anything.) The chaplain came and asked me if I wanted to sit in the office while they prepared to take Rob to surgery. I was able to go with them to the doors of surgery. Throughout this part of our experience, the ED nurse and PCA were very kind to my husband and me.

I called my family to let them know what was happening, and waited in the OR waiting room. The nurse liaison came out a couple of times to update everyone in the waiting room on their respective family member's progress. We were called into a quiet room, and the resident surgeon came out to tell us Rob's

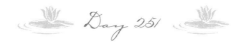

condition was grave. He had lost a lot of blood. He told us the surgeon would be out to talk to us as soon as surgery was over.

When the surgeon came out, he told us Rob's condition was still serious, and they would be monitoring him very closely for the next 24 hours. He said he would be there himself if Rob had to go back to surgery. The plan was to take him back to surgery in the morning if the bleeding did not start over, and close him. The surgeon was very attentive. He answered all of the questions from my family and me. He was patient and compassionate, and listened to us as if we were his own family.

Rob was in the Surgical Intensive/Neuro Intensive Care Unit (SINI) for 28 days. The doctors, nurses, and PCAs and the staff in respiratory, physical therapy, occupational therapy, and housekeeping were excellent. Their words of encouragement, respect for my family, and knowledge made the difference for us. The care was exceptional in the SINI.

My father-in-law (Rob's Dad) had many concerns and wondered if we needed to call in specialists. The doctors were not offended by his comment and reassured him he was getting the best care. When it was time for a tracheotomy to be done the doctors and nurses reassured me that this would be the best thing for Rob at the time and that they would eventually be able to take it out. They included me in all aspects of his care, keeping me up to date on everything, always showing compassion for my tears and fears.

Rob then was transferred to the Trauma Unit (4E/W) and stayed there for four days. The staff was phenomenal. Again, they always answered our questions, and treated my family with the utmost respect and dignity, while simultaneously helping my husband take more steps forward in his recovery.

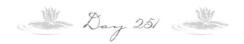

His next stop was the Rehab program (6 South). He attended therapy, and especially liked the transporters, who were friendly, courteous, and kind. He was determined to go home by my birthday. With the love, encouragement, and care he received from the nurses, PCAs, therapists, and physicians, Rob reached his goal. He was discharged on my birthday.

During Rob's stay, my in-laws had many meals in the hospital cafeteria. They said the staff was always friendly. The staff members got to know them and would always ask how Rob was doing. The staff in the parking garage also became their friends, and again, always gave them words of encouragement and showed they cared by asking about Rob.

I have not mentioned anyone's name in particular because I do not want to leave anyone out. After being in the hospital for a total of 48 days, it is hard to remember everyone's name, but I will always remember the kindness and the love we felt from the staff throughout his stay.

As I mentioned earlier, I work in the hospital where Rob received this great care. My peers were there for my family and me the whole time. You may be thinking, Oh, she works there and got special treatment—but I can tell you from sitting in many waiting rooms, talking with other families, and hearing their stories that mine is not the exception. Our stories were all the same. Not only were we getting the best care, we were all being treated by the most compassionate, caring staff in the world.

Our family still talks about how Advocate Christ Medical Center saved a husband, father, son, uncle, brother-in-law, and cousin. We talk about not only how grateful we are to still have him with us today but also about the excellent, exceptional care he received!

—*Submitted by Irene Tranowski, Advocate Christ Medical Center, Oak Lawn, IL*

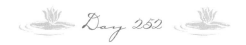

Good Samaritans

Last year, on Valentine's Day, an elderly Hispanic man was lying on the ground on a sidewalk near our hospital. Several people walked past him but did not stop. Soon a couple walking by him noticed that he was short of breath and asked if he needed help. He could not speak when they asked if he needed medical attention. Elicer (Elliot) Rivera, one of our Security Guards, was making rounds near the gates of the hospital. He too saw the man and came over to offer assistance. Elliot could see that the man was having difficulty breathing. He quickly called for another security officer to get a wheel chair. Together, they wheeled him from the street to our Emergency Department. He was subsequently admitted to the hospital in acute respiratory and cardiac distress.

Several weeks later, our CEO got a letter written by Captain Joe G., the head of Security at Temple University Hospital, located three miles away. The elderly man—"Mr. G."—was Joe's father. He had a long history of cardiac and pulmonary problems and was living with a pacemaker. He had been on his way home via public transportation. Shortly after exiting a bus he began to feel very ill and tried to get himself help. He could not make his needs known to the people around him since he spoke limited English. He then fell to the ground and was unable to speak.

Joe wrote that the Emergency Department physician had told him it was his father's pacemaker that had kept him alive while he was lying out in the street. If

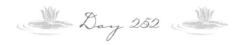

the couple and Elliot had not stopped to help him, he would have died there on the sidewalk.

Mr. G. was admitted to our medical surgical unit. He made a good recovery and was scheduled for discharge within a few days. He was able to walk down the unit on his own with Joe at his side. He made a point of thanking everyone and saying goodbye to the nursing, dietary and environmental services staff who had come to know him very well. Joe said they treated him like an old friend as he left the unit.

In the parking lot of the hospital, he told Joe that he was really amazed at how much Episcopal had changed from the community hospital it had been in the past. He stated that everyone was wonderful to him and was impressed with the care that he been given. He felt that all the staff had given him a second chance. He especially felt that way about Elliot.

Mr. G. was delighted to be home. The following Sunday he planned a big celebration with his entire family and invited everyone to his home. He died of a cardiac arrest, about one hour before everyone was scheduled to come for dinner—just in time for the rest of the family to be with Joe's mother.

Joe wrote the letter to express his appreciation for the care that his father had received. He said that Elliot had given the family more time with their father and allowed him to die with dignity. He also said that no one knew that the elderly man was his father; the care he received was excellent because the staff cared about all people.

Because of the couple, and Elliot, Joe's father was able to spend the last days of his life at home, surround by family and friends. You never know what lives you will touch when you care enough to get involved. Elliot's response to the letter was to smile and say, "I was just doing my job."

—Submitted by Doris Quiles, Temple University Hospital / Episcopal Campus, Philadelphia, PA

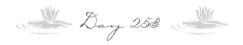

Last Rites

We had a patient on Cardiac Critical Care (CCC) who was convinced that she was going to die that day and wanted to have her last rites done by her priest. Unfortunately, her priest was not available—but wouldn't you know there was another patient on CCC who just happened to be a priest.

Sister Caritas went to the "priest patient" and explained the situation. He willingly got in a wheelchair and went to the other patient's room to give her the last rites.

Fortunately, our patient did not die that day, and was ultimately discharged home. However, she expressed to us how grateful she was to have had her needs met. The priest also told us how glad he was to be of service and said it felt good to be needed. All of our lives were touched that day, and we continue to be touched each time the story is related.

—Submitted by Loretta Franklin,
Mercy General Hospital's Continuing Care Center, Sacramento, CA

"Never underestimate the difference you can make."

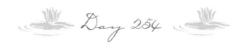
The King's Clothing

As a chaplain in the NJCU at Carle Foundation Hospital, I get to see nurses, doctors, a social worker, housekeepers and respiratory therapists go beyond their prescribed duties to provide individualized care. This highly protective staff, who serve infants and families, provide special touches such as pink or blue bedding, clean windows (so that no mommy or daddy had to peer through dirty glass), and bows to wee ones who might weight about one pound—humanizing the high-tech environment.

My story involves a quiet nurse who is very good at the technical aspects of her job. A baby boy was born with anticipated congenital defects not compatible with life. As the parents moved from hoping that perhaps all the medical technology was wrong to "accepting' the dire diagnosis, this nurse not only listened but helped them create meaningful memories.

Mom brought in a suit she bought for the baby three months before. One look at the ventilator tubing would have had most people asking, "Isn't there a different choice?"—but Kim gently and quietly changed him into his shirt, tie, and pullover vest. He looked so regal lying there as we took his picture. When the decision was made to disconnect life support, no family member could stay. At the end of her shift, Kim held him for the final 20 minutes of his life. She and the night nurse Kaci gave him his final post-death care.

Is this a rare occurrence in healthcare? No. As a chaplain, I could tell you many stories about physicians sitting at an elderly person's bed because no one should

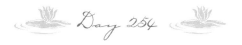

die alone…staff members who by request of a 17-year-old mom go to the morgue to put a pink bow in a baby's hair…nurses who weep openly in the face of a world view that often does not acknowledge the holistic wellbeing of employees. Why would a person continue to do this work where death is so common—work that society tries to avoid at all costs?

I believe the "Kims" of healthcare don't just come with fantastic knowledge bases. They come with a feeling of compassion planted deeply in their hearts and, daily, do something beyond the normal call of duty. It is as if they have the eyes, hands, hearts, and guts to know they care for royalty. Perhaps that is why Kim didn't complain about the outfit. Maybe she knew she was dressing a king.

—Submitted by Michelle Dragonlik, Carle Foundation Hospital, Urbana, IL

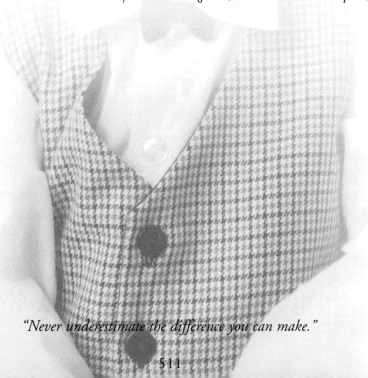

"Never underestimate the difference you can make."

511

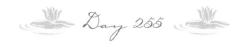

ANGELS AMONG US

*T*he night was as it would have been in a sad movie. Rain streamed down the windows. For one family at Arnold Palmer Hospital, the gloomy mood matched their emotions. For on that night, their child was losing her battle.

The twins had been born prematurely. One was gaining weight and growing and would soon be ready to go home. Her sister, however, had hit every obstacle imaginable and the battle had proven to be too difficult for her. The color of her skin and the numbers on all her monitors showed that she had only a little time left.

Her grandfather had just arrived to see his granddaughter for the first and probably last time. Bernie Conry, a night nurse, had developed a special relationship with the young family, and she knew there was not much time left. She pushed open the doors to the Neonatal Intensive Care Unit and asked, "Would you like to come in and a say a prayer for your little girl?" The child's father and grandfather entered and stood beside her Isolette.

The NICU team had taken every life-saving measure, but the baby was still declining. The therapist began ambuing the frail girl to give her family a few more minutes with her.

The two men looked at each other and the child's father said, "No Dad, you pray." Several nurses, respiratory therapists, and neonatologist Michael McMahan, MD joined the circle around the Isolette. The grandfather shifted his large frame,

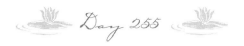
placed one hand on the Isolette over his granddaughter's heart, and lifted the other heavenward.

"God, we thank you for this child," he began as he prayed. They stood in a circle, holding hands as the grandfather uttered a soul-stirring prayer. In conclusion he said, "We give this child to You."

And then it was if the heavens had opened. The little girl's number started climbing and her color began to look pink. Within two hours, she had turned around. The grateful grandfather looked to Dr. McMahan and said a heartfelt thank you. However, Dr. McMahan said he could not accept, adding, "I didn't do this."

The twins went home. The little girls grew up side by side, and no one could tell which one had nearly lost her life. But the miracle did not go unnoticed by the grandfather. That night left a profound impression on him. He later returned with a watercolor painting he had commissioned. After hearing the story, the artist began to paint.

"I did not give him a picture of you," the grandfather told Bernie. "But that is you," he said as he pointed to the image of the angel moving to help. The thought took Bernie by surprise. She had no idea the impact her simple gesture had made. The grandfather then presented Bernie with the beautiful painting.

"I had not prayed in twenty years," he said. "But now I travel the world and share the story about the miracle that happened for my granddaughter here at Arnold Palmer Hospital."

Bernie and her husband Tom have donated the painting to Arnold Palmer Hospital to remind all that there are Angels among us.

—Submitted by Mary Tomlinson, as told by Bernie Conry,
Orlando Regional Healthcare, Windemere, FL

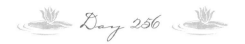
Day 256

Beyond Expectations

I called a patient who had recently been discharged to see how she was doing. Her daughter answered the phone and told me that her mother was doing fine. They had gotten her prescriptions filled and had made the follow up appointments but the home health nurse had not been out yet. When I asked if there was anything that I could do to help, she asked if I would come stay with her mother while she ran a few essential errands. I agreed to do so and went to stay with the patient and her spouse. My main role was to sit and listen to them as they told stories about their hospital stay, how they met, and other tidbits of their life.

While I was there one of their sons dropped by. He asked who I was, and when I replied that I was the manager of the CCC where his mother had recently been, he acted very surprised. He proclaimed that coming to stay with his mother was providing care above and beyond their expectations. Having the opportunity to help patients and their families in this way makes me proud to be doing what I do.

—Submitted by Loretta Franklin,
Mercy General Hospital's Continuing Care Center, Sacramento, CA

"Never underestimate the difference you can make."

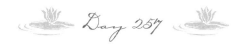

The Next Chapter

I have worked in Psychiatric Nursing for a number of years. This is a story from one of my days on the job. Allan was a 36-year-old man, six feet tall and good-looking. He had been very active most of his life until three years ago when he had a boating accident. This left him with severe back pain. He began using pain medications and became addicted to them. In the last year he had developed neurogenic bladder and other related problems, which resulted in multiple tests, procedure, and hospitalizations. Allan was hospitalized on BHS because he had major depression and had attempted suicide by overdosing on his pain medications.

I introduced myself to Allan as he lay in bed pale and disheveled, with a suprapublic and a Foley catheter in place. I said cheerfully, "Good morning, my name is Vera. I will be your nurse. How did you sleep? Breakfast will be here shortly."

I was met with no eye contact and monotone responses from a very depressed and defeated young man. He did not show up for breakfast, stating that he would rather eat when there were fewer people in the dining room. When I suggested that a shower before breakfast might be a good way to start the day, he immediately declined.

As I was doing his vital signs, I saw him looking at my scrubs with all the colorful "happy flowers." I joked with him: "It's so cheery it almost makes you

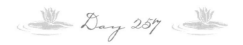

gag, huh?" He chuckled and said, "My thoughts exactly!" He said he wasn't hungry, but I brought his breakfast tray to him anyway and sat down with him. Our conversation was superficial, but at least he was making eye contact, and I began to see that he was more angry than anything. Though he wasn't coming right out with it, he *was* angry—he felt he had no control over his life anymore.

As he left the dining room, I reminded him that group therapy would be at 10 a.m. and he nodded. However, he missed group, sleeping instead. He also missed the 11 a.m. group.

After lunch, I was in his room supervising his roommate's shaving (for safety reasons). I asked Allan if he wanted to shave. He answered sarcastically and turned over in his bed. My immediate thought was *Whatever!* but instead of voicing it I said to him, "You are one angry man." He looked kind of shocked and then closed his eyes again.

I pulled a chair up to his bed and said, "Tell me about it." He pretended to sleep but I just sat there. To my surprise, he sat up, put his pillow behind him and started sharing. I listened as he vented and cried about his life before the boating accident, his life now, and the last 3 years, which he proclaimed had been "hell." He said he felt like giving up.

Fortunately, I had been to his staffing the day before, so I was aware of his medical conditions, prognosis, and so forth. We talked about how the catheters were not always going to be there. My heart did go out to him; he had been through a lot. I told him how we are all authors of a book, the Book of our Life.

We talked about how it is easy to have good character during the good times; it's in our trials that our true character is revealed. He shared with me about times in his life that he was proud of and times that he wasn't. I asked him how he would like this chapter in his life to read.

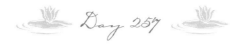

As I was leaving his room, he asked if he could take a shower. Later, I walked into the TV room and he was watching the Angels baseball game. I asked him who was winning. As I was leaving he called out to me "Who knows? Maybe the Angels will win the pennant during this chapter of my life!" Then, he winked at me.

As I walked to my car that night, I smiled.

—Submitted by Vera Trone, St. Joseph Hospital, Orange, CA

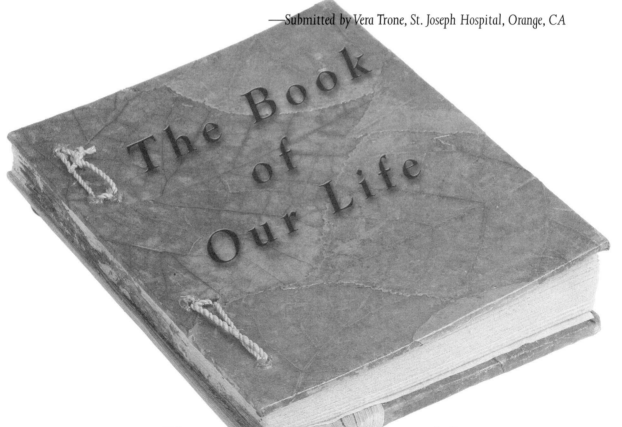

The Book of Our Life

"Never underestimate the difference you can make."

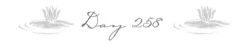

A THANKFUL MOTHER

The following letter was sent to give special recognition to a great nurse, Adele, who showed love and compassion to a young patient:

On April 3, I brought my 12-year-old daughter Mikeala to the Emergency Room at the Joe DiMaggio Children's Hospital. A boil the size of a golf ball had developed on her underarm. I was informed that she needed to have a surgical procedure done immediately. I quickly began to panic. My daughter was also quite upset and anxious, as this was to be the first surgical procedure she had ever had. Her face was completely filled with fear as the tears began dropping, one after the other.

As I entered the back medical rooms my anxiety continued to grow. That's when a woman with a smile that could calm a raging war approached me. Her name was Adele and she was surely an angel. She immediately took on the role of a nurturing mother to calm my daughter and me.

Adele talked with and comforted my daughter through the entire procedure. She was holding her hand and wiping her tears, and she spoke many comforting words. As for me, I never would have made it through the experience without Adele's kind support.

As we were leaving the hospital that day, my daughter said, "Mom I will never forget Adele. She will always be my friend." Adele is an angel walking the floor

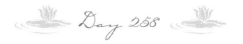

of the Emergency Room of Joe DiMaggio Children's Hospital. The management team should be proud to have her on the staff!

Thank you for your love and caring support!

A Thankful Mother

—*Anonymous Contributor, Joe DiMaggio Children's Hospital, Hollywood, FL*

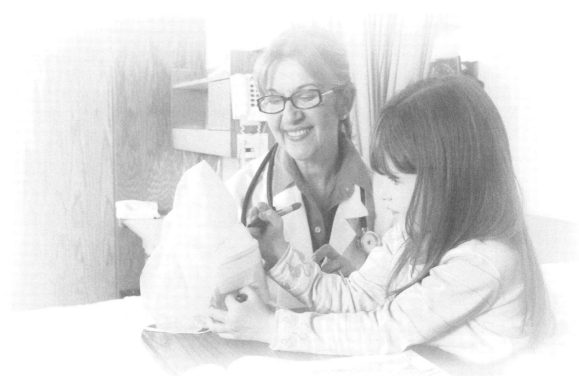

"Never underestimate the difference you can make."

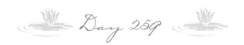

A Loving Touch

After years of working in healthcare I have so many stories to tell. Here's one that best illustrates why I love nursing.

In 1983 at King's Daughters Medical Center in Brookhaven, Mississippi, an 85 year-old patient of mine was dying from an inoperable glioblastoma. She was very demanding and, naturally, quite scared. I would often go sit with her when I was not busy on the floor. She loved to hold my hand while we would sit and just talk. One day she told me that I should never stop touching people because I have a very comforting touch. She then stroked my hands and passed away. Her words will forever be ingrained in my heart, and they still touch me today.

—Submitted by Loretta Franklin, Mercy General Hospital's Continuing Care Center, Sacramento, CA

"Never underestimate the difference you can make."

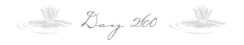
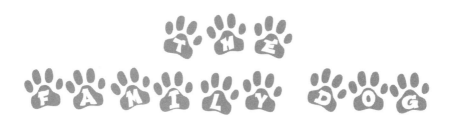

Mazzy Blue enters Orlando Regional Sand Lake Hospital* each week with a smile and a wagging tail. Sand Lake Spiritual Care volunteer Bill Baxter follows, knowing he will witness the amazing.

When Mazzy Blue graduated from obedience school, everyone recognized that she had a special skill. "I think Mazzy is a great candidate for a therapy dog," the trainer mentioned to Bill. She just needed to pass a certification test. After trial runs at a Publix and a local nursing home, Mazzy Blue proved she could handle rattling carts and crowds of people. Mazzy was never annoyed or spooked. She passed every test, including hair pulling and having a stack of books dropped near her tail. Bill knew she was ready.

So every Wednesday, Bill and Mazzy visit the hospital as part of Sand Lake Hospital's Mind/Body/Spirit program. Working with the clinical team, Bill and Mazzy visit patients who are in need of encouragement. Mazzy makes it easy for people to relax. Some share their stories. Others simply enjoy petting the beautiful dog. "For the few minutes we visit with someone, they are able to take their thoughts off their situation and think of something else," Bill says. "Mazzy Blue opens doors people can't open."

"Could I meet your dog?" a former military man once asked. After the familiar exchange, Mazzy Blue lay down across the man's feet. His disciplined personality was still evident and usually kept him from sharing with others. But

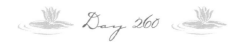

it was not long before the man began to share his story with Bill and tears began to fall. "Would you like us to pray together?" Bill asked. The man no longer carried his concerns alone.

Bill shares a story about a woman who had suffered a stroke. Her son had asked that Bill and Mazzy Blue stop by for a visit. The woman loved dogs. When they entered the room, Mazzy walked over to her bedside. The stroke had affected the woman's ability to speak and move her left side. Mazzy stood just beside her hand. "I watched for 15 minutes as that woman slowly moved her left hand," Bill recalls in amazement. Finally, she reached Mazzy's head and ran her fingers through her soft coat. "I sure am a believer in pet therapy now," said the nurse, also surprised by the woman's determination.

Another time, a woman stood crying in the hallway. Her husband was dying. Mazzy Blue walked over to her and she dropped to her knees, burying her face in Mazzy's neck. Immediately her tears dried up. "This is the best thing that has happened to me," she said repeatedly. "Will you come visit my husband?" she finally asked. As they entered the room, the frail man looked to Mazzy Blue. His eyes sparkled. "She looks like the golden retriever we once had," the woman explained. As a smile broke across her husband's face, she patted Mazzy on the head. "Thank you. You have no idea what this means to me."

But Bill does know. "Seeing or petting Mazzy Blue gives patients a taste of home. She reminds people of their pets. She brings comfort to those she meets," he says. The family at Sand Lake Hospital also knows. "I'm not sure who enjoys the visits with Mazzy more—the staff or the patients. Everyone feels better after a visit with Bill and Mazzy," a nurse shares.

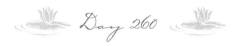

Bill and Mazzy also seek to encourage the team at Sand Lake Hospital. Bill watches nurses drop to their knees to hug Mazzy or feed her a treat. "I see them relax for a moment," he says. "In the middle of caring for so many others, they get a moment for themselves." With renewed energy, they return to caring for their patients. "I feel good when we get home," Bill says, "like we have accomplished something."

Sand Lake Hospital is known for its family feel. It is only fitting to have a family dog.

*Now known as the Dr. P Phillips Hospital.

—Submitted by Mary Tomlinson, Orlando Regional Healthcare, FL

"Never underestimate the difference you can make."

523

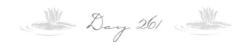

CARING FOR ONE OF OUR OWN

When one of our own employees faces serious illness, we often face special burdens trying to handle the practical and emotional consequences. When a member of the Emergency Department became seriously ill, her coworkers demonstrated not only teamwork, but compassion and care.

While many contributed, special praise goes to Lydia Schmidt, Camille Zengen, and Nicole Cron. Lydia took care of her coworker's personal needs, along with providing emotional support that only a true friend can supply. Camille Zengen has provided invaluable support throughout the past two years. She would often take her own time and visit the staff members at home, bringing her food and laughter. Nicole Cron was also a constant friend. When the staff member was hospitalized, Nicole would spend long hours in her room. When arrangements were made to enable the staff person to find specialized care near her family, Nicole took the long trip to the airport with her friend, providing care and companionship along the way.

All of this would not be possible without the administrative support given to this staff member. Administration went above all expectations to do the right thing for this person. It is heart-warming to work among great people.

—*Submitted by Gretchen Halstead, Vassar Brothers Medical Center, Poughkeepsie, NY*

"Never underestimate the difference you can make."

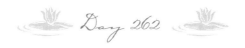

TAKING THE TIME

Several years ago I had a 62-year-old patient with small cell lung cancer. She was dying and needed a therapeutic paracentesis. She was afraid to do the procedure but agreed to have it done on the condition that I would stay there with her. My shift ended at 3:15 p.m. and the patient was supposed to have the procedure at 4 p.m. We waited for the doctor to arrive as the clock continued to march on. Finally the physician came at 6:30 p.m. and performed the necessary procedure.

One week later the patient died. About a month or so after her death, I got a phone call from Clifford Skinner, the Chief Medical Officer. He had received a letter from the patient's daughter telling him of the paracentesis and her mother's fear. Mr. Skinner sent me a copy of the letter with his comments, which I still have to this day. Truly, you can make a difference in the lives of others through little acts of kindness, touch, giving of your time and genuinely caring for others. This is why I know that nursing is my calling.

—Submitted by Loretta Franklin, Mercy General Hospital, Sacramento, CA

"Never underestimate the difference you can make."

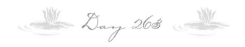

Robert's Wheelchair

This fall a patient named Robert, who had been hospitalized several times, was readmitted. He had been diagnosed with schizophrenia many years ago. This condition resulted in multiple psychiatric admissions and in the loss of his legs. Years ago, this patient had obeyed command-type auditory hallucinations telling him to lie down on train tracks and kill himself. While he was on the tracks, a train severed both of his legs. Now a double amputee, Robert had been dependent on a wheelchair for years, which also made his psychiatric disorder more severe.

When Robert was admitted he was very depressed and agitated. He was using an old wheelchair, which was hard for him to manage. It was torn in many places and held together with tape. Unit Clerk Maggie Torregrossa, who could see him from her chair in the nursing station, noticed his frustration as he went through the doors. She said, "He was trying to come through the unit doors but couldn't because his wheelchair was in such bad shape. It was coming apart. He wanted to do everything by himself and would get very upset when the wheelchair wouldn't go like he wanted it to go. He would become upset and punch the walls."

She felt very bad for him and wanted to do something. She asked his psychiatrist about the possibility of obtaining a motorized wheelchair for him. The psychiatrist and treatment team had some reservations that the client might

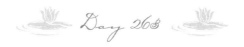

become aggressive while driving the motorized wheelchair, but ultimately decided that if they could obtain a new wheelchair, the patient's behavior could be managed.

Maggie took this task on as a challenge. While at home on her day off, she saw a commercial about motorized wheelchairs. She noted that the commercial indicated that if your insurance did not cover the cost of the chair, the chair would be free. She went on the company's website, and completed an online request for a new motorized wheelchair for the patient. Her request was denied because the patient's insurance was not valid in the state of Texas, where the wheelchair company was located. She was advised to seek help from a more local organization.

Within two hours of this response, however, the Chief Executive Officer of the wheelchair company contacted Maggie and asked for more information. She indicated that she had gotten a copy of the email from the service representative denying the request. She wanted to speak with her sales staff about the request and asked Maggie for further information, including the patient's height and weight both pre- and post-amputation. The Mental Health Workers on her unit helped her gather this information. Maggie then supplied it to the CEO who indicated that the patient would be given a free motorized wheelchair. She wanted it to be a Thanksgiving present for him.

Maggie was very excited, but several weeks after Thanksgiving the patient still had not received the chair. Maggie called the CEO. Her persistence paid off. The CEO had thought that the issue was taken care of, and immediately rectified the problem. The motorized wheelchair was delivered the next day via overnight mail.

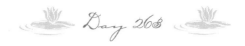

When it arrived, Maggie along with the rest of the staff from the unit entered Robert's room with the wheelchair. They told him it was a new motorized wheelchair that was his to keep. He started crying right away, stating that he could not believe what the staff had done for him. He got right into the wheelchair and started heading down the hallway.

Robert has not been aggressive in two months and has been participating in unit activities since he has received the chair. He takes great pride in cleaning it daily. Robert refers to Maggie as his "guardian angel" and thanks her daily for getting him his chair. Maggie was asked why, as a unit clerk, she took on the job of finding a motorized wheelchair for Robert. She said simply, "He didn't have a voice. I wanted to be his voice."

—Submitted by Doris Quiles,
Temple University Hospital/Episcopal Campus, Philadelphia, PA

"Never underestimate the difference you can make."

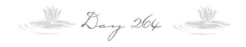

Saving a Life

Bryan Sleyzak is an operating engineer in the Plant Operations Department at Hackensack University Medical Center. On Saturday, February 10th, 2007 at 4:30 p.m., while he was working on the roof of the Medical Plaza, a vehicle that was parked on the roof of the main garage caught his attention. A hose ran from the vehicle's exhaust pipe into the rear window.

Brain left his work to investigate the situation. As he walked toward the vehicle, a man jumped out and disconnected the hose. As Brian continued toward the vehicle the man said, "I guess it's not my day," got back inside the vehicle and drove away. Brian quickly took note of the vehicle's make, model and license plate number and reported it to security. The information was relayed to the Hackensack police department. It was then learned that the man had been missing since Thursday, February 8th. The Hackensack police relayed the information to the man's local police department.

At 5:30 p.m., one hour after the man's attempted suicide, local police located him at his residence and took him into custody for a psychiatric evaluation.

Due to Brian's astute powers of observation, quick thinking and willingness to act, a suicide attempt was interrupted and a troubled individual was given a new lease on life.

—Submitted by Douglas C. Clark, Hackensack University Medical Center, Hackensack, NJ

"Never underestimate the difference you can make."

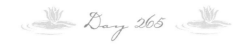

The Most Special Person in the World

This is a story about people who didn't know each other at all...but shared the values that make Vassar Brothers Medical Center the special place that it is.

The patient was a tiny woman who had suffered a stroke. The family knew the end was near, and gathered around her in her room on South Circle 5. She always loved having her family around her: her husband, all twelve children and their families. As the family got to know the staff, it was the little things that truly touched their hearts: the nurse who replaced the tape that held her IV in place because it "looked uncomfortable"...the case manager who kindly answered the same questions over and over, just because they needed to be sure...the staff who quietly washed her face and fixed her hair as the family came to terms with letting go of the gentle matriarch of their large, boisterous family...the food trays that appeared as if by magic.

When the shared memories caused laughter, the staff would simply shut the door, allowing the family to come to terms with their loss in their own way. And as the doctor removed her breathing tube, he gently explained the process to her, although she seemed asleep.

The staff treated this patient as if she were the most special person in the world...and they had no idea how special she really was.

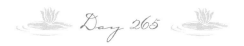

"Ms. F." graduated from Vassar Brothers Hospital School of Nursing in 1947. After raising her family, she returned to Vassar as a volunteer, mainly in Imaging. For almost 30 years, she was like a quiet angel who would appear out of nowhere to offer comfort to a waiting patient who looked lonely or afraid, or a blanket to someone who seemed cold.

It was very scary for her when she found herself not recognizing the staff that she had worked with every week for years, or losing her way in the familiar hall leading to Imaging. She finally made the decision to stop volunteering…and it broke her heart.

She was a nurse to the very core of her being, always thinking of others before herself. When at Vassar for a procedure, Ms. F. would express concern for the people she passed in the waiting room, saying that she "hoped they weren't alone."

The staff on South Circle 5 could have treated her as "just another patient," but their actions proved that there is not such thing. Each person they care for is treated with respect and dignity. Ms. F. lived these principles…and thanks to the staff on South Circle 5, she died surrounded by them.

—Submitted by Gretchen Halstead, Vassar Brothers Medical Center, Poughkeepsie, NY

"Never underestimate the difference you can make."

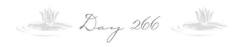

TAKING TIME

O ver the years while working in nursing I have learned to be more flexible with each day, no matter how controlled I would like my shift to be. About a month ago, I had a 23-year-old male patient from CV-ICU transfer to our floor on 4 East after having an atrial septal defect repaired. His wife accompanied him to his new room and both of them just seemed to be so full of energy. I received my patient from ICU about two hours before my shift ended, so I was running around trying to get my other tasks done so I could finish on time. When I was doing his assessment, I just wanted to get it done as quickly as possible, but then he asked if he could borrow my stethoscope. He said he wanted to use it to listen to his heart. I handed him my stethoscope. He took it and used it to listen to his own heart. He closed his eyes as he listened and a big smile followed. He said, "My heart used to sound like a washing machine. Now I finally have a heart that sounds normal."

That was such a moving moment for me, to see this young man so grateful after waiting 23 years to have something that the majority of us would usually just take for granted. This introduced him to a life he had never known before. I thought to myself, *This is the reason I went into the field of medicine. I get to be a part of other people's life journeys by working along beside them and I get to witness miracles like this.* The everyday things that may seem like another "to do" item on our list may actually have the potential to be a life-changing event. That's what I like about being a

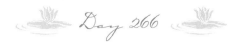

nurse—it's moments like this one that make me stop to take a breather from the busyness of the day and teach me to be thankful for what I was called to do in my life. We need to take time to reflect on the uniqueness of every patient we take care of—to take time to really *listen* to them and allow interruptions in our organized routine. This way we can make room for little moments like this one to shine in their own little way.

—Submitted by Aileen Ingles, St. Joseph Hospital, Orange, CA

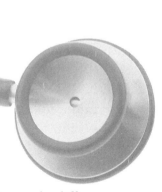

"Never underestimate the difference you can make."

A (Not) Forgotten Vet

A 60-year-old patient died of cancer on South 5 in late May. He had no known family and no visitors while he was in the hospital. After his death, no one came. He had only been a patient on one or two prior occasions, but staff found him to be a gentle and kind person, and did their best to relieve his suffering at the end of his life.

Ruth Recchia was the nurse who cared for him those last days, and she contacted Peggy Kraft, the case manager on South Circle 5, after his death. Ruth was upset that he would have a "pauper's burial" with no one present to honor his life. Peggy contacted John Simon, the Director of Pastoral Care, who quickly agreed to help with a burial service.

Peggy also investigated other sources for help, and it turned out that the patient was a Vietnam veteran and was eligible for some benefits through the Veteran's Administration. He was also a native of Poughkeepsie and there was a family plot at St. Peter's Cemetery. A local funeral parlor provided a discount, and the Friday before Memorial Day, Ruth, Peggy, and John held a service for our patient at the gravesite. Peggy cut flowers from her garden to put on the grave and John provided several readings. One of them—"What Is a Vet?"—had special meaning to Ruth, who has a son in the military, stationed in Iraq.

Our patient did not die alone—and his death did not go unnoticed. Vassar Brothers Medical Center's caregiving team worked hard to honor a "forgotten" vet on our national holiday.

—Submitted by Gretchen Halstead, Vassar Brothers Medical Center, Poughkeepsie, NY

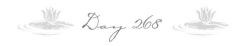

A GREAT FIRST IMPRESSION

The following letter very effectively describes two people who give a very positive "first impression" of Vassar Brothers Medical Center:

Dear Dr. Aronzon,

Recently, my mother was hospitalized for a week at VBMC; a week after her discharge, my husband was a patient for two weeks. During that time, it was necessary for me to take advantage of your valet service.

Rebecca Oakley and Vicki Spoletti handled that service, and I give them my heartfelt gratitude for their kindness, help, courtesy, and efficiency. Because of their caring attitude, friendliness, and professionalism, the stress during those three weeks was lessened for me, and every day I knew that when I arrived at Vassar they would help in every possible way so that somehow everything seemed a little brighter and a little more hopeful.

They handle their job so efficiently, effortlessly, and pleasantly that patients and their family members are given a feeling of confidence in VBMC. They are the first people that many of the patients and their families are in contact with, and they are truly most deserving of praise and acknowledgment of their excellent work ethic.

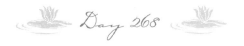

They are very caring young women and Vassar Brothers Medical Center should be duly proud of them. Thank you for your time and consideration of this matter.

> Most respectfully,
> Barbara T.

Rebecca and Vicki receive many positive comments in our patient satisfaction survey, and greet everyone, patients, visitors, and their fellow employees, with warmth and kindness. We are very fortunate to have such high caliber individuals at our front door.

—Submitted by Gretchen Halstead, Vassar Brothers Medical Center, Poughkeepsie, NY

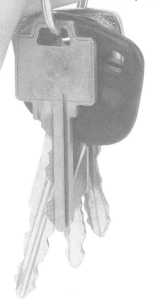

"Never underestimate the difference you can make."

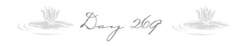

Barshella

We had recently completed a Studer seminar, and we were focusing our health care providers on the importance of introducing themselves and shaking hands with their patients to make them feel cared for right away.

We find that lots of times ICU patients are ignored because there is so much care going on for them that the actual one-on-one care—like talking with them or shaking their hands to let them know we care—gets neglected.

With the seminar lessons fresh in her mind, Barshella, one of our GI technicians, was setting up the GI equipment that would be necessary for a procedure on an ICU patient. When Barshella noticed that the patient was awake and alert, she extended her hand and said, "Hello, I'm Barshella, and I'm going to take great care of you today."

After the procedure, as Barshella was packing up the equipment, the lady thanked her for acknowledging her and gave Barshella a hug goodbye.

—*Submitted by Tillie Balliet, Roper St. Francis Healthcare, Charleston, SC*

"Never underestimate the difference you can make."

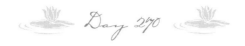

THE LETTER

Dear Son,

I want you to know that I love you.
Be a good boy and be a good man.
Know that I will always love you.

Love,
Your Mom

This letter was dictated by a 46-year-old mother to her 10-year-old son. She was about to undergo a surgical procedure and realized that she may not survive. She dictated the letter to her nurse, Kim Russell, RN, ONC, and asked that it be read to her son if she died during surgery. The mother survived the procedure, and so the letter became a part of her medical record.

A short two months later, the mother succumbed to cancer while she was a patient on South Circle 5. Two days before she died surrounded by her family, the mother asked Reverend John Simon if he would "give the sermon." As the funeral was planned, Reverend Simon asked the family if they had a copy of the letter, as it would help the son in his healing process and would be cherished as he grew into manhood. The family could not find the letter and gave permission to John

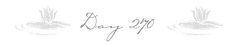

to try and obtain a copy. John was unsure what to expect since the letter was part of the medical record. Pam Singh in Health Information Management went out of her way to help John, and within the hour he had a copy of the letter.

At the patient's funeral, where there were over 200 persons present, Reverend Simon read the letter as part of the eulogy. Thanks to Kim and Pam, John was able to provide personal comfort and a copy of a mother's loving words to her sad little boy. Kim and Pam's single act made a difference and it will help in untold ways in the years to come.

—Submitted by Gretchen Halstead, Vassar Brothers Medical Center, Poughkeepsie, NY

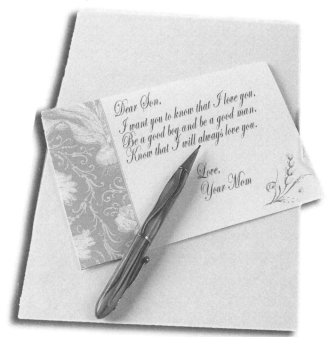

Dear Son,
I want you to know that I love you.
Be a good boy and be a good man.
Know that I will always love you.

Love,
Your Mom

"Never underestimate the difference you can make."

Share Your Own Story

Please share an experience that connected you back to purpose, worthwhile work, and making a difference. You are a big part of what's right in health care!

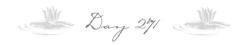

All About Bob

He arrived on our hospital-based care unit during the worst part of an Indiana winter. He was like most eight-year-olds: loud, silly, and full of energy. He had a lopsided grin that warned you of the "ornery" in him. However, the difference between most eight-year-olds and Bob was that Bob was 6 feet 4 inches tall and weighed in at 245 lbs. You see, physically he wasn't eight anymore, but because he was the result of an incest relationship, developmentally he was still an eight-year-old.

Bob had gotten into an argument with his mom and had left his home the night before. They found him in an old barn the next morning with frozen feet. Bob would be joining us for several weeks of whirlpool treatments.

As the days passed, Bob became harder and harder to entertain. He had no visitors. He would wheelchair through the unit, shouting at the top of his lungs, "Attention all nurses and staff, party in my room at 2:30 today!" At least one of us would always try to show up at his room to join his party, which usually consisted of his TV and radio blaring simultaneously and whatever snack he had kept from lunch.

The longer Bob stayed, the more bored he got. He would bark and growl at the CNAs. Instead of bathing, he would jump on his bed completely naked, shouting nonsense phrases. He was becoming more aggressive each day, and I started to become a little concerned for the staff's safety.

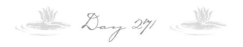

The staff became so frustrated that no one wanted to be assigned to him. It was such a relief to see the therapy techs twice a day; at least then you knew you would have a couple of hours of peace.

So, imagine my surprise one day as I witnessed two CNAs blocking Bob's door and arguing with the PT tech. As I approached, the frustrated tech stormed off. The CNAs called me over and shushed me as I looked in Bob's room. In the middle of the bed sat this gentle giant, holding very still. He was talking quietly,

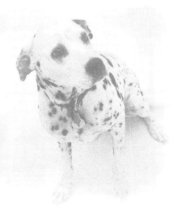

with tears streaming down his cheeks. It turned out the CNAs had called a service which provided pet therapy. In the middle of Bob's lap sat the roundest speckled pup I have ever seen. The little pup appeared content to hear Bob's woes. The argument with the tech had ensued when she wanted to interrupt the scene.

When I asked one of the CNAs what had prompted this change of heart, she said that she had heard Bob crying in his room the day before. Though she had been sure she would be sorry, she went in to see if she could comfort him. In the process she found that Bob did not miss his family, but he very much missed his best friend and companion: his dog. After talking with the rest of the crew, they called the pet service, and they came with this pup.

We realized Bob had only been acting out because he was lonely and afraid. We all did some self-examination that day and realized we had no idea what it was like in Bob's world—a world in which no one came looking for you in the night, a world in which your best friend had four legs and fur. I know that this pup made a positive difference in this man-child's recovery. I could not have been prouder of my staff than I was on that day. They gave him the therapy that would best help him heal.

—Submitted by Denise Renkenberger, Indiana Surgery Center Kokomo, Kokomo, IN

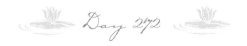

Well-Rounded Care

Administrator Nina Tucker received this wonderful letter from a patient:

Dear Miss Tucker:

We didn't want to let the year end without telling you how terrific Joe DiMaggio Children's Hospital's neonatal care unit is.

This July, while on a business trip in Florida, I gave birth to our son Benjamin three months prematurely. Ben was hospitalized at Joe DiMaggio Children's Hospital from July 19 to October 8. I stayed with Ben while my husband, Rich, regularly flew in from our home state of New Jersey. Many family members and friends also visited to spend time with Benjamin and me. However, since we had no immediate friends or family in Florida, it was really the NICU staff that served not only as an excellent medical team for Ben, but also as our onsite support. I would like to thank a few of the people who were so dedicated to our wellbeing.

Ben's triumvirate of primary nurses—Mika Weidlich, Jennifer Williams, and Linda Owens—always made sure Ben got the best care. However they also went way beyond the call of duty by ensuring that I had three new friends. Mika wound up doing Ben's laundry a few times and helped secure a place for me to stay during one of the summer's hurricanes. Jennifer was always so gentle with

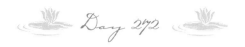

Ben and even brought me lunch on occasion. And Linda's NICU knowledge and kindness was amazing.

Dawn Hawthorne motivated me and countless other new mothers to pump breast milk for our preemies. Rich and I credit this with Ben's great growth rate both at the hospital and since we've been home. Dawn even bought us dry ice so my breast milk would remain frozen during our trip home.

Daphne Pryce made sure our journey home was a good one by tirelessly arranging for oxygen and monitors in Florida and at our home in New Jersey.

In addition, we wish to thank all the NICU doctors, nurse practitioners, day- and night-shift nurses, and respiratory therapists as well as Ben's physical therapist, Joan; speech therapist, Cathy; and social worker, Shawna Smith. All of these people should get credit for how well Ben has done to date. Ben's New Jersey doctors always comment on how healthy he looks despite his premature arrival and tell us how lucky we were to land at such a great NICU.

Thank you for having taken such good care of our son!

Sincerely,
A Happy Mother

—Submitted by Nina Tucker, Joe DiMaggio Children's Hospital, Hollywood, FL

"Never underestimate the difference you can make."

MORE THAN A NURSE

Sandy Viola is an experienced nurse in every area of the Labor, Delivery, Recovery and Postpartum (LDRP) suite. She is very capable of running the nursery and triage area, and provides excellent care for women in labor and after their deliveries. Finding someone who is comfortable and reliable in all of these areas is quite rare. She is a woman to be admired.

In addition, Sandy has been invaluable to the perinatal bereavement program at Vassar Brothers Medical Center. Bereaved parents have very little to remember their babies by. We've found that one of the best ways to remember a stillborn baby is to create memories for the family to keep. Sandy consistently offers her time and talent by taking digital pictures of these babies, very often on her own time. She then enhances the pictures on her home computer, often personalizing them with names and dates. She gives the parents multiple pictures of their child as well as a DVD or CD to keep. Sandy personally purchased the digital camera on LDRP for this purpose, and she also buys all of the supplies she uses.

Sandy is a very talented individual and has done many other projects on her own time and at her own expense. She spent many hours setting up the slide show for last year's "Ceremony of Remembrance," which is an annual event for families that have suffered a perinatal loss. She also designed and created a beautiful brochure for a new Care Center program called "Centering Pregnancy," and has created posters for other clinics and Care Center events.

Sandy is a multitalented woman, a strong advocate for her patients, and a valued member of the LDRP team. Thank you, Sandy, for all that you do!

—Submitted by Gretchen Halstead, Vassar Brothers Medical Center, Poughkeepsie, NY

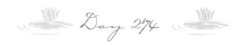

CLOTHED IN COMPASSION

$\mathcal{S}$helly Sturgill, in the Cardiology Outpatient Clinic, as an excellent example of what's right in health care. This story illustrates why. E.A. is a woman in her forties who was employed, had health insurance, and owned a home and a car. She was being treated by another cardiology group in town for congestive heart failure. In November of 2000, her condition had deteriorated so much so that she could not continue to work and subsequently lost everything: her job, health insurance, home, car, and almost all of her belongings. She began living in a homeless shelter and had only two sets of clothing and one pair of shoes. In late June 2001, she was admitted to Saint Joseph Hospital and was seen by Creighton's Family Practice and Cardiology physicians. Upon discharge, E.A. was referred to The Cardiac Center's Health Improvement Therapy Clinic for patients with congestive heart failure and her condition began to improve. With weekly monitoring of her physical status and medications, she proceeded to lose three dress sizes. This loss of weight was brought about by the much-needed loss of fluid which had accumulated during her acute heart failure incident.

E.A. was late for an appointment one day and Ms. Sturgill asked her if everything was all right. E.A. said she had been at a secondhand store trying to find clothes that fit, since her two outfits were now too large. Ms. Sturgill went home that night and purchased new clothing, shoes, undergarments, a winter coat, and snow boots for E.A. When E.A. was presented with these items at her

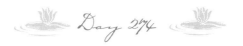

next visit she began to cry. She has relayed to us that the Creighton physicians and staff have "saved her life" and thanked everyone for their care and compassion.

—Submitted by Susan Walsh and Dr. Syed M. Mohiuddin,
The Cardiac Center of Creighton University Medical Center, Omaha, NE

"Never underestimate the difference you can make."

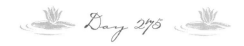

THE EXTRA SHIFT

On a recent Friday morning, I scheduled myself for an extra shift so that I would be able to come in and take care of a friend of mine who was scheduled for a repeat cesarean section. When I came in that morning, I glanced at the labor and delivery board and noticed that it was extremely busy that day. One of the nurses had called in sick and the rest of the staff was relieved to see me come in. I saw that there was a postoperative patient in the recovery room and I offered to take care of this patient so that I could finish her recovery and transfer her to the mother-baby unit in order to be back in time to admit my friend at 10 a.m. Unbeknownst to me, I missed the word "transfusion" next to my patient's name and was clueless as to the situation that lay ahead.

When I arrived in the recovery room, I found quite a few people at my patient's bedside. The primary RN, our anesthesiologist, the obstetrician, and two other nurses all surrounded N.R., the patient. Her husband was at her head talking to her quietly and attempting to keep her relaxed. Another family member was also sitting quietly in a chair nearby. I introduced myself to N.R. and her husband and then quickly received the report from the night shift RN.

N.R. had had four previous natural labors and had been admitted in labor with a spontaneous rupture of the membranes the day before. She had undergone a primary cesarean section at 3:30 that morning and had been in the recovery room ever since. At about 4:30 a.m. her blood pressure had started to drop

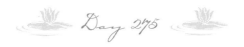

drastically. The nurse caring for the patient had called our anesthesiologist. They had been trying to manage her hypotension for the past two hours by continuously replacing her fluids.

After we ran several tests and performed a thorough examination, it became obvious that N.R. was bleeding internally from somewhere in her body. I felt that we were wasting time by pumping fluids into this patient when we should have been taking her back to surgery. Hemorrhage is the number one cause of death in an obstetrical patient, and we had already been in this situation for more than two hours. However the obstetrician felt that N.R. was not stable enough to take back to surgery. Just prior to her shift change, she had requested that the interventional radiology team be mobilized so that they could perform a uterine artery embolization on the patient to attempt to stop the uterine bleeding that appeared to be the cause of her hypotension.

At 7:30 the interventional radiology team was in-house and ready for us to bring the patient down to the radiology department. I bundled N.R. into the elevator with two anesthesiologists, the obstetricians, and my friend Debbie, a second nurse who had been assigned to assist me with my patient. The patient's family followed in a second elevator. When we arrived in interventional radiology, we escorted the family to the waiting room and went on with N.R. to the operating room where the IR team was waiting for us.

We quickly transferred the patient to the OR table while the team bustled around her trying to get everything ready as fast as possible. Debbie and I felt somewhat out of place, but there did not appear to be a nurse in the room to whom I could give a report about the patient, so we both jumped in and tried to help as much as we could. We had a new anesthesiologist in the room who had assumed care of the patient. Debbie continued to help by running to the blood bank and picking up more blood products for the anesthesiologist.

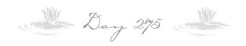

We were so busy rushing around that I almost missed it when N.R. called out my name. She grabbed my hand as I reached her bedside. She was very agitated and moving around on the table. She told me that she was experiencing a lot of pain and asked if I could please hurry everyone up. I tried to reassure her that everyone was working as fast as they possibly could. She continued to look up at me desperately and tightly clasp my hand. In that moment I realized that the person who needed me the most in that room was the patient—not the medical personnel. I concentrated all of my attention on N.R. I stayed with her at the head of her bed and stroked the hair on her forehead while still continuing to hold her hand. I talked quietly to N.R. and worked to keep her focused on me, holding her attention with my eyes.

She remained very agitated, moving her knees up and down and disrupting the area where the IR team was going to be working. I looked at N.R. and told her to think about something nice. "Like what?" she asked. I suggested she tell me where she liked to go, thinking maybe she would say "the beach" or "the mountains"—somewhere that would allow me to try some guided imagery with her and allow her to be distracted from what was going on in the room at that moment. To my surprise, N.R. replied that she liked to go to church. I asked N.R. if she would like for me to pray with her, and she shook her head "yes." I put my head close to hers and for the next five minutes I prayed quietly with her as people in the room continued to work around us. We both felt God's presence in that room. N.R. immediately became calmer and less agitated. When I was done, there was a tear at the corner of her eye. She looked at me with relief and said "thank you."

It wasn't long until we put N.R. to sleep and completed her procedure. We moved her to the recovery room and I gave a report to the post-anesthesia care

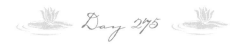

unit nurse and returned to labor and delivery. Two hours had passed since I had assumed N.R.'s care but I felt as though I had already worked an entire shift. As I continued through my day, I couldn't help thinking about N.R. I realized that it should have been *me* thanking *her*. She had provided me with one of my more memorable moments as a nurse. What N.R. needed from me that day was not my medical expertise, but my personal experience that comes from being a Christian. What a blessing that God had placed me in just the right place at the right time to provide N.R. with the spiritual comfort that she needed the most! What a blessing for me that God has allowed me to work in an environment where there is no fear in offering to pray with a patient to meet her non-medical needs!

I continued to check on N.R. throughout the day. She continued to bleed in PACU, which required a second trip back to interventional radiology. When that second procedure did not stop her hemorrhage she was finally taken back to surgery by her attending obstetrician. The cause of her bleeding was finally discovered and the surgeons were able to ligate the bleeding vessel. The patient was taken to the ICU after her recovery and placed on the ventilator. Most importantly, she was alive.

I went to see N.R. the next day in the ICU and was amazed to find her sitting up in bed using the breast pump to express milk for her baby. I will never underestimate the power of the human body. This woman had received over 17 units of blood to keep her alive and just 24 hours later she was trying to do what was best for her baby. The nursing staff from the mother-baby unit had even brought the baby up to the ICU that morning for N.R. to see. She was discharged to go home the following Tuesday…and I breathed a sigh of relief that the collaborative efforts of several units in our hospital had saved N.R.'s life.

—Submitted by Caroline Price, St. Joseph Hospital, Orange, CA

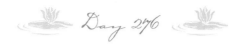

Help in a Hurry

A grateful hospital employee wrote this note to express her appreciation to personnel in the Emergency Room after her father's visit there.

Just a few minutes of your time to tell you how great the ER is. My name is Lori Leach. I work in X-ray. I just have to brag about your staff and the Cardiac Cath Lab/Acute MI team.

My dad, Gary M., was brought into the ER on December 21, 2006, with chest pain. He is a healthy 55-year-old with no major health issues.

He walked in and told triage that he had some chest pain and was taken back to Acute Care, where he then collapsed. He was immediately put into Acute Care Room 2 where he started to aspirate. The quick work of the ER staff and the Cardiac Cath Lab team saved his life. He was shocked somewhere around 18 times and given all the meds he could be given.

Dr. Wheeler and Respiratory did an amazing job as well as the nurses and other staff. I would like to thank them all, but I could never begin to know who all was there. That day was a big blur.

Dr. Horton came in and put a balloon pump in the ER and took him to the Cath Lab and stented him. He walked out of the hospital 12 days after coming to the ER. He is still doing well with minor bumps in the road, but I would not have him at all without the advancements and the staff at Southern Ohio Medical Center.

—*Written by Lori Leach, Submitted by Mary Kate Dilts-Skaggs,*
Southern Ohio Medical Center, Portsmouth, OH

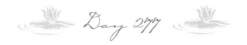

Baby Timmy

Over the past 14 years, my job as a breastfeeding consultant has allowed me to be a part of many families' lives. On a cold January day in 2000 I stopped by a room to visit with one of our new moms, whose baby was in the Neonatal Intensive Care Unit. The baby had been born the night before, a full-term baby boy who had some breathing problems at birth and was put on the ventilator to help him breathe. I entered the room of this mother, knowing beforehand that she would be anxious and afraid. I was aware that she would most likely not be ready to hear my talk on breastfeeding and pumping milk for her baby while he was in the NICU.

Much to my surprise, this young woman quickly recognized me, as I had helped her learn how to breastfeed her daughter when she was born at the hospital three years earlier. She was so glad to see me and so eager to begin collecting her breast milk for her ailing baby. She told me the story of her baby, Timmy, and his birth. Her pregnancy had been uneventful, with no problems at all, and she was so concerned and scared now that her baby was very ill. We talked for quite awhile about all of her feelings, and I let her share her fears with me. She was very happy to begin the pumping process so that she could begin collecting the "liquid gold" for her baby.

As the days passed, I saw her many times in the hallways of the hospital and I continued to visit baby Timmy in our NICU. I would always talk to her to get

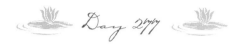

an update on Timmy's condition and the progress of her milk collection. She always seemed glad that all of our staff, including myself, had taken such an interest in her baby. She visited frequently and often brought her three-year-old daughter with her. Timmy was not making significant progress but he had many toys and darling baby boy outfits during his stay in the NICU. It was obvious that he was so special to his family.

After two months of being hospitalized there was not much progress in the baby's condition. The results of some special testing revealed that Timmy suffered from a very rare neuromuscular condition. Most babies born with this condition die right after birth. The family was devastated. It was likely that Baby Timmy would never be able to breathe on his own and would not be able to move his arms and legs due to lack of strength. Despite all of these disabilities he would have normal brain development and would be as intelligent as his development would allow him to be. He would be fully aware of his condition but would be totally dependent on others for his care.

His family was crushed by this news. They researched the Internet and read all of the medical information that they could find on this dreadful disease. They prayed to God and asked over and over why this had to happen to their little baby. They finally found one family in Colorado that had a 10-year-old child suffering from this condition. They decided to go and visit this family so that they could see what may lie ahead in the future for Timmy.

After returning from their trip they had many long talks with other health care professionals. After probing the situation and getting all of the information they could on this condition, they decided to let God decide what should happen to Timmy. On a Friday afternoon in April I was called in to talk to the family. They had decided to remove Timmy from the ventilator over the upcoming weekend.

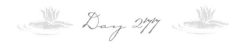

They had talked to many professionals about this and now wanted some information about how best to handle the situation with their three-year-old daughter. She had been such a part of Baby Timmy's life and they were at a loss as to what to tell her. Because of my work with grief and Journey of Hope, the children's grief center in our city, I was asked to talk to the family about their concerns. We went over several possibilities of what might happen when the life support was turned off. Then we discussed how to best handle the situation with their daughter. Since I was going out of town that weekend I was not sure if I would see Timmy or his family again. I stopped by his crib on my way out of the NICU to see him and say goodbye.

On Monday when I returned to work I went to the NICU. Baby Timmy and his family were in one of our parent "rooming-in" rooms. The ventilator had been removed on Saturday but the baby continued breathing without assistance. I walked to their room so that I could talk to the family and see if they needed any additional support. Timmy and his mother were alone in the room. The father had gone home to shower and clean up, and so the mother was enjoying some time alone with Baby Timmy.

We talked about their daughter and how she had been there during the weekend after the ventilator was removed. Then she began to speak about all of the things she was going to miss doing with Timmy that she had enjoyed so much with her older daughter. He would never go to the park, she explained, and she would never get to take him to the zoo. She had read to him and played music for him to listen to, but she continued to lament the fact that he would not have the chance to go to preschool or to dance around to music and sing songs. She revealed to me her devastation that Timmy would never know what it felt like to be outside—he wouldn't see the blue sky, hear the birds, feel the grass, or see the

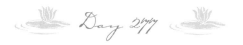

flowers. I felt something come over me and I immediately said to her, "Would you like to take Timmy outside?" She was overwhelmed at the thought. I told her that I would check with the physician and I would return in a few hours to accompany her and her husband as they took their baby out to see the world. She was so happy about this idea. Timmy's breathing had become more labored that day, and she wanted to make sure that he would be able to see the world outside of the NICU before it was too late.

As I left the room I saw the physician in the hallway, and she immediately agreed to what I had proposed to the family. I began to plan how I would take this family outside with their baby. I had never done this before, nor had it ever been done at our hospital. I decided that the courtyard between our two buildings would be an ideal place for us to take the baby outside.

Three hours later I returned to the Parent Room. Timmy and his parents were waiting for me so that we could go outside. His mother had bathed and dressed him and swaddled him in blankets in preparation for the big adventure. Although Timmy's breathing had become slower he was alert. His mother whispered to him, explaining the big adventure that lay ahead. We called the nurse who was caring for Timmy that day and the five of us took the baby outside.

As we walked into the courtyard the world seemed to stand still. All that we could hear were the birds singing and the movement of the leaves on the trees. The smell of fresh green grass wafted through the inviting April air as an airplane flew overhead. I went to a bench and sat down so that the family could enjoy this time alone with their beloved baby. The mother kept telling her baby over and over about all of the things he was experiencing for the first time: the singing of the birds, the movement of the trees, the airplane overhead. Then she sat down on the grass with Baby Timmy, her husband right next to her. They unwrapped the blanket from around Timmy and his mother removed his tiny socks. She wanted to be sure that Timmy could feel the grass between his toes. She continued singing and talking to the baby as her husband hovered close by. I sat with the nurse and watched the precious scene from a distance.

All of a sudden Timmy's mother called for the nurse. The baby had stopped breathing. Diane took her stethoscope and checked the baby's vitals. She confirmed what we had feared. The baby was gone.

We accompanied the family back to the Parent Room so they could spend a 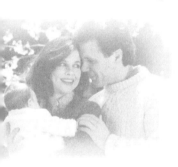 little more time with their baby. As she sat down in the chair with him, his mother looked up at me and said, "You knew this would happen, didn't you?" I was totally overwhelmed with so many feelings. I looked at her and said, "No, there is only one person who knew when this was going to happen and it wasn't me." She thanked me profusely for allowing her to have this experience with her baby. It was the one thing she had wanted for Timmy before he died, and she was amazed and thankful that this wish had been fulfilled.

As I left the room I walked down the hall and slumped into the chair in my office. This experience had been the most profound moment in my entire nursing career. I knew for a fact why I had chosen nursing as a career. I knew that I had been placed in this family's life for a reason, and that the talents I had been given had all come into play that day to make this a memorable experience for them. The ability to help families in a time of crisis is one of the most crucial attributes we all share as health care professionals. However, just being in the right place at the right time can be a powerful gift. It is something that none of us control, but something that we all hope will happen as we perform our daily tasks of caring for families.

—*Submitted by Ginny Robinson, Medical Center of Plano, Plano, TX*

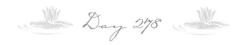

Recognizing Maritza

A traveler who was assigned to work in our ED had these words to say about Maritza Vasquez:

Maritza Vasquez deserves recognition for her SPIRIT. I have never seen Maritza without a smile on her face. She is always so helpful to the patients and their families, often turning some of the most difficult situations into moments of hope.

Maritza worked with me on a case involving finding further health care solutions for neurological intervention that was unavailable in our area. Here's what happened:

As a result of my niece having a Cerebrovascular accident (CVA) at age nine, I knew my sister had knowledge in the area and many direct connections to a neurological institute in New York City. Commonly referred to as a stroke, a CVA occurs when the blood flow to the brain is impaired by blockage or rupture of an artery and the subsequent lack of oxygen to the brain causes the sudden death of brain cells.

To find the information and solutions we needed, I went home and researched CVAs with my sister. I then returned to Vassar and gave many pages of information to Maritza, educating her on pediatric CVA. She was most appreciative for this information as she knew others would benefit

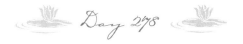
greatly from it. We then discussed ways to help disseminate the information to others in need.

Maritza never tires of helping patients and their families. She goes above and beyond on a daily basis. I hope she is appreciated by others as much as I appreciate her.

People like Maritza give VBMC a good face and give them a positive memory of their experience here. She sets the bar high for health care workers everywhere.

—Submitted by Gretchen Halstead, Vassar Brothers Medical Center, Poughkeepsie, NY

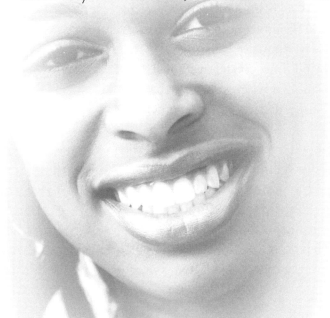

"Never underestimate the difference you can make."

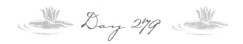

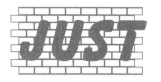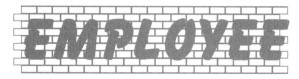

JUST AN EMPLOYEE

When the phone rang, I quickly checked caller ID and smiled when I realized it was my dear friend, Helen. Her voice sounded strained so I immediately knew there was a problem. She had tripped while working in her garden on a slope at the side of her house.

"I think I have broken my ankle," she said. I assumed her assessment was most likely correct, since she had broken an ankle several years before. Helen had osteoporosis and despite a concerted effort to improve her bone density, her readings still indicated dramatic bone loss.

I rushed the several miles to Helen's house. She was sitting in the kitchen, leg outstretched. She laughed when she saw what I had dragged into the room—a set of crutches from some distant athletic injury one of our kids had sustained a decade earlier.

Helen had grabbed a pack of frozen cut veggies and laid it on her ankle, which was rapidly swelling. "I read that little tip in the Harvard Medical Newsletter," she said, pointing to the bag. "And just think—if we get stuck at the hospital, we'll have something for dinner!"

I found an Ace bandage and strapped the veggies to her throbbing ankle.

I gathered up Helen's possessions and struggled to help with her jacket. Helen tried to balance with the crutches but it was nearly impossible for her to navigate

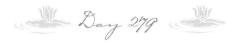

to my car. The crutches were much too large and the combination of pain and awkward movement brought tears to Helen's eyes.

The Kansas sky had been threatening a downpour all morning, and as we drove the six miles to Overland Park Regional Medical Center, the storm finally broke. By the time I arrived at the Emergency Department, water was swirling in the parking lot and along the curbside. I was baffled as to how we were going to get Helen into the ED without falling again. I put on the emergency lights and ran inside and asked if someone could help me with a wheel chair.

I was told I needed to go to another entrance. And then someone else said, "Well, I don't even know where a wheelchair is right now." I had to chuckle, knowing that every hospital deals with disappearing wheelchairs. But my amusement at that thought quickly changed to aggravation when I realized no one was going to help me.

"I need to get a lady inside who has most likely broken her ankle," I said. Still, no one was doing a thing to assist me.

Then suddenly, a young man touched my elbow and said he would help. I glanced at his name tag and realized he was a Radiology Technician.

"Don't you need to be someplace taking Xrays?" I said. "Isn't there a transporter around somewhere?" He just smiled.

"Yes," he said, "but right now, I am here and you are here and your friend needs help, so let's see what we can do."

I began to explain my situation and the young man simply pointed out the door and asked, "Is that your car?"

I had hardly responded affirmatively when he said, "Bring the umbrella and come on."

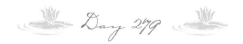
We dashed to the car, I opened the door, positioned the umbrella, and the young man swooped Helen into his arms and sprinted inside the building.

"How's that for transport?" he said once we were inside. Helen and I were shaking off the rain, trying to get her settled in a chair, and as I turned away, he was already rushing down the hall.

"Thank you! Thank you so much!" I yelled to him as he hurried down the corridor. "But I didn't catch your name!"

He lifted his hand in the air in a salute and shouted back at me.

"I am just an employee!" he said. And then he was gone.

—Submitted by Ann Beard Hornberger, Charlotte, NC

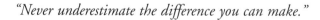

"Never underestimate the difference you can make."

Exceptional Care During Trying Times

After her husband's stay at the Medical University of South Carolina Medical Center, where she is also employed, Sheila Griner wrote this letter about their experiences.

My husband, Benji Griner, was a patient on the 8th floor, in the Bone Marrow Transplant area. The total hospital experience was excellent. Starting off in Admissions, we were greeted and told who would be assisting us, given an estimated time before they would be available, and how long it would take once we were called back. We felt we were registering into a nice hotel, not a hospital.

Once the elevator opened onto the 8th floor, Karen, from Guest Relations, welcomed us, introduced herself, looked over our papers, helped with our belongings and escorted us to our room.

The nursing staff was awesome. Jill, Sonia, Sandra and Lucy—all were very competent, attentive and compassionate. What an excellent group of care givers. They never entered the room without first knocking, and always explained what they were doing, how long it would take, what will happen next. They did not leave the room without saying "Is there anything that you need?"

The CA's were also competent and caring. Monica and Mathie took especially good care of Benji.

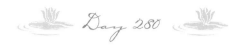

Ms. Cash knocked on our door each day, introducing herself, explaining what she would like to do (mop, clean the bathroom, empty trash, etc.) and would ask if this was a good time for her to come in.

We had visits from the Pharm-D each day. Dr. Kristi Lenz discussed in detail the medications Benji was taking (prescriptions and over the counter), the treatment that he would be receiving, and the symptoms he could expect. Benji takes a lot of different supplements. Dr. Lenz introduced us to a Pharmacy student, Jimmy, who researched and presented us with a detailed supplement comparison report. Benji was advised to stop taking some of the supplements during chemotherapy.

When released on Saturday morning 5/5, Benji hugged Sonia his nurse, and Monica his CA, and said "I enjoyed it." Did he actually enjoy three days of chemotherapy? Of course not. But he did have an excellent experience throughout the hospital and felt he was in the best place for his treatment.

Am I proud to be associated with MUSC? Absolutely! Would we recommend coming to MUSC as a patient? You bet we would.

Thank you.
Sheila Griner (Hospital Human Resources)

—*Submitted by Sheila Griner, MUSC Medical Center*

"Never underestimate the difference you can make."

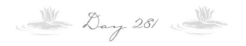

The Best Care for Baby Aaron

Our hospital received this letter of gratitude from the parent of a new baby:

Dear Ms. Tucker:

I would like to compliment you on the outstanding Neonatal Intensive Care Unit that you have. My son, Aaron, was admitted at two days old because he required emergency surgery. This was an unbelievably frightening situation, but we were comforted and cared for every step of the way.

Every person whom I came into contact with was compassionate and dedicated. Aaron's surgeon, Dr. David Drucker, was professional and approachable throughout the entire course of his stay, as were the other surgeons looking after him. The neonatologists were always quite informative as to Aaron's condition.

However, it was the nursing staff that really takes the cake. From the first night, Aaron's nurse focused on his post-operative needs, and the nurse manager focused on our needs as parents. Getting us a room at the Conine Clubhouse was so beneficial for our family in so many ways. The intense care that Aaron received after his surgery from his nurses, especially Jackie and Penny, was astonishing. It was so comforting any time I called (mostly late at night) to speak immediately to his nurse and know he was receiving the best care. These people really work hard for 12 hours a shift!

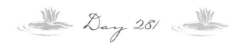

As Aaron continued to improve, we were introduced to more excellent nursing from Rob, Vanessa and Sue. I appreciated the support given by Dawn concerning breastfeeding and Aaron's special needs. Actually, all his nurses were concerned, but Dawn led the charge. The support meetings were helpful, especially for family support. Also, family and friends all over the country and even internationally were able to keep up with Aaron's progress through the care pages that Rob helped me set up. Finally, these nurses did not forget that I was postpartum and always made sure that my recovery continued.

Let me end this just by saying every person that I came into contact with in the NICU blew me away with their compassion and dedication to my son and every baby there.

Sincerely,

An appreciative parent

P.S. Aaron is doing great at home!

—Submitted by Nina Tucker, Joe DiMaggio Children's Hospital, Hollywood, FL

"Never underestimate the difference you can make."

A Good Call

On January 28, 2003, a patient, who was also a Creighton University student, had palpitations and was sent to the Cardiac Center for an event recorder. Nancy Weber, a Cardiac Technician II in Cardiology's Monitoring and EKG Services Section, received his first transmission on March 1st. The patient complained of his "chest fluttering." His recording was evaluated as normal and he was encouraged to continue to record events as his symptoms recurred. The next day he called again with symptoms of right-sided chest pain, right arm weakness, right leg weakness, and shortness of breath. Again, Nancy took the call and his recording was normal. Concerned that the recording was normal, but the symptoms seemed significant and he sounded short of breath, Nancy contacted the cardiologist on call who recommended the patient go to the Emergency Department. The patient was found to have a spontaneous pneumothorax.

Nancy visited the patient on March 4th as he was recovering from his surgery. As soon as she started to speak, the patient said, "You must be Nancy." Although he found it difficult to speak, he wanted to thank Nancy for her help. She used her common sense and perception skills to ensure her patient was cared for even when his symptoms did not fit the protocol. Her "above and beyond" efforts may very well have saved this patient's life. This is only one example of Nancy's tenacious spirit and dedication to our patients. She is a valuable staff member who has taken her job-related responsibilities to a higher level and incorporated

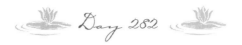

the values that embody Creighton University. Her actions are an example of her continuous efforts to "live" Creighton's mission and move the School of Medicine toward 100 percent customer satisfaction.

—Submitted by Susan K. Walsh and Dr. Syed M. Mohiuddin,
The Cardiac Center of Creighton University Medical Center, Omaha, NE

"Never underestimate the difference you can make."

The Best Reward

I have been a nurse for 45 years and have worked in many areas. We have seen many changes and advances during my career but the one constant is that we still have sick patients. And those patients still need competent, caring, dedicated health care workers to meet their needs.

Patients are expected to absorb so much when they experience a life change or receive a diagnosis that affects them and their families. If we can keep it in mind, that we may be that patient one day and need support and understanding, our job becomes much easier. And as we experience success, we feel the ongoing desire to make a difference.

Although nursing has provided me the security of knowing I could always find a job and help support my family, I can honestly say the greatest thing about nursing is that it is a profession of giving as well as receiving. I feel one of the biggest rewards the nursing profession has afforded me is the opportunity to work with great people who also want to help people feel better.

As I look toward retirement, I truly feel I have gotten back a wealth of things that have no material or monetary value. I can't think of anything I would rather have done in the workforce. I am proud to be a nurse.

In many situations I have encountered, the look on the patient's face, a grateful family member or being with someone in the last minutes of their life–those things are my rewards.

—*Anonymous Contributor, Capital Region Medical Center, Jefferson City, MO*

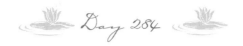

A Momentous Walk Down the Aisle

My dad was taken care of by the staff at Martinsville Memorial Hospital in Virginia. I would like to share a story about how his health care providers went above and beyond their call of duty to make sure my dad had the best care possible. The story about my dad was so inspiring to the employees of Martinsville Memorial that his nurse, Wendy Nuzum, was voted as Employee of the Year. I hope that this heartfelt story will be an inspiration to all.

Wendy Nuzum is not only an exceptional nurse; she is an exceptional person. She is dedicated to her profession, her co-workers, and especially her patients. Serving in several patient care areas, she has a caring attitude that's apparent with each and every patient and co-worker she sees…by the smile on her face, or how she greets you by name.

One particular example of Wendy's loving kindness spoke to the hearts of all of our employees and made her a clear candidate for Memorial Hospital's 2002 Employee of the Year. This year, Wendy had an oncology patient who had been given six weeks to live. Even though this news was overwhelming on its own, his family was even more devastated as they were planning his daughter's wedding day. This patient's final wish was to be able to walk his daughter down the aisle to give her away, but this was a difficult task, given that the wedding was three hours away from Martinsville and the man needed specialized care. On Friday afternoon, Wendy and Dr. Arthur Sleeper clocked out, packed their bags and

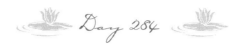

picked up their patient, hydrating him with IV fluids to ensure that he realized his goal of being part of his daughter's special day.

Because of Wendy's dedication and compassion, every family member could celebrate the joyous occasion together. On the following Monday, the patient was admitted to our Hospice program. Although she was not a nurse on that unit, Wendy spent her time off with the family to ensure that their needs were being met as they made difficult decisions about their loved one and his care. She was there when they needed a hand to hold, there when they needed answers about his care, there when they needed a shoulder to cry on, and there to surround the family with love and support as he took his last breath.

We are very fortunate to have Wendy Nuzum, and others like her at Memorial Hospital. They serve to inspire us all to be everything we can be and more, not only as health care providers, but as employees and individuals.

As a final note: an oncology patient in our community once commented to a staff member that other larger cancer centers can offer treatments that Martinsville cannot, but no one else can offer Wendy Nuzum.

—Submitted by Jessica E. Read, Martinsville Memorial Hospital, Martinsville, VA

"Never underestimate the difference you can make."

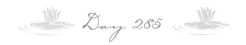
New Equipment

We have an amazing story to tell. Winchester Hospital Hematology/Oncology Center is an offsite cancer treatment facility. This past September, a 64-year-old woman with lung cancer was coming to receive her first chemotherapy treatment. As is customary, the patient had a nurse assessment, which was normal, and was waiting in an exam room to see the physician.

Alerted by a patient in the corridor, staff was called to the exam room and found the patient on the floor. The patient was quickly assessed with a weak pulse and respiratory effort. Shortly thereafter, no pulse or respiration was evident. CPR was started, and 911 was called. When the paramedic team arrived on the scene, the patient was shocked and she quickly resumed normal sinus rhythm. The patient's family was notified and appropriate support given to them.

After the patient was safely transported to the hospital, the staff agreed that the clinic needed an AED, and requested a response from their nurse manager. Immediate contact was made to advocate for a unit at the oncology clinics at Baldwin Park and Montvale Avenue. Shortly after, a relative of a Baldwin Park patient who had been at the clinic and witnessed the event contacted Winchester Hospital administration requesting AED for the center.

Aileen Day received immediate support for the AEDs from Donna O'Brien, Emergency Room Nurse Manager, and Sean Ahern, Associate Director of the

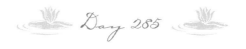

Cardio Pulmonary Department. Both assisted in the efforts to obtain a unit. A presentation was made to the code committee, which subsequently decided to equip all outpatient areas with an AED. The decision was brought to Winchester Hospital senior management, and twenty-two AED units were purchased in less than a two-month period.

As for the patient, she continues to come to the clinic for ongoing treatment. She has no recall of the actual events, but no member of the clinic staff will ever forget it.

—*Submitted by Winchester Hospital Hematology/Oncology Center, Woburn, MA*

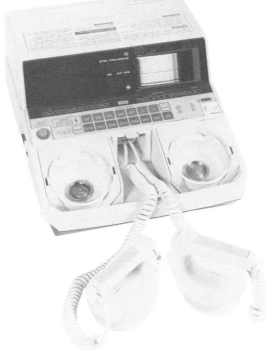

"Never underestimate the difference you can make."

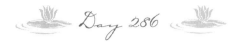

TIMELY RECOGNITION

We began working with Studer Group in 2004. One of the directives specifically recommended was recognizing those among us who have done good things for our organization. So in November 2004 we presented our first Physician of the Month Award to Dr. Chikere Agadaga, an internal medicine physician from Nigeria. Dr. Agadaga was a well-loved member of our medical staff, known for his outstanding care for his patients as well as his work in the ER.

Dr. Agadaga brightened our lives with his wonderful sense of humor and a great smile that shone brightly from his dark, round face. His attitude was upbeat and positive. When asked to attend a hospital meeting, he would quickly reply that he planned to be there "unless the Lord comes." Dr. Agadaga was very touched and honored by the award and mentioned it several times over the following weeks.

On January 11, 2005, Dr. Agadaga was killed in an automobile accident while on his way to the airport to fly to Nigeria to bury his father. We are so glad we implemented our physician recognition award. It allowed us to express to Dr. Agadaga how much he meant to us. The award he received remains as an enduring legacy of the positive impact he made in our lives.

—Submitted by Charlotte Burns, Hardin Medical Center, Savannah, TN

"Never underestimate the difference you can make."

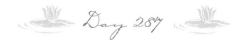

Inspiring Commitment

Rita Craig truly loves working as a home health aide for Home Nursing Agency. In fact, her enthusiasm for her profession has influenced her daughter, Melissa, who is pursuing her baccalaureate degree in nursing at Mount Aloysius College in Cresson, Pennsylvania and enjoying her clinical rotation at an area nursing home.

How has Rita transferred her passion for caring to her daughter? She says that she believes it's not necessarily her *words*, but rather her *actions* that had the greatest influence on Melissa's career choice.

"There were so many days I could have taken off work, but I wouldn't because my patients were like family and I knew they needed me," explains Rita. "I could not let them down."

Rita is candid about the challenges of raising a daughter as a single mother and also of overcoming an ankle injury four years ago—an injury that nearly ended her work as a home health aide.

While performing a home improvement project, Rita was replacing cement slabs when she broke both ankle bones. At the time, she was given a grim prognosis about her future mobility. Her job required travel throughout the rural mining towns of Central Pennsylvania. Injuring her ankles could have made this nearly impossible, but Rita worked hard to overcome her injuries to return to the job she so enjoys.

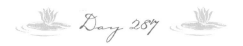

Rita believes adversity only makes a person stronger. She fervently holds on to her belief that God doesn't give her more than she can handle—and that He'll provide the way and the means to overcome.

Rita cherishes the close-knit, personable atmosphere of her hometown of Carrolltown, Pennsylvania. "People are like family here," says Rita. Unsurprisingly, Rita's patients echo this sentiment when discussing their relationship with her.

Rita's attitude is one reason her peers bestowed her with the "Extra Effort Award" at the Agency's annual employee recognition brunch.

Following are a few excerpts from what Rita's colleagues wrote about her:

"Rita has exhibited a strong commitment to the patients and families of Home Nursing Agency...She is an individual with unbelievable flexibility with her schedule to accommodate and achieve the utmost in patient satisfaction. We admire her willingness to put in the extra time and in never turning down assignments. She has shown extraordinary dependability through her excellent attendance record...Patients never hesitate to praise the quality and compassion she places in her work...Rita has distinguished herself as a dedicated, genuine and compassionate employee...She has a strong commitment to the ideals of Home Nursing Agency and goes above and beyond to make sure those entrusted to her care get the attention and services they need and deserve."

These from-the-heart words are truly a testament to the inspiring commitment level of an extraordinary health care professional!

—Submitted by Nicole Fedeli-Turiano, Home Nursing Agency, Altoona, PA

"Never underestimate the difference you can make."

BRINGING BACK ALBERTA'S SMILE

"No man is an island, entire of itself; every man is a piece of the continent." There are few places where John Donne's quote is more poignant than a cancer treatment center.

Alberta is a 67-year-old African-American woman who came to our center on a warm summer's day. Alberta had been diagnosed with breast cancer in 2005 and less than two years later, she learned her cancer had returned. A petite woman at 5 feet 5 inches tall and only 100 pounds, Alberta made up for her small stature with her enormous courage and dancing eyes. She had a beautiful spirit about her and brightened the room with her warm personality.

Alberta had endured many hardships during her life, including growing up in an impoverished neighborhood as one of six children. Her mother and maternal grandmother both died from the very cancer that she faces today. Her father died from lung cancer. Alberta has four children, all of whom she raised alone.

Never one to allow for self-pity, Alberta has continued to work at a local YWCA through her current diagnosis and surgeries. Her meager wages don't afford her many luxuries. She doesn't own a car and came to her appointment today by way of a cab. She has minimal health insurance, but no dental insurance.

When I first met Alberta, she used her hand to cover her mouth and hide her smile whenever she was greeted. Alberta has no teeth. Years of poor diet and no

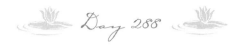

dental care continued to destroy her oral hygiene until, eventually, all of her teeth were gone and her overall health began to deteriorate. She stated that she had such a difficult time eating that she had lost 20 pounds since losing the last of her teeth. She also said she hadn't eaten meat of any type in over two years.

Helping Alberta was a true team effort. The assessment nurse contacted Social Services to see what services were available to her, and Karen from the American Cancer Society made a phone call to a local orthodontist who generously offered his services to help cancer patients in need. When I went to the room to tell Alberta we had found a way to address her dental needs, she cried. I held her hand and we lifted our voices in praise to God for the wonderful blessing He was about to bestow.

After several visits to the orthodontist's office, Alberta presented herself to our office with a brand new set of dentures. She was absolutely beautiful with her brilliant new smile! When I reached out to offer her a hug, she said to me, "My mother always told me I had the most beautiful smile and now thanks to all of you, God has let me smile again."

—Submitted by Terrie E. Mellington, St. Joseph Cancer Center, Warren, OH

"Never underestimate the difference you can make."

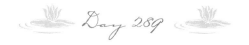

Keep on Paddling!

Early in my career as a nurse, I worked on a Medical/Oncology unit. The nurse manager of the unit, Dianna Paustian, was a wonderful nurse. She was one of the most dedicated nurses–to the practice of bedside nursing–that I have ever met. She taught me many things.

Dianna was well respected by her staff. She had a marvelous way of making sure we knew exactly what the priorities were. Always, the patient was Number One. Then, once the patients were cared for, she had a way of being sure we were aware of the stuff that came down from the organization in the way of memos, policies, and procedures.

And then there were the things that we really "needed" to know. Those things she would post in the bathroom. Any time we took a three minute personal needs break, we were instantly updated by reading the bathroom walls! We would wash our hands, initial the information on the wall, and in a very efficient way–we were all in the know.

When I went into nursing, I knew I wanted to specialize in Peds/NICU so I only stayed on Dianna's unit for less than two years, but I got a great foundation from a leader who still is a nurse leader 22 years later. I know she is still focused on the patient, still prioritizing information for her staff, and still making impressions on nurses like me.

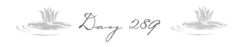

Years later, when I was in a different position, I would occasionally go up to the bathroom on her unit to read the walls because I knew I would leave "updated."

Dianna had a quote on the bulletin board that I still think of often. It said, "Nurses are like ducks. Calm and serene on the top, but paddling like hell underneath."

In my 23 years as a nurse, there has never been a day when that hasn't been true. To all the nurses, and nurse leaders, if you are reading this, keep paddling!

—Submitted by Lyn Ketelsen, Studer Group, Coal Valley, IL

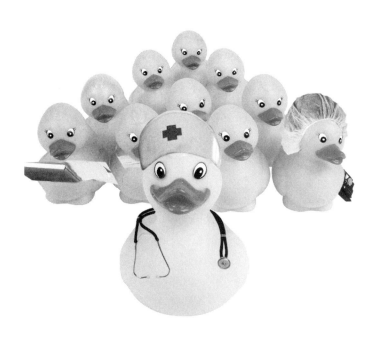

"Never underestimate the difference you can make."

Connecting to Purpose

When I tell people I work in Hospice, I often get an "Oh, how depressing!" response. People seem genuinely surprised when I tell them I don't find it depressing at all, but instead, find it very rewarding. I point out to them that short of helping to bring people into this world, I can't think of a more significant event in someone's life than when they leave this world. My goal is to help them to do so with as much dignity and comfort as possible, and to help their loved ones as well.

My first nursing experience with death and dying occurred when I was a young Army Nurse. I had been stationed at a large medical center for about three years. The first two years were spent on an orthopedic unit where I had been somewhat sheltered from death. My third year there, I was moved to a general medicine unit and my world was no longer sheltered.

We had admitted a retired officer a week before for some tests for urinary retention problems. I found myself forming a bond with him because he reminded me in so many ways of my own father with his humor and wit. His daughter was a regular visitor and we would frequently laugh and joke about our dads.

One evening, during shift report, it was noted that this gentleman's biopsy results had come back positive. He had advanced prostate cancer which had apparently metastasized. I felt awful about it. I asked if the patient had been told

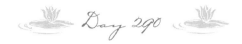

yet and was told no, but that his doctor would be coming in that evening to meet with the patient and his daughter to discuss the results.

All evening long, I dreaded the daughter's arrival on the unit. I found myself avoiding the patient's room because I didn't want him to see on my face that he was dying.

At the usual time, his daughter arrived, obviously eager to hear the test results. I dodged her questions by saying the doctor should be up "any minute" to talk to them, and then I ducked into the med room.

An hour went by and still no doctor. The patient's daughter came to me at the nurses' station and asked if I could try paging him to find out when he would be coming. When I reached the doctor and informed him of the daughter's request, I could tell he had been dreading the conversation as much as I had. He sighed and said something about being really busy, but he would be up when he could. I told the daughter he was tied up but would come as soon as he could. She waited another hour and then came back out to the front desk. She had small kids at home and the sitter was getting impatient. I called the doctor again and this time he told me to "just handle it."

I was terrified. How was I supposed to tell this patient he was dying? What if I screwed it up? I had just about decided I wasn't going to do it when the daughter came out to the station again and noticed I was upset. She asked me if I was okay. That was when I realized that no matter how uncomfortable I was with the situation, the patient and his family deserved better treatment than they were getting from us. I told her that no, I wasn't okay, and asked if she'd mind joining me in the lounge where we could talk.

We went in and sat down and I began by telling her how I had formed a kinship with her father and that made the news I had to give her that much more

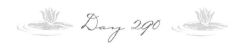

difficult. I told her what I knew of the test results and prognosis. She seemed a bit stunned and asked if there was any chance of a mistake. Then she began asking questions about treatment options. Even though I had already told her that the disease was too far advanced for curative treatment, I realized she needed to go over this information again to assimilate it. We discussed chemo, radiation, and surgery and what the likely outcomes would be.

When she began to cry, I handed her a box of tissues and grabbed a handful for myself. At first I was embarrassed to cry in front of her, but when I apologized to her she responded, "Nonsense…it just shows how much you care."

Amazingly enough, the world had not come to a screeching halt because I had mentioned the "d" word. More importantly, the family had not fallen apart because I was less than perfect in delivering bad news. We talked some more and eventually the doctor arrived on the floor to have his meeting with them. I went in to the room and held the daughter's hand during the talk.

The patient took the news much as I expected he would. He was very stoic and seemed more concerned about maintaining control and not being a burden to his family than he was about his own impending death. I think we were all relieved when he responded that way, as it made it easier on us.

I look back now and wonder if we did him a disservice by encouraging that stoicism. I can only hope that he and his family were referred to Hospice and received the right kind of support.

I realized at that point that, as healthcare professionals, we were not trained well to deal with death. Death was viewed as the enemy, something to be fought against, and to have your patient die meant you had somehow failed them. Since then, I have worked in ERs, sub-acute care ventilator units, and long term care. I have seen that there are things that can be worse than death.

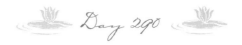

During the past nine years that I've worked in Hospice, I've seen that when handled correctly, death does not have to be painful or even feared. Feeling sadness is just an indication that you care and it doesn't need to be viewed as a negative emotion.

For all the tears I've shed, there have been ten times the smiles and laughter which I've shared with my patients and their loved ones, as well. I would say I have been quite blessed.

—Submitted by Pam Edwards

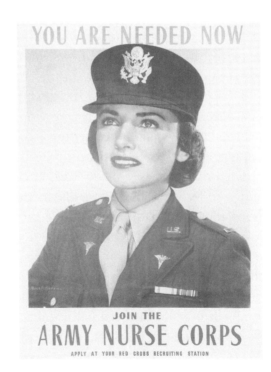

"Never underestimate the difference you can make."

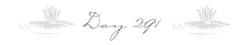

Professionalism Makes Big Impression

Sometimes, it's the little things that carry the most weight in how a patient perceives her care experience. D.B.'s outpatient laparoscopic cholecystectomy (gall-bladder removal) surgery was hardly dramatic, but the kindness and compassion she experienced at St. Vincent Mercy Medical Center made a tremendous impression on her.

"This was the first surgery I've had since having my tonsils out at age eight, so I was a little nervous," D.B. admits. "I had been prepared for the hospital staff to be detached, busy and to not trust me to understand what was going on well enough to bother explaining anything to me. I was pleasantly surprised to find the opposite is true at St. Vincent."

D.B. says she received excellent care and service from the moment she registered through her discharge.

"The third-year medical student assigned to my case was especially open and informative," she says. "He talked to me while I was waiting for Dr. Rosol (Stanley Rosol, DO, FACOS), and he explained the entire procedure in detail, in a way that I could understand and without once sounding condescending or irritated that I was asking so many questions. I am extremely grateful to him for taking the time to talk to me and treat me not only with respect but also as an equal."

D.B.'s positive experiences continued throughout her surgical and post-surgical experiences.

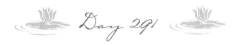

"Dr. Rosol and his surgical team were all immensely good-natured and terrifically skilled," D.B. says. "I left surgery on Nov. 17, 2006, with just four tiny scars, and today only two are slightly visible. I had a little bit of tenderness and fatigue after the surgery, but I was amazed at how quickly I recovered."

D.B. spent about an hour and a half in the hospital post-surgery and says she credited the "gracious concern and outright good humor of everyone there" with helping her immediately start to feel better. She may not remember the names of her care providers, but she will never forget their compassionate, quality care.

"Thank you all for everything you did for me," she says. "The entire staff went well above and beyond the call of duty in making me feel comfortable, relaxed and at ease. I sincerely hope I never need to have anything else removed, but if I do, I will definitely return to St. V's to have it done. You are all truly amazing."

—Anonymous Contributor, St. Vincent Mercy Medical Center, Toledo, OH

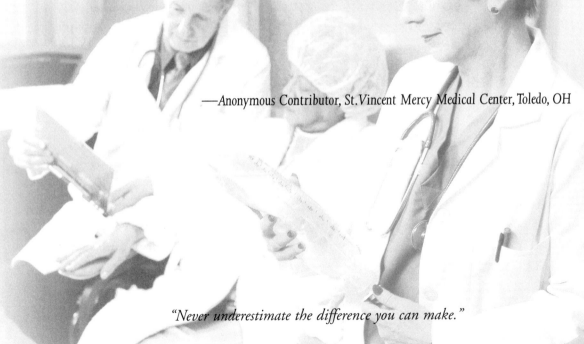

"Never underestimate the difference you can make."

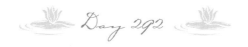
MAKING A CONTRIBUTION

Ursula reclined in bed at the Ambulatory Care Center waiting for surgery in her fight against breast cancer. The woman, originally from Germany, recalls being anxious and in pain. "I didn't feel good. And then…Jim Baynes came over," she begins.

When Jim Baynes, a World War II Veteran, retired from working at Boone High School as an assistant coach and boys' guidance counselor after 29 years, he had nothing to do. "I was not making a contribution and I felt horrible," Jim shares. With an excitement that lit his face, Jim explained what happened next:

"One day, a former neighbor and long-since-graduated student of mine stopped by for a visit. At the end of the conversation, the man told me to be ready at eight o' clock the next morning. He said he would come get me. The following morning I waited and exactly at eight, Clarence Brown, MD, President/CEO of M.D. Anderson Cancer Center Orlando, picked me up and drove me to the volunteer office at Orlando Regional Medical Center. 'Do something with him,' he requested, 'and start him now.' I have been here ever since." Jim concludes his story with a proud smile on his face.

For nine years, Jim has worked every weekday morning in the Ambulatory Care Center (ACC) totaling 12,218 hours so far. One morning in the spring of 2005, Jim began talking with Ursula and relating with her in his compassionate and light-hearted manner. He joked with her and shared his personal experience with breast cancer in 1980. "He even had me laughing," Ursula continues. "He made my experience wonderful and my waiting period so much better."

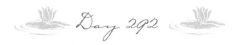
Day 292

Jim credits the team at the ACC for the wonderful job they do while still relating with patients and making them feel better. "Give them all the credit. It is because of them that I am here," Jim always insists. "My contribution is only possible because of their reputation."

"I forgot about my pain. I forgot about the concerns I had about surgery. Jim diverted my fears to something so delightful and made a big difference," Ursula praises.

"I like making a difference in someone's life; it is why I volunteer," Jim says.

"He really is an amazing man and is an inspiration to us all," explains the manager of Volunteer and Guest Services. "We are very lucky to have him; he has made such a difference in so many lives."

"I wake up and want to be there," Jim says. "It is selfish, I know, but I like making a contribution."

—Submitted by Mary Tomlinson, On Purpose Partners, Winter Park, FL

"Never underestimate the difference you can make."

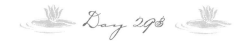

Making Wishes Come True

At 20, Desmond had been in and out of the Oncology/Vascular Unit at St. Charles for eight years. Desmond was once again a patient, admitted for radiation therapy. He was bored and obviously unhappy, and staff members at St. Charles wanted to find a way to put a smile on Desmond's face.

"He was burdened with so much pain and a very difficult-to-accept diagnosis," said Director of Case Management Maria Johar.

Case Manager Dianne Shetley, Social Worker Greg Frankforther, and many of Desmond's nurses, including Jessica Showaker, Jennifer Fryman, and Peggy Margraf, worked to develop a positive relationship with Desmond. He expressed an interest in watching movies, provided a list of favorites, and Dianne Shetley found those movies for him to view. Once the nurses learned of his interest in video games, they began bringing those to him, also.

Desmond perked up when he heard about the new Nintendo Wii gaming system, so the staff thought procuring the new system might do a lot to make Desmond more comfortable. However, the system had not yet been released, so despite Dianne's phone calls to locate one, it seemed the impossible task.

Angie Powers, a nurse in Palliative Care, took up the search, and after explaining Desmond's situation, found a Wal-Mart willing to donate a Nintendo Wii before it was released for sale to the public.

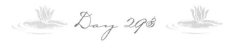

"It's moments like this that make nursing worth it," Angie said.

Maria Johar picked up the game system and several SCMH staff members surprised Desmond with the gift.

"I woke up today and had a feeling something out of the ordinary was going to happen," Desmond relayed, "but I didn't know what."

Touched by the effort made on his behalf, and grateful for the new system, Desmond said he was blessed to be surrounded by people who truly cared about him.

"I know they care about me here," Desmond explained. "They don't just say it; they show it, so I know they mean it. I really love them here."

—Anonymous Contributor, St. Charles Mercy Hospital, Oregon, OH

"Never underestimate the difference you can make."

590

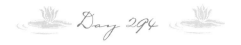

FAR-REACHING REPUTATION

We have experienced very good results from our implementation of Studer Group's principles. We received improved patient and employee satisfaction scores right from the start. Our patients have never received better care! We found out how far our efforts had gone when one of our employees told us about a call from her brother-in-law, Casey, a riverboat captain who lives in Pensacola and works out of Houston.

Casey had lost most of his eyesight and couldn't work. He had been referred by his employer's insurance company to a specialist in Houston for surgery, but the procedure did not correct the problem. He was then sent to a specialist in Miami, who told him there was nothing to be done. Casey's company was desperately trying to find help for him.

After much research, Casey received a call recommending a doctor in Jackson, Tennessee. Casey told them he was familiar with Jackson. They explained that the Jackson physician recommended that he have the surgery performed not in Jackson, but at Hardin Medical Center in Savannah, Tennessee, because of the facility's low infection rate. Casey laughed as he explained that his brother lived in Savannah and that his sister-in-law actually worked at that very hospital!

We are pleased to report that Casey had his surgery here and is doing great. He's back at work, and he can see! Our "Port of Excellence" initiative reached all the way from our small west Tennessee town on the banks of the Tennessee River to Texas. How wonderful to know we were able to help another river traveler continue his journey!

—*Submitted by Charlotte Burns, Hardin Medical Center, Savannah, TN*

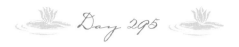

Noticing the Little Things

About three months ago, Ryan Miller, Van Driver for Cardiology, noted scratches on the marble floor of our front entryway. He thought the scratches looked as if a walker may have caused them and began visiting with the patients who used walkers. Mr. Miller found Mr. W, a 79-year-old widower who comes to our Cardiac Rehabilitation Program three times a week. Mr. Miller talked with Mr. W and told him he noticed the rubber tips of his walker were worn out. He asked if he could get them replaced for him. Mr. W quickly agreed and thanked him for his concern. Mr. Miller went to a friend's medical supply company (on his own time) to ask for a donation of the rubber tips for Mr. W's walker during his next visit to Cardiac Rehabilitation. Needless to say, the patient was thrilled by their concern and assistance.

Mr. Miller does not have any type of medical training or higher education in his background. He has worked for the division of Cardiology for only ten months. He is not a well-compensated professional, but rather an individual who makes an hourly wage and demonstrates an innate caring for people.

—Submitted by Susan K. Walsh and Dr. Syed M. Mohiuddin,
Creighton University Medical Center, Omaha, NE

"Never underestimate the difference you can make."

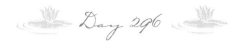

My Daddy, My Hero

It started out just another sticky summer evening in central Florida. It was 1973, I was 13, and my one true love was an oversized strawberry roan with a Roman nose and a four-beat canter. So when Daddy called to say he was stuck at the hospital and would be late picking me up, I was glad to have the extra hour in the barn with my horse Fritz.

Daddy is a radiologist and I knew that meant he was some sort of doctor, even though all he seemed to do was sit alone in a dark room all day. It was a tiny room with a wall of lighted panels displaying X-ray films, which Daddy pored over hour after hour as he dictated gibberish into a tape recorder. I knew what real doctors were. I'd seen plenty on TV. They worked at inner city hospitals with big ER departments filled with gunshot victims, prostitutes and drug dealers. Doctors were superheroes who said things like "Bring me the clamp!" and "I'm going in!" as they crammed a breathing tube down a patient's throat. Doctors were moody and authoritative, and when they bellowed "Stat!" everybody jumped. My father, on the other hand, was a kindly small town radiologist who worked in a one-hospital town where the most exciting event was another Florida retiree breaking a hip. Daddy spent his days sitting in a dark room talking to no one. I loved him. But I was not impressed.

The Ford station wagon finally rolled through the barn gates. I got inside, smelling like horse and sweat and hay, and we set off on the long ride home

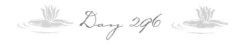

down a two-lane country road. There were scattered farmhouses in the distance and a few humble homes alongside the road, but mostly there were rows of orange trees with the occasional oversized oak covered in dangling Spanish moss. We drove and drove down that dark country road, the only break in the monotony coming from the occasional flash of headlights from an oncoming pickup truck. One had pulled behind us and was attempting to pass just as a car was coming from the other direction.

I heard the high pitch of screeching brakes followed by the shattering of glass and two loud thumps. Then there was silence. We pulled over and got out of the car. The moonlit road smelled of burned rubber and I saw an overturned car and a crumpled pickup. Some kids had run up to the scene.

"Stay here," Daddy said as he ran to the accident.

"Go back to the house and call an ambulance. Now!" he barked to one of the kids. "Give me your shirt," he said to another.

"Stay here," he said to me again, and I retreated back to the station wagon. I waited as Daddy walked calmly back to the overturned car and then to the truck. When he finally returned to the station wagon, he was holding a baby in his arms. He opened the passenger side door. "Hold him. We can't wait for the ambulance. We're taking him to the hospital."

The baby wasn't crying. He had cuts all over his face and head and he was bruised. He looked like he was asleep and he was breathing. I kept checking to make sure he was breathing. I held the baby tight on my lap as we drove the 20 minutes to the only hospital in town. Neither of us said a word.

My father and I never spoke about that night again. I never found out what my father encountered when he stepped up to help the victims of that horrible crash. And I don't know what happened to that baby. But I do know what happened to Daddy. Right there before my 13-year-old eyes, my father became a doctor. My father became a hero.

I've thought about that night a lot over the last 30 years. Maybe most doctors and nurses and others who've dedicated their lives to the healing arts aren't as glamorous as the actors who portray them on TV. But they are all heroes to someone. They are all heroes to me.

—*Submitted by Nancy Wollin, Sarasota, FL*

"Never underestimate the difference you can make."

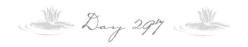

HAPPY REUNION MADE POSSIBLE BY DEDICATED STAFF

George and his dog enjoyed a happy reunion when George returned home upon discharge from St. Charles Mercy Hospital Acute Rehabilitation Center. Had it not been for the efforts of the staff at St. Charles to work with the Lucas County Commissioners' Office and the Dog Warden, his dog might have been euthanized when he was not claimed by the end of his initial "hold period."

In March, George and his dog were walking to a neighbor's house when George was attacked. Robbed and shot in the knee, he underwent surgery at St. Vincent Mercy Medical Center, and then transferred to the St. Charles Mercy Hospital Acute Rehabilitation Center.

"When I woke up in a hospital bed, the most important thing to me was knowing if my dog was OK," George said. "I know that might sound kind of silly, but he's more than just a dog to me. He's my best friend."

George, a Vietnam vet who survives on his Veteran's Affairs pension benefits, suffers from post-traumatic stress disorder with avoidance.

"I pretty much keep to myself, so it's usually just me and my dog," he said. "He goes everywhere with me."

George has had his dog, which is now 15 years old, since he was a puppy. "At first I thought—no one is gonna adopt him," George said. "He's an old guy, like me. He's not gonna know what happened. I was despondent."

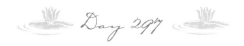

The staff at St. Charles intervened.

"We have the creative freedom in Acute Rehab to go to our bosses and say, 'I think the patient would get better if we could do this,'" said Julie Coyle, social worker. "We knew that in the course of the attack, this gentleman had lost his dog, so it was only natural to ask if anyone had found the dog, and if so, how could we get the dog and owner reunited.

"When someone lives alone, a pet can be everything to them. So, in this case, even though it wasn't a normal part of the hospital treatment, we were allowed to go forward and do it—to spend the time, to make the phone calls."

George did not have a current license for his dog, and, according to law, an unlicensed dog may be sold or euthanized after three days of impoundment by the Dog Warden.

The staff at St. Charles Acute Rehab worked with the Lucas County Commissioners and the Dog Warden to have the dog's hold extended indefinitely, until George could be discharged from the hospital.

George said that hearing his dog would be returned to him renewed his resolve to complete his therapy and get better.

"You get to a point where you just don't care," he said. "But, when I found out he was alive and OK, I really threw myself into this program here."

In preparation for George's discharge home, the staff of Acute Rehab arranged for him to have the walker and wheelchair he would need to get around on his own and even got the hospital to donate a television. While George was in the hospital, someone had broken into his home and stolen his television, stereo and computer.

The burglar had broken a bathroom window, and George had not yet reported the damage to his landlord. Greg Welch, director of Acute Rehab, went

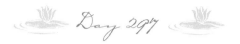

out to George's house and taped up the window. Meanwhile, staff members continued to try to reach the landlord on George's behalf.

When George returned home in April, so did his dog.

"I think everything's going to be OK now, especially now that I see him," said George. "Since my attack, it has been a lot of ups and downs, but since I have been at St. V's and here, most of it has been up. Everyone here has been great. They've given me the tools to go on and help myself get better. Knowing my dog would be waiting for me was icing on the cake."

—*Anonymous Contributor, St. Charles Mercy Hospital, Oregon, OH*

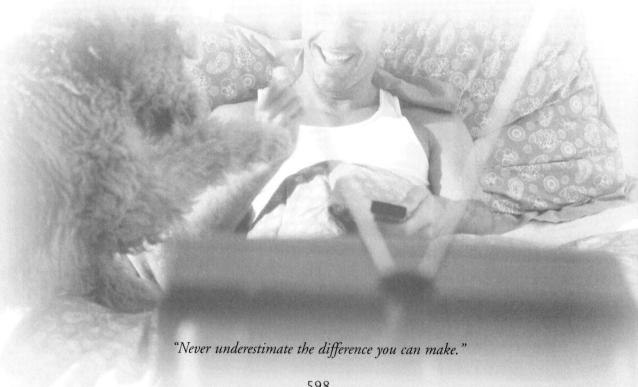

"Never underestimate the difference you can make."

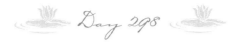

Mending a Broken Heart

F ive or six years ago, I was working at St. Charles. It was time to go home, and when I got to my car in the parking lot, I discovered I had a flat tire. I was worried about finding somewhere to get help, since it was a holiday.

I headed back to the hospital and stopped the first person I saw walking out. His name was Dave, and he worked in the Pharmacy. I asked if he knew of anywhere nearby that I could get help with my tire, and he said he would help me himself.

I had a trunk full of pottery, because my husband is a potter. As Dave helped me empty the trunk, he asked me about the pottery. Then he told me that he had lost his wife the year before. When she was in Hospice, they had her put her hand in cement to make an imprint, but when she pulled her hand away, the impression left behind was that of a heart. The pottery was now crumbling, and Dave asked if I thought my husband might be able to help restore and preserve this cherished memento.

Of course, my husband helped him.

I never would have met Dave had it not been for my flat tire—it was like the Lord put me in his path.

Recently, at St. Anne, I was assisting a patient, and the man with her looked familiar. It turned out to be Dave. It was one of those moments that gave me pause—it really is a small world. It also reminded me that the Lord works in mysterious ways.

—*Anonymous Contributor, St. Charles Mercy Hospital, Oregon, OH*

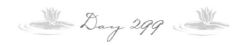

Dialing the Wrong Number to Reach the Right Person

arta Watson from the Cardiology Medical Records Section is an excellent example of what's right in health care. A Spanish-speaking mother, MCJ, took her son to the Creighton University Emergency Department on Thursday, March 28, 2002. Her son had a painful lump on his genitals. MCJ was told at the time of discharge that her son would need to be seen on Friday by Dr. Chiou and to call for an appointment. When MCJ called to make an appointment, she dialed the wrong number and, by accident, called Cardiology Medical Records instead. Kim Brouse answered the telephone and quickly thought to ask Marta to assist this Spanish-speaking caller. Marta told MCJ to hold while she found the right person to make the appointment.

Even though Marta encountered multiple wrong numbers, transfers, and voice mails, she persisted because she recognized the mother was upset, concerned, and having urinary symptoms, too. Marta finally reached Regina in Urology, explained who she was, the situation, and that she had a Spanish-speaking mother on the line. Instead of stopping there, she offered to interpret for Regina so the mother could make her appointment.

Regina verified the son had been seen in the Emergency Department, and that she would need to get the medical records, and said she would need to call the patient back. Marta continued to be MCJ's advocate and informed her that she would call her back after Regina had obtained the records.

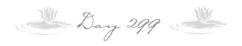

Regina promptly called Marta back and both MCJ and her son were scheduled for 3:15 that afternoon. Regina also told Marta she would arrange for the Spanish interpreter to meet MCJ at the front desk of Creighton University Medical Center to make sure she found the Urology clinic and had an interpreter for the appointment.

Because of Marta's tenacious spirit and dedication to our patients, she helped to ensure a Spanish-speaking mother navigated a confusing system. Marta is truly a caring person and this is just one example of how her actions make a difference.

—Submitted by Susan K. Walsh and Dr. Syed M. Mohiuddin,
Creighton University Medical Center, Omaha, NE

"Never underestimate the difference you can make."

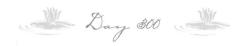

CRYPTIC CALL TRACED TO SUFFERING PATIENT

O ne evening in December of 2006, Little Company of Mary Hospital's Admitting and Central Scheduling staff received a cryptic voicemail from a frantic man who did not leave his number, but seemed to be in the middle of an emergency.

The man's name was Stephen. On the voicemail, Stephen sounded short of breath. He said he was bleeding, that he had three types of cancer and that he needed help because he couldn't reach his physician. Stephen also said he had a reservation at the hospital. Stephen then handed the phone to his wife, who evidently thought he was talking to a live person. His wife said, "Hello, Hello," and when she didn't hear a response, she hung up the phone.

Little Company of Mary's Patient Access Specialists, Bridget Galbraith and Sheila O'Neil, heard the message. They tried to find Stephen's phone number. It turned out that Stephen had a common last name, but Bridget and Sheila didn't have the correct spelling. His physician, a Dr. Shah, also had a common last name. So Bridget and Sheila began calling local hospitals to find out if Stephen was due to be admitted to any of them. He was not.

Then, Bridget and Sheila called every "Dr. Shah" with privileges at Little Company of Mary. They finally reached the correct physician's office, but Dr. Shah was in another country on vacation. They spoke to the physician filling in for Dr. Shah while he was away. The physician was not familiar with Stephen.

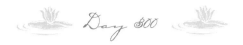

Sheila and Bridget began searching phone directories for Stephen, but to no avail. Finally, Sheila tried spelling Stephen's last name differently and suddenly, they located his information in Little Company of Mary's Patient Information System. The physician on call for Dr. Shah then found records on Stephen and directed him to the Emergency Room.

Bridget made the return phone call to Stephen and urged him to come immediately to Little Company of Mary's Emergency Department. "From what the physician said, it seemed he had little time to live," Bridget explained.

Stephen was resistant, but finally heeded Bridget's recommendation and later that day he was admitted to the hospital.

Bridget and Sheila didn't have to go to these extraordinary lengths to contact this patient. After all, he didn't initially leave a phone number. They didn't have to call all the local hospitals on the southwest side of Chicago. They didn't have to try to locate Dr. Shah. But they did.

These persistent, dedicated employees made a difference that day for Stephen and his family but they work to make a difference every single day, for each patient they encounter. Bridget and Sheila are not required to go to these lengths to assist patients; they do it because they believe it is an expression of their healthcare ministries.

—Submitted by Marjorie Ritchie,
Little Company of Mary Hospital and Health Care Centers, Evergreen Park, IL

"Never underestimate the difference you can make."

Share Your Own Story

Please share an experience that connected you back to purpose, worthwhile work, and making a difference. You are a big part of what's right in health care!

ONE SMALL GESTURE

O ne day, when I came to work as a nurse in the OB Department, we had a low patient count, so I went to work on the Med-Surg floor of our hospital. While there, one of the nurses asked if I would help her give a bed bath to a terminal cancer patient. She said, "Let's just both go in and get him done as quickly as possible, so he can rest."

So we worked together and in no time at all, we had the gentleman bathed and put clean sheets on his bed. The other nurse gathered the linens and hurried out of the room. I went to follow her but stopped by the doorway and looked back at this frail, elderly gentleman lying in his bed and I thought, *there has to be more we can do than just bathing him.*

Not knowing what to say, I approached his bed and took his hand in mine. I looked into his eyes and said, "I'll pray for you."

Immediately, he squeezed my hand and tears began to run down his face. He said, "No one knows how much it hurts."

"Thank you, thank you," he repeated over and over. At this point, no more words were necessary, as we both knew he was terminal. With tears in my own eyes, I continued to hold his hand for a few more minutes. Then, before I left, I assured him I would talk to his doctor about getting more effective pain medication.

This was one of the most profound moments of my life, and I will never forget it. Sometimes, the smallest gestures or words mean the most to our patients.

—*Anonymous Contributor, Mercy Hospital of Tiffin, Tiffin, OH*

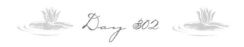

St. Charles Cancer Center to the Rescue

One of the patients we have been treating in our Cancer Center was robbed just before Christmas. He is in his eighties, and thankfully, he and his wife weren't harmed when their home was broken into. Still, they were quite shaken up about it. They lost about $350 in the robbery.

My staff heard about what had happened and knowing that this couple had no money to spare, they jumped into action to help out. They took the initiative and pulled some money from the fund that they use for mission projects and for which they fundraise all year. Then, they all started pulling money from their own pockets, until they had almost enough to cover the couple's loss.

Then, they went to Sr. Dorothy (Sr. Dorothy Thum, Vice President of Mission and Values Integration), and she approved a donation from the Sr. Phyllis Gerold Fund to make up the difference so we could give the full $350 back to our patient and his wife.

I was so impressed that my staff took it upon themselves to do this—it was just one of those great reminders that we work in a really special place and that we have a wonderful team.

—Anonymous Contributor, St. Charles Mercy Hospital, Oregon, OH

"Never underestimate the difference you can make."

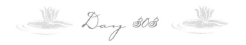

Dad, I Love You. It's Okay.

A patient had recently received a terminal diagnosis and was admitted to the hospital for an extended stay. He was faced with a cascade of physical, emotional, psychological, and spiritual needs as he moved toward the end of his life. Our nursing staff spent time comforting and caring not only for him, but for his family as well.

When the patient's death became imminent, his 16-year-old son was in school, but the patient's wife was afraid her husband would die while she was in transit to pick up their son. She didn't want her husband to die alone.

Sandy Montgomery, an RN on 5 Main called the school guidance counselor and arranged for the son to speak to his father on the phone. The son was told that his father could not speak but could hear him.

Sandy held the phone to the patient's ear so the son could talk to his father one last time. She could hear the son's words—"Dad, I love you. It's okay." The patient died while his son was telling him that he loved him.

A few weeks later, the wife and son returned to the hospital to visit with the nursing staff. The son wished to personally meet Sandy and thank her for the opportunity to talk to his dad before his death. The son said, "My dad died knowing I loved him."

—Submitted by Cyndi Baxter, Central Baptist Hospital, Lexington, KY

"Never underestimate the difference you can make."

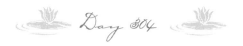

Full of Heart

A. is a patient who was hospitalized at Creighton University Medical Center in December 2003 with a heart condition. She was frightened by her diagnosis. She feared that after her discharge from the facility, she would go home, fall asleep, and never wake up again. Her fears subsided when Tami Ward, APRN, and Renae Hohnstein, RN, visited with her about the Heart Failure Clinic at The Cardiac Center of Creighton University Medical Center. After meeting with Tami and Renae, A. no longer felt alone in her fight to survive, and she knew she had people on her side who really cared about her.

During the next few months, A. found the strength and courage to turn her life around. Once Tami and the rest of the clinic staff got to know the beautiful person A. was inside, they came up with a plan to help her see herself the way they saw her. They decided a makeover would be the perfect way to accomplish this. One of the nurses just happened to know someone from a local salon who was kind enough to donate a complete makeover for A. The patient was thrilled by the offer and touched by the caring nature of the staff. Later, A. spent four glorious hours at the salon and came out a new woman.

This story shows how the staff at The Cardiac Center did more for A. than just help her manage her heart condition. They helped restore her spirit and revive her outlook on life. In a letter to The Cardiac Center, A. wrote, "I'll never be able to express how thankful I am to have Tami Ward and everyone else at The Cardiac Center by my side, I truly love them with all my heart."

—*Submitted by Susan K. Walsh, The Cardiac Center of Creighton University Medical Center, Omaha, NE*

Graduation Day

Reverend Sherry Schermbeck is a chaplain at St. Charles Mercy Hospital (SCMH). Here is her story:

In spring 2005, I was blessed to share in a very special graduation ceremony for the daughter of a patient I had been in contact with during her four-year struggle against cancer. Deanna was a divorced mother, and her only child was scheduled to graduate from Genoa High School at the end of May.

During one of Deanna's many treatments, I asked her where she'd gotten her strength. She said her strength came from God and everyone's prayers, along with her desire to "make it to June" to see her daughter, Jaclyn, graduate from high school. During Deanna's last admission to St. Charles Mercy Hospital, Deanna was deteriorating rapidly, and her nurses and physicians did not feel she would be able to attend Jaclyn's graduation ceremony, which was being held two weeks later.

I mentioned to Diann Lento, RN, and Dr. Rajender Ahuja that it would be nice to have some kind of graduation held in Deanna's room to fulfill her heart's desire. Dr. Ahuja, along with Dr. Dean Bernardo, felt that this was a good option. We also approached Deanna, who gave her approval to move ahead with the graduation plans.

Diann, Angie Knannlein, RN, and Avis Johnson, LPN, got swept up in the excitement of the moment and added their presence and good wishes,

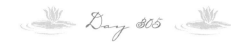

along with tears of joy, compassion, and physical and emotional support for Deanna and her family.

Within approximately two hours, we put together a lovely ceremony that could not have been more perfect if we had planned it for two months. One of our nurses contacted Audrey Milbrodt, RN, Cancer Center, and told her that the school principal could not be reached.

Audrey personally went to the school and found the Superintendent of Schools, Dennis Mock, at a track meet. She explained the situation, and he immediately put things into action. He arrived at the hospital a short time later in his suit and tie and carrying the graduation certificate and two long-stemmed red roses, one for Deanna and one for her daughter.

Our graduate's grandpa had driven her home to get her cap and gown and returned with several students and friends of the family. In the meantime, Carolyn Gladney, unit clerk in the Intensive Care Unit, explained the circumstances to Dietary and requested that they bring a cake. Cindy Kortze in our gift shop donated balloons and flowers to make it a festive occasion, and I purchased an owl that played "Pomp and Circumstance."

As everyone assembled in Deanna's room and spilled out into the center nurses' area, Mr. Mock asked that I begin the ceremony with a prayer. He noted that we couldn't have begun with a prayer at the school, but we surely could pray that day as we gathered together at St. Charles. Darshana Pandya from Dietary realized what an important occasion this was for this family and saw how many people were present. She brought up a larger cake than the one her department initially provided, some cookies, and cans of Pepsi. She made sure that the utmost in hospitality was extended, not only to the patient's family, but also to each of the

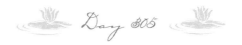

families present in the Critical Care waiting room. All of the families joined in the celebration, and some even gave small gifts and cards.

I told our visitors in the waiting room how our staff had all come together for this family, and I told them about the many departments that were involved. The visitors applauded St. Charles several times and affirmed their positive feelings and experiences with SCMH. I believe we have wonderful, compassionate staff at St. Charles, and I am so thankful to be a part of the Mercy system.

Editor's Note: Shortly after the special graduation ceremony, Deanna's family sent the following thank-you note to the hospital:

The family of Deanna S. wishes to thank everyone at St. Charles Mercy Hospital for all the excellent care, kindness, and thoughtfulness shown to her during her illness. We would like to especially thank the ICU staff for the wonderful graduation they let us have there for Deanna's daughter, Jaclyn. We would also like to thank Dietary for donating a cake, cookies, and soda.

And a special thank you goes to the Gift Shop for donating flowers and balloons. A very important thank you goes to Rev. Sherry Schermbeck for all of her support, for always being there when we needed her, and for everything else she's done for our family throughout Deanna's illness. We can never put into words the thankfulness we feel in our hearts for St. Charles Mercy Hospital.

God bless you all.
Family of Deanna S.: her daughter, Jaclyn, and her parents, Jan & Glenn S.

—Anonymous Contributor, St. Charles Mercy Hospital, Oregon, OH

A Small Act of Kindness

Tori Bailey is an office assistant in the Rehab and Wellness Center at Mercy Hospital of Willard. Here is the story that Tori shared with us:

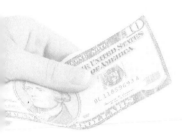

We had a patient who was coming in for occupational therapy, normally three times a week. During his first visit, he told his therapist, Lynne Bailey, that he was going to have to cancel his other appointments until the beginning of the following month, which was a full week away.

When Lynne asked his reason, he replied, "Because I don't have the money for gas to get back and forth to therapy."

Lynne went above and beyond the call of duty by giving the gentleman gas money out of her own pocket. When she gave him the money he was so appreciative, and he said he was going to pay her back. Her response to him was, "Don't worry, it's a gift."

Lynne's patient came back in for therapy the first week of the following month, and he offered to pay the money back. Again, Lynne told him not to worry, it was a gift. She told him everyone needs help from time to time and said someone, somewhere along the way, had helped her out and now it was her turn to pass a favor on to someone else.

Something like this might be a small gesture, but it made this patient's day, and it made her coworkers feel "warm and fuzzy."

—*Anonymous Contributor, Mercy Hospital of Willard, Willard, OH*

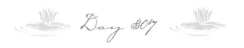

QUICK THINKING

Judi Johnston, an administrative assistant at Cassano Health Clinic, part of the Kettering Medical Center Network, has demonstrated her willingness to go beyond the "call of duty." A seemingly normal workday last year is an ideal example of her commitment. When Judi arrived at work at 6:30 a.m., a pregnant woman was waiting for the clinic to open at 8:00 a.m. The expectant mother only spoke Spanish, but Judi was able to determine the situation—the woman was in labor with her third child, and had taken the bus to the clinic. Judi tried unsuccessfully to get a cab, so she put the woman in her own care and drove her to Southview Maternity Center. This quick thinking is typical of Judi's outstanding service.

—Submitted by Sherri Herrick, Kettering Medical Center Network, Dayton, OH

"Never underestimate the difference you can make."

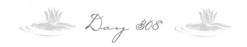

Art of Nursing

There is an art to nursing that can't be learned from a textbook. It comes from a keen sense of being able to read a patient's mood or body language and knowing how to respond to those subtleties. Judy Hatch, RN, BSN, and other nurses like her, practice that art every day.

A major part of Hatch's job as an oncology clinical coordinator is to sit in when a doctor consults with a patient about their disease, treatment plans, and choices. There's usually a vast amount of information for a patient to absorb and many emotions at play, so Hatch stays after the doctor leaves in order to give the patient a chance to ask additional questions and assure them that she will provide them with written information that's specific to their condition.

One day, Hatch was participating in one of these consultations—this particular time she was with a woman in mid-life who was coping with a cancer recurrence. Her treatment had required additional surgery, which resulted in a post-operative drain to remove fluid from the area of surgery. The patient arrived for her appointment expecting the drain to be removed, but after assessing her, the doctor decided the drain needed to remain in place a bit longer.

"I noticed that she seemed really disappointed when he said the drain had to stay in," said Hatch. "She just briefly mentioned that she was scheduled to go to a camp in Georgia, but she didn't really pursue the issue with the doctor. It was like she was giving up on her trip because she had the drain, and she needed to stay near her doctor because of it."

Picking up on the patient's mood change, Hatch decided to inquire further about the planned trip after the doctor left the room. The patient shared that she had won a stay at an art camp in Georgia. She had already missed the first week of the camp and had counted on being able to leave for the second week of the camp after this particular doctor's visit. Now, it seemed, with the drain still in place, she wouldn't be able to go.

Hatch soon learned that art was very therapeutic to the patient and had helped her cope with her cancer. It was obvious the patient had been really looking forward to going to the art camp. Hatch excused herself and stepped outside the patient's room to find her doctor.

After explaining the situation to the doctor, he agreed that there was no reason why the patient wouldn't be able to attend the camp. If there was a problem with the drain while she was in Georgia, a local physician could remove it or plans could be made to take it out when she returned.

Hatch returned to the patient's room and shared that the doctor didn't have a problem with her going on her Georgia adventure, and of course the patient was elated.

For Hatch, this situation reaffirmed that assessment is not just about vital signs it's also about picking up on a patient's subtle communication and acting upon it.

"That's what I call the art part of nursing," explained Hatch. "It comes from being present. You're not going to pick up on it if you're already thinking about the next patient coming in or the schedule or even something that happened yesterday. It's about being in the present with the patient and really listening to them and watching them."

—Submitted by Cyndi Baxter, Central Baptist Hospital, Lexington, KY

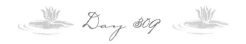

Christmas for a Coworker

Three members of the Radiology Department—Kathleen Wilkins, Bill McGeorge, and Tracey Cowan—decided not to let a deadline for the Christmas Adopt-a-Friend program lapse in the midst of a busy holiday season. Instead, they decided to help out Bill Massey, a fellow employee.

Bill has worked in Environmental Services since 2000, mostly around the Radiology areas in the ground floor. But 2005 was not a good year for him as health problems caused him to miss a lot of work. As the holidays neared, Christmas for the Masseys—who have four children, one with Cerebral Palsy— was not looking bright.

Unbeknownst to Bill and his wife, the Radiology Department took up a collection, found out clothes sizes and the kids' wish lists, and filled every one and then some. On December 9 they then filled the Radiology Conference Room, and surprised Bill and his wife with a Christmas they surely will never forget.

"All I could see was a Christmas tree," Bill's wife Joyce told the Delaware County Daily Times. "There was a room full of people—and half of these people I don't even know. I'm in tears; my daughter's in tears; (Bill) is trying to hold back the tears."

"All the generosity…and all the support that he was given in the hospital. They must have spent thousands on us. It was amazing," she said.

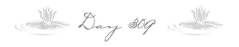

Time and again, the Radiology Department demonstrates compassion for both their coworkers and their patients. While the employees who organized and contributed to this special event were not looking for recognition, the power of their story demonstrates the genuine respect they shared with a valued coworker and friend.

—*Submitted by Terry Lynch, Crozer-Chester Medical Center, Upland, PA*

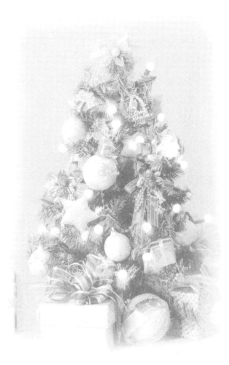

"Never underestimate the difference you can make."

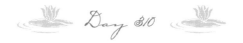

Spirit and Dedication

S ue Deyke, Nurse Manager at Cardiology's Columbus Office, is an excellent example of what's right in health care. Several months ago, Sue received a call on a Sunday morning from a patient who told her the leads on his event recorder were broken and needed to be replaced. Ms. Deyke decided she had time before church to run into the office and replace the leads for him. Later that day, the patient experienced symptoms and called our toll-free number to transmit his tracing. The tracing showed the patient was in complete heart block. Our technician told him to go directly to the nearest Emergency Department where he was evaluated and then transferred to Creighton University Medical Center for a pacemaker insertion.

Sue helped to ensure a patient was cared for on a Sunday morning and her "above and beyond" efforts may very well have saved this patient's life. This is only one example of Sue's tenacious spirit and dedication to our patients and their families. She is an RN who has taken her professional responsibility to a higher level and incorporated the values that embody Creighton University.

—Submitted by Susan K. Walsh and Dr. Syed M. Mohiuddin,
The Cardiac Center of Creighton University Medical Center, Omaha, NE

"Never underestimate the difference you can make."

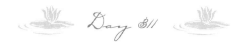

YOUTH DEVELOPMENT PROGRAM

B ased in Community Hospital, the Youth Development Program addresses multiple risk behaviors of high school students in the Chester-Upland School District. Each year, the program involves 40 high school students and provides them with training to be peer leaders to sixth grade students, while also offering enrichment activities to help develop the participants.

The goal of the program is to train these high school students to be leaders in their community. The program trains peer leaders on adolescent health topics such as interpersonal violence, teen pregnancy, and sexually transmitted infections. The peer leaders then work with an average of 450 middle school students. Peer leaders are offered a number of positives, such as student resume writing workshops, college tours, tutoring, career presentations, job shadowing opportunities, and public speaking engagements.

This year, the Youth Development Program won an achievement award from the hospital and the Healthsystem Association of Pennsylvania.

Led by Rina Himelstein, M.D., medical director for the Wellness Center and director of adolescent medicine at Crozer-Chester Medical Center, and Kate Blackburn, director of the Youth Development Program, the program's results have been impressive: Program leaders outperform those not in the program

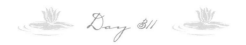

with better school attendance and performance. Of the 121 high school students who have been enrolled for more than one year since 1996, 120 have graduated.

The team has been able to create and sustain interest in the Youth Leadership Program for nine years, all while achieving its health-related objectives. The program is an example of true community collaboration, identifying and effectively addressing the shared interests of the health system and the surrounding community.

—Submitted by Terry Lynch, Crozer-Chester Medical Center, Upland, PA

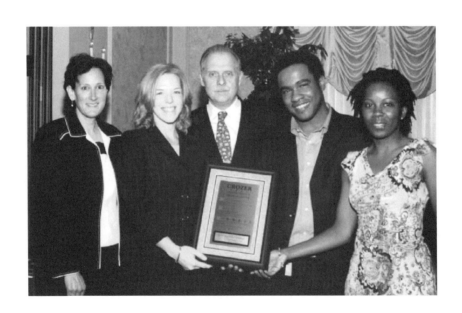

"Never underestimate the difference you can make."

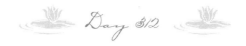

A Little Extra Effort

The following is an excerpt from a speech to employees by Tom Strauss, president and CEO of Summa Health System in Akron, Ohio:

There are many stories I could tell you about the wonderful caring leaders who work in this organization, but this story is about an employee who does not have the title of a leader. See, we believe that a title does not make you a servant leader; your actions do. I'd like to read a short excerpt from a very moving letter we received from a patient. She tells how one employee changed her life by paying attention to the needs of the heart. Here is the letter:

Please recognize the outstanding employee you have working at the desk in nuclear medicine at Akron City Hospital. Her name is Linda. In November, my husband and I were both scheduled for a stress test. My husband is physically challenged and unable to walk any distance, and I use a walker. The secretary, Linda, noticed we were scheduled to return on Friday and Monday for more tests and also to go to St. Thomas Hospital on Tuesday. She took it upon herself to change the schedule and get every test done that day at Akron City Hospital! She saved us so much physical stress and hardship. We thanked her profusely. Her comment was, "Kindness is free—and I'm sure you would do the same for me. It's the least I can do for you." I am still reeling from being told last Friday that I do not have much time left to live—lung cancer is causing my death as early as the next few weeks. When I returned to Summa in January, I had my lungs drained of fluid. Linda could see I was upset. She came around the

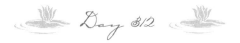

desk, comforted me, and reassured me the procedure would go well. She pushed my wheelchair herself and told the volunteer, "I need to take her myself—I need to hug her and talk with her."

—Submitted by Charles Elliot, Summa Health System, Akron, OH

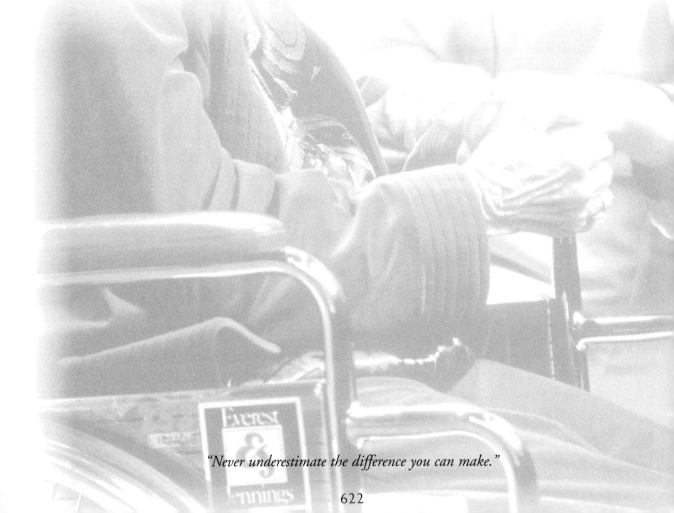

"Never underestimate the difference you can make."

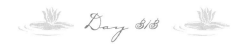

Pranee Richardson

*I*f you have an inpatient stay at St. Mary Medical Center in Apple Valley, California, and if you're on our Medical/Surgical North or Main units, you may be blessed to have Pranee Richardson as your housekeeper.

Pranee was born in Phet Buri, Thailand, in 1947 and came to California in the 1960s after marrying her husband Dwayne, an American serviceman. She came to work with the St. Mary Environmental Services (EVS) Team in 1993 and has been a mainstay of the department ever since.

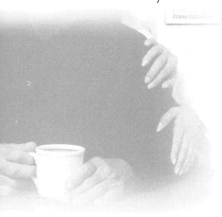

Over the years, Pranee has self-defined her role to include elements of patient care and customer service. She quickly forms relationships with the patients' spouses who spend long bedside vigils with their recovering loved ones. When a local man recently had an eight-day stay, Pranee ministered to the man's wife each morning, bringing a hot cup of coffee and a fresh pillow. "You need to have your strength!" Pranee said. "When your husband gets discharged, you will be working hard at home to help him." Pranee explains this part of her role, "Right now, in here, the doctors take care of the patient, but who will take care of the wife or husband?! That's where I can come in." When Pranee spots a visitor

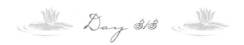

or family member having difficulties or moving slowly down the hall, she offers to locate a wheelchair for them.

She also keeps an eye out for nurse call lights, especially when the units get busy. "Many times, those call lights don't need a nurse. I can bring blankets, new linens, fresh towels, boxes of tissue, ice, water, washcloths, soap. I tell the patients, 'Anything you need, I can get it for you.' This helps the nurses, too, if they don't need to answer every time a call light goes off. Then if the patient says they need their nurse, I tell them, 'Today is very busy on this unit. Your nurse is Jennifer, so I will go get her for you right away and come right back.'" It's no wonder that when our nursing units began displaying team bulletin boards with snapshots of the unit team members, Medical/Surgery North and Main were two of the first to include a picture of their EVS worker, Pranee, in their team display.

Pranee is a St. Mary high performer and is frequently nominated by others in the organization to receive one of our annual "Values in Action" awards for exemplifying the hospital's core values. She's a smiling face to anyone in the hallways, and to us she's a great example of an empowered team member expanding and re-shaping her own role in the organization to better serve our patients and guests.

—Submitted by Bob Diehl, St. Mary Medical Center, Apple Valley, CA

"Never underestimate the difference you can make."

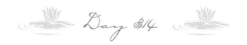
St. V's Gives Micropreemie a Fighting Chance

Chase H. tipped the scales at just 1 pound, 12 ounces and was only 13 inches long when he was born at St. Vincent Mercy Medical Center on April 10. Thanks to the excellent care he received in St. V's Level III Neonatal Intensive Care Unit, his mom, Noelle H., says he was doing great when he was discharged from the hospital 86 days later. When Noelle and her husband, Tony, took their bouncing baby boy home on July 5, he weighed 6 pounds, 1 ounce, and a week later he was bursting out of his preemie outfits. Today, he weighs more than 8 pounds and is about 21 inches long.

Noelle had been due to deliver on July 7, but she developed preeclampsia during her second trimester and was admitted to the Labor and Delivery Unit at St. V's at 26 weeks gestation.

"They did everything they could to treat the preeclampsia and keep her from delivering in order to give the baby more time before birth," said Noelle's father, Steve Larrow, a transformation specialist in Information and Process Services at Mercy Health Partners. "But, her blood pressure kept spiking, and it became clear that they wouldn't be able to delay things much longer. They began treating the baby to prepare him for the birth. After he was born, he went into the NICU.

"I can't say enough good things about the nurses there or the unit itself. I am very proud of our new NICU and the remodeling project they did. Working in IS,

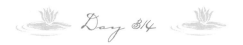

I had done a couple of projects in the old NICU. The difference between old and new is night and day, and the changes are all good."

Having worked in a sleep lab, Noelle already was somewhat comfortable with being in a medical environment when her son was born. But, she still had a lot of questions.

"My husband and I were very impressed with the nursing staff," Noelle said. "They really took time to answer our questions and never made us feel as if they were in a hurry to do something else. I know they are very busy, but they never rushed with us."

Noelle added that while all of the nurses were professional, courteous, and thoughtful, some went above and beyond the call of duty.

"The third-shift people in general were especially outgoing and friendly," Noelle said. "One night, I called to check in, and a nurse named Gina told me that Chase had looked like he needed a little extra love that night, so she had picked him up and carried him around with her all night.

"I couldn't be there with him all the time, so to know that she did that for him meant so much to me—I was so touched by that I nearly cried. I know that Chase was in a medical environment, and I expected great medical care, but I never expected people to show that kind of love for my baby. It really did feel almost like a second family there. I definitely would recommend the NICU at St. V's to other mothers, and I would certainly go back and have another baby there myself."

—Anonymous Contributor,
St. Vincent Mercy Medical Center / St. Vincent Mercy Children's Hospital, Toledo, OH

"Never underestimate the difference you can make."

Helping Hospice Hands

"A." entered hospice with a diagnosis of metastatic breast cancer. She was divorced, living on public aid, and estranged from her family members. A friend had provided a place for her to stay but wasn't able to offer the many other types of support she needed.

Over the next five months, Evanston Northwestern Healthcare Hospice staff and volunteers came together to assist A. on her end-of-life journey. While hospice staff and volunteers are used to offering support to patients and families, A.'s grace in the face of devastating circumstances made a profound impact on those who assisted her.

Social worker Denise Zicher recalls, "Even as A. was declining physically, I was impressed by her vision, by the way she became the leader of the hospice team that was caring for her." For example, A. was a Reiki Master, very spiritually minded, and interested in alternative approaches. She challenged her physicians and pharmacists to find medications she was comfortable with. At the same time, A. showed immense gratitude for the hospice staff and volunteers who became her primary source of support.

"She called us her 'angel team,'" said Zicher—referring to the cadre of physicians, pharmacists, RNs, nursing assistants, social workers, spiritual care coordinator, bereavement counselor, and volunteers. This team did everything from providing medical care, case management, and emotional support to baking cookies, running errands, and driving A. to church and appointments. A.'s

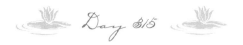

physical and financial resources were severely limited, but her capacity for caring was undiminished.

"As much pain as she was in, she went to the effort of providing a Christmas gift for a needy family at her church," said Zicher. "I was driving her around to visit nursing homes, and she asked me to stop at the church so she could drop off the gift." Hospice chaplain Maureen Martin took A. to run errands, often stopping at a coffee shop on the way. "She loved café mocha with lots of whipped cream," said Martin. "When she couldn't get out any more, I would bring the café mocha to her house, and she was always a little disappointed that the cream had melted on the way. As she was choosing a nursing home, one of the things she commented on was that it was close to a coffee shop."

A.'s delight in small pleasures was in contrast to the great challenges she faced. "She had been married but was single at this time. She didn't have any children, didn't have a support system," recalled Martin. "It was fascinating to see how she handled it all with extreme grace." For example, fluid would build in A.'s lungs, and she had a catheter in her side that had to be drained periodically. Usually, a family member would take care of this. In A.'s case, she learned the sterile procedure and did it for herself until shortly before her death.

Bereavement counselor Thom Dennis recalls, "A turning point in A.'s care came about when three hospice staff members and a volunteer participated in an anointing service, along with a priest and some friends. It was an hour-long service, in which we offered A. strength for her final journey." Shortly thereafter, A. moved to a nursing home and, with Zicher's assistance, was able to reconcile with a family member, allowing her closure and peace of mind in her final days. "I know the team made a significant positive impact on this patient," said Dennis. "But I also believe the patient had an impact on the staff, reminding us of why we choose to work in hospice and the value of the work we do."

—Submitted by MaryAnn Lando, Evanston Northwestern Healthcare, Evanston, IL

Under the Big Top

*I*n December 2006, 15 children were told they would need to spend the Christmas holiday in the "Big Top" pediatric unit of Brooks Rehabilitation Hospital, a 143-bed acute physical rehabilitation hospital located in Jacksonville, FL. These children endured numerous traumatic events in recent weeks and many were suffering from brain injuries.

After finding out about the situation, several employees and contractors of Brooks decided they wanted to make sure this holiday was memorable for the children, even though they would be away from home.

The Brooks maintenance manager and two local paving company and site construction business owners began planning a way to bring Christmas to the hospital. They obtained a list of the kids who would be spending Christmas at the facility, along with a wish list of gifts they would enjoy.

On the morning of Christmas Eve, one of the business owners dressed as Santa Claus and visited the pediatric patients with a bag full of gifts. Santa also brought his two helpers—his grandchildren—to help him distribute the toys door to door. That morning, Santa gave out over $500 in toys and iTunes gifts to the excited children, but he didn't neglect the families of the patients. Santa also delivered $300 in gas cards and gift certificates to visiting parents.

The marketing manager for Brooks came along to take pictures of the children with Santa. Visiting parents were as excited as the children when they

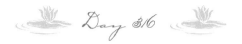

realized they would have their annual photos with Santa. All of the pictures were later developed and presented to the families.

Even though it was a stressful time in the children's lives, these exemplary employees went above and beyond to bring some fun and happiness to the children and their families, truly demonstrating what's right in health care.

—*Anonymous Contributor, Brooks Rehabilitation Hospital, Jacksonville, FL*

"Never underestimate the difference you can make."

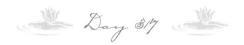

Angels Among Us

I am a "case manager" at Shepherd Pathways, an outpatient and residential program for people who have sustained brain injuries. I have worked with people with brain injuries for 25 years, and the work has never become mundane for me. I am inspired by the perseverance and persistence that my clients and their families display. It is inspiring to see that our clients—and often, their family members—faithfully arrive for therapy day after day. I am surrounded by miracles.

Due to the nature of brain injury recovery, time with us can be long. Because Shepherd Center is a Southeast catastrophic care hospital, we are fortunate to work with people within and outside of Georgia. Although we see clients from the metro Atlanta area, many of our clients are from much farther away.

I am honored to be with my clients and their families as they struggle with this "life interruption." Typically, people will come together in a crisis and we all celebrate even small progresses. Each work day, I witness a change in attitude as people deal with how their lives have changed. Our clients become more in tune with the moment while setting goals for the future.

I see these basic aspects of human nature occurring in my own life when something "interrupts" my life as I know it. I am truly blessed and honored to be with my clients and their families and to witness the adjustment and recovery process in them. They teach me even as I am teaching them.

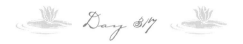

There is a Biblical verse of scripture from Hebrews that comes to mind each day I am at work. "Be not forgetful to entertain strangers: for thereby some have entertained angels." I feel I experience this every day. We, in health care, have a unique opportunity and the good fortune to be a witness to those around us, regardless of our job title or job description.

—Submitted by Kendra Moon, Shepherd Pathways, Atlanta, GA

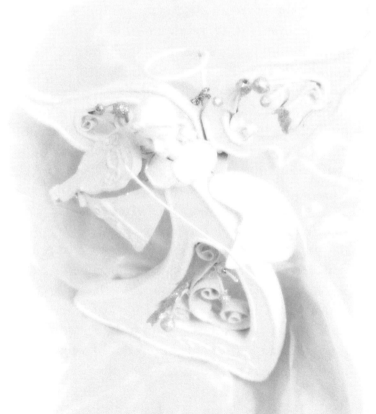

"Never underestimate the difference you can make."

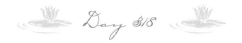

Emotional Connection Speeds Recovery

I began working at Frye Regional Medical Center in December 2001, in a non-patient-care area. I knew this was a good hospital, with a solid reputation in the community. I had no idea, though, just how awesome the facility and the staff are at Frye until my grandma became a patient.

In January 2003, during a snowstorm in the North Carolina mountains, my 75-year-old grandmother caught the toe of her slipper on a vent in her kitchen floor and fell. She knew immediately that she was injured. My family found her an hour later, and she was transported by ambulance to the local hospital where, unfortunately, the physicians weren't sure how to treat her injury and even recommended sending her back home. My family stood their ground—after all, the roads were treacherous at this point and Grandma couldn't walk or even sit up—and eventually, she was moved from the ED to a room.

For the next few days, the staff at the local hospital did several x-rays but were never quite sure what to do with her. Eventually, a surgeon determined she needed to see an orthopedist who specialized in spine surgery. He spoke to Alfred Geissele, MD, in Hickory, North Carolina, and Dr. Geissele accepted Grandma as a patient. She was transferred by ambulance to Frye Regional Medical Center, over an hour away from her home.

The evening that she was transferred to Frye, Dr. Geissele met with my family and explained to us that she had fractured her spine and that considering her

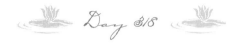

history, he would prefer not to do surgery immediately. It was his hope that by keeping her immobile, the fracture would heal on its own. He spoke to us with a great deal of kindness and compassion and patiently answered all of our questions, even though it was late in the evening. He treated Grandma as if she were his only patient. We all left in tears that night, but knew that she was in good hands.

For almost four months, my grandma was a patient at Frye. She ended up having two surgeries, which included numerous rods and screws being placed in her back. She spent time on almost every floor in the hospital. We joked that the only unit that didn't have her as a patient at some point was Labor and Delivery! For the majority of her time at Frye, she could do nothing for herself. The nurses and nursing assistants would roll her over every two hours, feed her, bathe her, and take care of all her physical needs. However, what they did for her emotionally is what was so amazing about her care.

My grandma has a great sense of humor, but naturally, she was somewhat depressed. She was independent and had lived alone for several years, and now, she was totally dependent on others to take care of her. The nurses really made an effort to get to know her, and she quickly became friends with everyone involved in her care. She spent many weeks in the Restorative Care Unit. The nurses on RCU would take their breaks in Grandma's room to just chat with her, and you could always hear laughter coming from her room. The unit secretary didn't want Grandma to get bored, so she would bring her little craft kits and show her what to do. The family started joking that once we did get her back home, we were going to have a hard time entertaining her like these nurses did!

There were so many little things that they did for her each and every day that really made a difference. I'm sure that the emotional connection helped with her

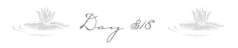

recovery. There were times we did not know if she would survive, and if she did, if she would ever walk again. The day that she took her first steps, every nurse on the unit was there cheering for her. When she was transferred from RCU to Rehab, the nurses brought her a big heart-shaped pillow with a pen and all of them autographed it for her. She still treasures that pillow.

Today, she is once again independent and living alone. So many people at Frye contributed to her recovery. I wish I could name each one and thank them individually.

—Submitted by Cathy Jones,
Frye Regional Medical Center, Hickory, NC

"Never underestimate the difference you can make."

635

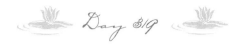

Time Out

We hold two major social events for our families every year—a Christmas party and a summer ball game. We invite all Mercy Children's hematology/oncology patients, former patients, and their families. It is a chance for the kids to just be kids and for the families to be surrounded by others who can relate to what they are going through.

We average 100 to 150 people at each event. Some children and parents have just learned of the diagnosis, some are survivors who have been off therapy for 10 years. It is a wonderful mix of people in a non-threatening, non-medical environment. The kids start talking; the parents start talking.

For some of these parents who are still reeling from the news that their kids have cancer or whose children are in the midst of their first round of treatment, it is reassuring to see the survivors—to realize that, yes, kids do make it through this, their hair does grow back, they do return to school, and the family can return to normal.

These events do for those parents what all the positive statistics in the world cannot. It is one thing for us to tell them how good their children's chances of beating cancer are—but often, in the back of their minds, they are always wondering if their children will fall on the short end of the statistics. Seeing so many children who had cancer and are now healthy increases their ability to believe their own children will survive.

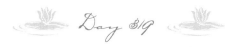

We take the kids to the baseball game at Fifth Third Field and hold the Christmas party at COSI. In both cases, it is a fun atmosphere, and, thanks to a grant we get via Children's Miracle Network, we pay for everything, providing an opportunity to experience activities some of our families wouldn't otherwise be able to afford.

Simply put, it is a really happy time. It gives the children something to look forward to—they talk about it all year. It's a chance to be away from the needles and medications. It's like a mini-vacation from pain and the often harsh realities of each family's personal situation.

We deal with a lot of difficult situations, and we often see people in their darkest hours. It is so great to spend a joyous, carefree time with everyone. I think I look forward to and treasure those two nights a year as much as any of our kids and families do.

—*Anonymous Contributor, St. Vincent Mercy Children's Hospital, Toledo, OH*

"Never underestimate the difference you can make."

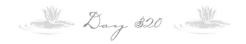

Moving Mountains to Make a Wish Come True

Our patient was in palliative care, dealing with the final stages of a five-year battle with ovarian cancer. She was a champion dressage rider and fervently wished to see her horse one last time. Her deteriorating condition made it impossible for her to leave the hospital and visit the stable.

On Valentine's Day, the University Health Network, Gynecologic Surgical Oncology team of the Toronto General Hospital Unit 6A West put a plan into place. The team, known for its dedicated approach to meeting patients' needs, decided to work with the family to make her wish come true. If she couldn't go to visit her horse, maybe the horse could come to her.

After much planning, the horse arrived at the TGH receiving dock. For Sherida Chambers, clinical nurse specialist, honoring the patient's wishes was part of the patient-centered care dimensions of "respect for patient's values, preference, and expressed needs" and "involvement of family and friends." The staff was able to facilitate what was most important to the patient and to contribute to something that made a real difference to her and to her family.

During the visit, the patient was surrounded by her husband, three children, family, friends, and of course, her horse. Sherida recalls, "It was a very special moment." Sadly, the patient passed away a few days later, surrounded by her family on 6A West.

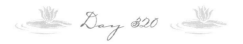

Linda O'Leary, the nurse manager for 6A West, is incredibly proud of the team effort to help this patient fulfill her last wish. Indeed, even the TGH Security team played an integral role, ensuring safety during the horse's visit.

"What a great example of patient-centered care," Linda says. "This is truly what UHN is all about."

—Submitted by Jim Natis, University Health Network-Toronto General Hospital, Toronto, ON

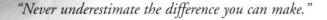

"Never underestimate the difference you can make."

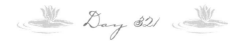
Every Patient Has a Story

Ultrasound technician Lani Moon ordered a carotid ultrasound for an elderly patient. She began by greeting and explaining the exam. Noticing the patient was cold, she offered her an additional blanket. After completing the exam, Lani placed the woman in a more comfortable position and told her she would be going to the MRI department for the next test.

Suddenly, the woman became extremely agitated and in a European accent began asking questions about the MRI "tunnel." Lani answered her questions and, sensing her fear, accompanied her to the MRI.

Once there, Lani gently touched her arm to wish her well. As she did, the patient reached for her hand, squeezed it tightly, and said tearfully, "I will never forget you."

The reaction was more extreme than usual and Lani was somewhat concerned and perplexed by the woman's fearful affectation.

It was then that Lani noticed the numbers tattooed on the woman's wrist and suddenly she realized—this lady was a Holocaust survivor. In that moment, Lani fully understood the woman's despair as well as her deep gratitude for the small acts of kindness that Lani had shown her.

Every patient has a story; we just don't always know what it is.

—Submitted by Darlene English, Lake Hospital System, Painesville, OH

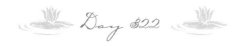

An Agent of Change

Liver and onions—you either love it or hate it. Mr. F loved it. His wife hated it. She hated it so much that she couldn't bring herself to fix the dish for him. So when Mr. F became a patient at Falls Memorial Hospital, he jumped at the opportunity to order it from the hospital's new patient choice menu.

Unfortunately, there were still some small problems with the new menu selection system, and Mr. F did not receive his much-anticipated dinner. Mr. F was not happy and he did not hesitate to let everyone know about his displeasure.

Because of a chronic condition, Mr. F was a frequent patient at FMH. The staff knew him well; he was known to have high expectations regarding his medical care.

"There wasn't a stay that didn't involve an opportunity for improvement," says Kim Kucera, Director of Nursing. Mr. F took issue with the cleanliness of his room, the freshness of his sandwich, the quality of the meal trays, his care, and more.

At one point, he made an appointment to talk to the hospital CEO. "He felt we had not met his health care needs as a member of the community," Kim says. The entire hospital staff had to make a choice: greet Mr. F's comments with a smile and a nod and do nothing, or embrace him as an engine for change.

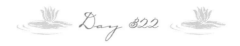

Falls Memorial Hospital got it right. "It took us a long time to understand that Mr. F wasn't just complaining for the sake of hearing himself talk," says Laura Hopkins, FMH VP of Patient Services. "He sincerely wanted us to succeed. He wanted Falls Memorial Hospital to be the best, and he helped move us in that direction."

Mr. F inspired some small changes, such as dating the sandwiches in the family pantry refrigerator to ensure freshness. But he inspired larger changes as well.

Kim recognized the value of patient rounding, which she had just begun when she met Mr. F. "The decision to move into an administrative role was an easy one for me," Kim says. "I had been in health care so long, I felt like I needed a change. However, the longer I was away from direct patient care, the more I began to feel I didn't really make a difference with patients anymore. Mr. F gave me that back. He touched my soul."

When Kim arrived at the hospital December 11, 2006, her first thought was to visit Mr. F, but when she arrived in his room, the bed was empty. "He had passed away over the weekend," Kim explains. "I had so badly wanted to be there for him."

Several days later, Kim attended Mr. F's funeral. Toward the end of the eulogy, Mr. F's daughter-in-law spoke of the impact the staff at Falls Memorial Hospital had on Mr. F. The nurses and ER physician, Dr. Gillette, who had sat with him the night of his death, and Kim were all mentioned by name.

"It was an awakening for me," Kim says. "When I heard how highly Mr. F thought of the hospital, I knew we had brought the relationship with a wonderful man full circle."

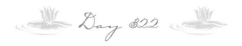

Mr. F's wife felt the same way. She, too, had formed a bond with Kim and the rest of the FMH staff. "I couldn't be at the hospital with my husband all of the time," Mrs. F says. "But when I left, I knew he would be okay. The FMH staff didn't just take care of him, they cared for him."

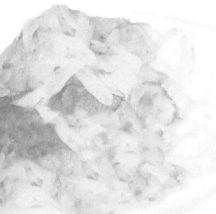

Before Mr. F's death, Kim had a chance to make amends for his missed liver and onions lunch. Although it was not on the menu for dinner that night, Kim, along with Environmental Services Director Margaret Hyatt and Administrative Assistant Kim Nelson, made sure he received his meal by ordering it from a local restaurant.

"The surprise on his face when I brought that dinner in could have tipped you over," Kim says. "He was so impressed we would do that for him."

The transformation of the hospital's relationship with Mr. F and his family is an example of what's right in health care. Through the lens of service excellence, employees recognized an opportunity for improvement and growth. Although Mr. F is no longer here to guide FMH in its pursuit of excellence, the impact he made has remained.

—Submitted by Sage Hemstad, Falls Memorial Hospital, International Falls, MN

"Never underestimate the difference you can make."

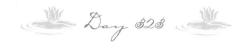

The Cutting Edge of Teamwork

A patient arrived at the East Emergency Department with a four-foot threaded rod impaled in his abdomen. It was necessary to cut the metal piece down before he could be transported via Life Flight to another hospital.

Workers from the Painesville City Fire Department, who brought the patient in, started to use a large chainsaw for the rod removal, but Harry Vaught of Plant Operations offered a grinder, which was a smaller, more efficient tool.

First, it was necessary to turn off the oxygen in the ED to avoid ignition of the sparks. The Plant Operations team promptly handled the situation, and the nurses transferred patients to the use of portable tanks. Harry then recommended applying ice to the patient's abdomen and cold wet towels to the patient's face to prevent any burning during the hot pipe cutting procedure. For safety reasons, he also suggested clearing the room of nonessential people.

Tony Van Gils of the Plant Operations team was a former fabricator, so he took over and cut three feet off the metal rod. This enabled the ED to complete the transfer with Life Flight.

Amazingly, the patient remained awake during the process and witnessed the exceptional teamwork taking place around him. Thanks to Plant Operations working hand-in-hand with the Emergency Department, the patient made it through this unusual ordeal—and eventually was able to return to work.

—*Submitted by Darlene English, Lake Hospital System, Painesville, OH*

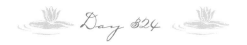
breaking the rules

We had a 35-year-old man who came in after collapsing at work. He had sustained a massive heart attack. It seemed nearly unbelievable for such a thing to happen at age 35 and to someone with no risk factors.

We were attempting to stabilize him at our hospital to transfer him to a larger facility where he could get cardiac catheterization. His beautiful wife and daughter were sobbing and scared. They asked for a priest.

The priest came and performed the Sacrament of the Sick. The patient was very unstable, with blood pressure dropping, then sky-rocketing. His heart rates were wildly varying, too.

As we were getting ready to load him into the ambulance, the priest came over and said "Wendi, the wife is not sure he was ever baptized. I need you to baptize him."

"I can't do that!" I exclaimed. The priest said, "Yes you can, and here is how."

I have been an ED nurse 15 years, and I believe I can do most anything I need to do but never have I been asked to baptize anyone. And I am far from being eligible to be a nun!

But I decided I had to do what was needed, so I went into the ambulance, dealt with the drips, the ventilator, etc., and then I did it—I baptized this patient.

We transported the patient to the other hospital. He had a rough next 24 hours, and he was barely holding on.

I went to visit him. His wife hugged me immediately and then introduced me to the twenty or so people in the waiting room as the nurse who baptized her

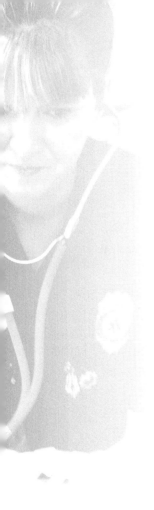

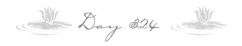

husband. She went on to tell me how that act alone helped her believe that her husband was going to make it.

Five days later, he walked out of the hospital, holding his daughter's hand on one side, and his wife's on the other.

Isn't it amazing what can be done through the power of prayer and the willingness to break the rules for what is right for the patient?

—Submitted by Wendi Thomas,
Petaluma Valley Hospital, Petaluma, CA

"Never underestimate the difference you can make."

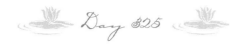

WHEN SECONDS COUNT

Barbara "Rosie" Rosenbarger, RN, is a nurse at Floyd Memorial Hospital. With 25 years of experience, she knew something was wrong when she began experiencing troubling symptoms on her day off.

"I was home straightening up the house when I felt what I thought was indigestion," Rosie relays. "I wasn't worried at first, but when my fingers got numb and my jaw began to ache, I thought I'd better get help."

Rosie called her next-door neighbor, Michael Scott, and told him she needed to go to the hospital. She doesn't remember the whole trip to the hospital, however, because she passed out shortly before they reached Floyd Memorial's Emergency Department.

"She was in total cardiac arrest when she arrived," says Srini Machi, MD. "Through CPR and defibrillation, the ER team was successful in getting her heart back into rhythm. Because her lungs and respiratory system had also shut down during the cardiac arrest, they put her on a ventilator. The EKG showed she was having a heart attack."

The hospital team quickly moved Rosie to the cath lab for tests. One of her arteries was totally occluded and the other artery was 90 percent blocked. Rosie had emergency balloon angioplasty and stents were inserted.

In cardiac cases, minutes count. Rosie knows that in those crucial moments, a team of professionals was making decisions that would affect the outcome of

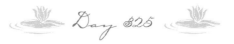

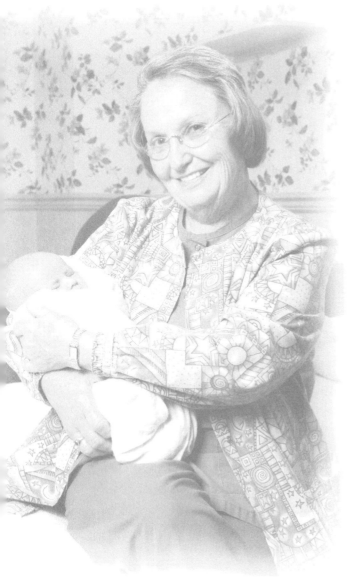

her future health. Rosie credits the expertise of her coworkers at Floyd with her rapid recovery.

"I went into cardiac arrest on a Friday in June, got two stents the same day, and was discharged from the hospital the following Tuesday," Rosie says. "I was able to come back to work the first of August!"

Rosie has always been enthusiastic about her nursing career, even though at nearly-64, she could retire. With her recent personal health care crisis, Rosie is even more convinced about the exceptional quality of care available at Floyd Memorial Hospital.

"It's a wonderful place to work," she explains, "and a wonderful place to receive care."

—Submitted by Darlene O'Bryan,
Floyd Memorial Hospital, New Albany, IN

"Never underestimate the difference you can make."

Small Hospital, Big Results

Mike R. was a patient at Mercy Hospital of Willard and St. Vincent Mercy Medical Center. Here is his story:

I was mowing my lawn on May 15, 2005, when I experienced chest pain. At first, I tried to convince myself and my wife that it was nothing. But my wife insisted we go to the hospital. Having lived and worked in Norwalk most of my life, I had always gone there for my medical care, but Willard was closer and my pain was intense at this point, so I told my wife we'd better go there.

When we got to the ER at Mercy Hospital of Willard, they put me on a gurney and took me into an advanced care treatment room where care was begun immediately. In a few short minutes, all I remember was seeing Dr. Miller's nametag (Albert Miller, MD) and asking him if I was having a heart attack. He said, "I believe you are." I asked if I was going to make it, and he replied, "That's certainly the plan."

I remember them telling me to settle down and cooperate as they were struggling to get me hooked up to tubes and monitors, which I guess I was trying to pull out. The final thing I remember was hearing a call for "Code Blue."

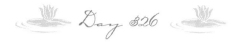

I woke up in Toledo two days later, and my wife helped to fill me in about what had happened. I learned that my heart had stopped and they had used the automated external defibrillator on me once in Willard and twice on Life Flight on the way to St. Vincent Mercy Medical Center. I'm sure I am not the only patient to say that Mercy was instrumental in saving his life, but for me, it was absolutely the case. I would not have made it to the hospital in Norwalk, and had I not received such professional, rapid treatment at Mercy that day, I would have sustained a great deal of heart damage, had I lived.

I had two stents placed on May 15, and on June 14, I had the third one installed in Toledo. When I was on the operating table, Dr. Kabour (Ameer Kabour, MD, FACC, FSCAI) came into the room and said to the three nurses there, "This is one lucky man." I said, "To what do you attribute that, Doc?" He replied with one word: "Willard."

I believe that said it all. He said they did all the right things on May 15, and as a result, he said he could not see any damage to the heart muscle, which, with the massive heart attack I had, is nothing short of incredible.

Not only did Mercy Hospital of Willard provide excellent care, they were caring and compassionate as they did so. A nurse, Carol Niedermeier, sat with my wife while the ER team was working on me. She even called a week later to see how I was doing! I told her I wanted to meet Dr. Miller, and she helped to arrange an introduction. I felt it was important to meet the man who, without a doubt, not only saved my life but spared me much damage and a drastically different lifestyle in the years to come.

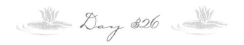

In fact, I received such amazing care that just five weeks after my heart attack, I came out of retirement and took on what was intended to be an interim role as a Chief of Police. To be able to take on a full-time job such a short time after my attack shows just how great the care was—they saved my life, and they saved my heart from permanent damage. I am still working full-time as Chief of Police today, and I feel great.

From my own observations as well as everything I have heard, Dr. Miller is an outstanding, very caring physician, and Mercy is fortunate to have him. I can also say the same thing about the entire staff on duty when I went into the ER, because my wife told me everyone was just terrific and helped her through a very difficult day. My wife and I have already sung the praises of Mercy Hospital of Willard to dozens of friends. We shall be forever grateful.

—*Anonymous Contributor, Mercy Hospital of Willard, Willard, OH*

"Never underestimate the difference you can make."

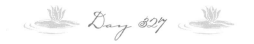

Healing a Heart Far from Home

A lot of stories have come out of the Hurricane Katrina experience. This case study also has a connection to the storm. Charles was raised in New Orleans, as one of nine siblings. He currently resides in California with his wife, Jan. Most of his siblings were displaced by the storm and are now living across Louisiana.

Charles flew to Louisiana to see his family and visit a brother who was gravely ill. After his visit with the family, he flew into Houston to conduct business. While here, he suffered a heart attack and was brought to MHMC.

It was determined that he required immediate coronary artery bypass surgery. His wife was notified and she made arrangements to fly to Houston from California. I first met Jan in the surgical waiting room while Charles was in surgery.

There were two of his siblings there as well; the other siblings were in Louisiana conducting funeral services for the brother who died following Charles's visit. Needless to say, everyone was in a state of crisis.

Jan was extremely nervous and apprehensive about her husband's surgery. I told her that I would be there to assist her and the family in any manner possible. Her first request was simply for something to write on and something to write with. She realized that in her current emotional state, she needed to write down even the simplest things in order to remember.

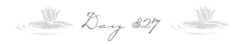

During our conversation, she stated that, being from out of state, she knew nothing about Houston and did not know where she was going to stay. I obtained the names of two hotel/residence suites in this immediate area and provided her with this information, along with a map of the area surrounding the hospital.

During the first post-op day, I visited with Charles in the Surgical Intensive Care Unit. At that point, his recovery was unremarkable. Jan had found a suite nearby and was less apprehensive than on the previous day.

On the second post-op day, I received a phone call at about 7:30 a.m. from Jan. She was in a state of panic and stated, "Charles is doing okay, but I am falling apart." She told me she was on her way to the hospital. I told her I would meet her there and we could talk.

We sat together and she told me that her father had bypass surgery eight years earlier, and following his surgery he and her mother came to stay with her. On the second day following his discharge, her father went into cardiac arrest and died in her home.

Jan was so afraid that the same thing would happen to her husband. She said to me, "I can't go through this again. I should have been able to save my father. I can't lose Charles, too." I reassured her that we would give her all of the instructions and assistance she would need to be prepared to care for him at the time of his discharge. This seemed to help her.

On the third post-op day, Charles was moved to the Cardiology/Telemetry Unit (7 East). He was complaining of pain in the incision area; this made it difficult for him to cough and tolerate respiratory therapy treatments. I visited with them about four times that day and left the hospital at 3:30 p.m.

Upon arrival the following morning, I saw that he was no longer on the unit (my heart stopped). I had a message that Jan was anxiously looking for me and

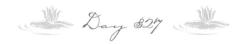

her cell phone number was there. Around supper time the preceding day, Charles's incision opened and the sternum had separated. He was rushed to surgery and then back to SICU.

Jan was afraid she would not be able to contact me. I told her I did not normally give my home number to patients, but I gave it to her since she was in a strange town where she knew no one. I told her to call me day or night anytime she needed to talk or if she needed help. Charles stayed in the SICU for about two weeks before being moved back to 7 East.

He, too, was extremely anxious and afraid. Slowly, he was allowed to move about more. His chest incision was showing less signs of infection and his mental status was improving. Of course, as he improved, so did Jan. During this recovery period, I was with them the entire time. Fortunately, his room was located across the hall from my office, so I was close enough for them to contact me whenever they needed me.

By this time, we had formed a bond based on trust and understanding. I continued to provide as much post-op teaching and home care information as I could. After 35 days, Charles was discharged; he was not going to be able to travel back to California for at least another three weeks.

They both expressed their gratitude for the excellent care he received here at MC and told me they would call me and update me on his recovery. I did visit with them in person several times prior to their return to California.

The rest of the story: One morning in August I received a phone call. From the other end of the line I heard, "Judy, guess where we are? (It was Jan.) We are on a cruise in Alaska…we were talking about you and said that had it not been for your love and concern, we would not be here today."

Two months later, I received another call, "Judy, guess where we are? We are in our motor coach in Jackson Hole, WY! Your picture is on our refrigerator and we wanted to tell you we would not be here today, either, had it not been for you."

This is what holistic nursing is all about! There could be no greater reward!

—Submitted by Judith Farmer,
Memorial Hermann Heart & Vascular Institute-Memorial City, Houston, TX

NOTES

"Never underestimate the difference you can make."

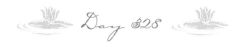

THEY MADE IT EASY

Christie S. is the mother of Meguire, a five-year-old boy who has been battling leukemia since June 2003. Here is her story:

It has been so hard to see our son so sick. When you have a child facing a life-threatening illness, the last thing you have the energy to cope with is figuring out how you are going to pay the medical bills.

When Meguire was first diagnosed, our insurance coverage was great, so we had no worries. But about six months after his diagnosis, our coverage dropped from 100 percent to 90/10, and then it dropped again to 80/20.

We were getting a lot of bills. Then a wonderful woman by the name of Mary Helen Desko, a Mercy Health Partners financial counselor, contacted us. I don't even know how she got a hold of our case—we hadn't yet even thought to apply for any assistance—and she said there might be financial help available for us, and she would send us some forms to fill out. We filled them out, and then she just took care of everything. She got us qualified for Mercy's Financial Assistance Program.

Even when we had to go to Columbus Children's for Meguire's bone marrow transplant, we had the help we needed from Mary Helen. I called her when I had questions, and she always took time to go over things

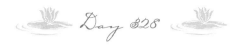

with me. I was in Columbus with Meguire for four months, and when I came home, there was a big stack of bills waiting for me. I just took them to Mary Helen, and she reviewed them all, and then told me they'd already been paid. I didn't have to deal with any of it—it was wonderful.

We have been to another hospital with our older son, who was treated for asthma in the past, and we like Mercy so much better. Beyond the help they have given us with all of the financial worries, Mercy has provided excellent care to Meguire. The doctors and nurses at Mercy Children's are second to none, especially Ellie (Eleanora Ducey, RN)—I hope she stays there for a long time.

They all really make an effort to include the family in everything and keep us informed about what is going on. From the very beginning, they have explained things really well and have been really helpful. They just do a wonderful job.

—Submitted by Melissa Shay, Mercy Health Partners, Toledo, OH

"Never underestimate the difference you can make."

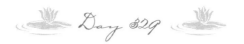

The Gift of Dignity

A mother from an outlying county was transferred to the hospital in premature labor. Given the emergency situation of her delivery, the mother had only the clothing she was wearing during the ambulance ride and had arrived at the hospital with no shoes.

The mother delivered her baby and was scheduled to go home. It was very cold outside, and an inch of snow had fallen since she had first arrived at the hospital.

Paula Lyons, RN, who works in the Neonatal Intensive Care Unit, overheard the mother fretting over her bare feet in such weather. Paula went to her locker, retrieved her own snow boots, and offered them to the mother.

"Take these," Lyons said. "They were left here by another mother who didn't need them, and she thought there might be someone who would."

Lyons maintained the mother's dignity and sent her home with her own snow boots. Lyons went home from work that day in her nursing clogs, with a heart that was much warmer than her feet.

—Submitted by Cyndi Baxter, Central Baptist Hospital, Lexington, KY

"Never underestimate the difference you can make."

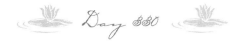

Flossie's Goal

Upon entering the cozy home in Shelby, NC, a rural town of 20,000 people about 30 miles east of Charlotte, you can't help but be drawn toward the high-pitched, constant, jovial cackle coming from the living room. Inside resides a 17-year-old and a 95-year-old, one of whom sits quietly on the couch, the other continuously talking, grinning, and laughing, discussing plans for college and the spring though winter has barely hit its stride.

But the one who speaks of such a promising future is the one who lives day-to-day with a life-altering disease. Flossie is a 95-year-old who suffers from congestive heart failure (CHF), a condition in which the heart can't pump enough blood to the body's other organs. It's the cruelest of ironies for a woman whose heart seems to be stronger and larger than that of anyone you'll ever meet. Specialists say that, in terms of her disease, which she has suffered from for four years, she's in stage four, or the "end stage," a term that means exactly what it suggests.

Statistics show that the average person of Flossie's age at this stage of the disease lives for less than a year. Flossie has one goal left in life—to see her grandnephew Phillip, a high school senior whom she has raised since birth, off to college. Flossie's goal is within reach. She has lived three years longer than statistics suggest she would survive, and she feels that she would not be around had she not been able to stay at her home with Phillip.

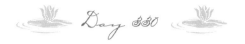

Both credit this important factor to the care that she has received from the staff at Cleveland Regional Medical Center (CRMC), a proven leader in CHF and a participant in the HQID project. In Flossie's instance, by following the suggested processes of care for congestive heart failure, which include adult smoking cessation advice and counseling, left ventricular systolic (LVS) assessment and detailed discharge instructions, CRMC has helped her to live longer, as well as at a much higher quality. Prior to HQID best practice measures being in place at CRMC, Flossie experienced four CHF hospital readmissions for a total of 17 days in the hospital over a six-month period.

At this rate, over the course of 21 months, she would have endured 14 readmissions and 60 days in the hospital. But, with HQID best practice indicators in place, Flossie has since experienced only two CHF readmissions over the course of 21 months for a total of seven days in the hospital.

Flossie was born in 1911 in a home less than 100 yards from her current one. She spent over 40 years living on her own in Brooklyn, NY, supporting herself as an electrician. She regularly attended Brooklyn Dodgers games and was a mourner at Jackie Robinson's funeral. She crossed paths with Coretta Scott King on multiple occasions. Flossie also lived in Philadelphia and Camden, NJ, where she worked on an assembly line at the Campbell's Soup Company worldwide headquarters. She returned to Shelby in the 1980s to raise Phillip, whom she has cared for since birth.

Phillip is six feet two inches tall, weighs 250 pounds, and looks like he should be a starting offensive tackle for his high school football team. And though he loves the game, this is not so. He simply doesn't have the time or the resources that the normal high school senior has. In fact, he had a Game Cube video game system but had to sell it to make ends meet.

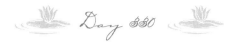

Phillip prepares breakfast for Flossie each morning as well as many of the evening meals and is a constant companion to her. Flossie says, "Phillip is lucky to have me," which is one of many examples of the good-natured ribbing that she is constantly pushing on her grandnephew.

Meredith Morehead, a registered nurse with Care Solutions, says that every time she goes to see Flossie, she goes with the intent of helping her but comes away with a special blessing. Flossie is an incredible woman, and you can't help but smile when you're around her.

—*Submitted by Ginny Starnes, Premier Inc., Written by Alven Weil, Premier Inc.*

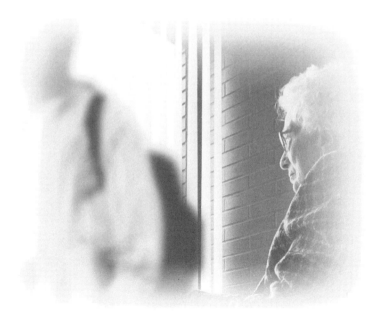

"Never underestimate the difference you can make."

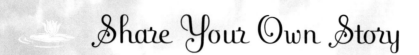

Share Your Own Story

Please share an experience that connected you back to purpose, worthwhile work, and making a difference. You are a big part of what's right in health care!

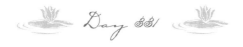

Christmas Fellowship

*I*t was a few days before Christmas 2003 when the staff in 4 ICU North and 4 ICU South realized that they would probably have a house full of critically ill patients for the holiday. Debbie Purcell, RN, thought it might be nice to bring a bit of Christmas cheer to the families of those patients who would be spending the holiday in one of the last places they would like to be.

With the approval of her supervisor, Norma Lake, RN, BSN, Debbie made plans to provide a home-cooked meal for the patients' families. About 20 staff members from the two ICU units brought ham and turkey as well as loads of side dishes and desserts. When the meal was announced on Christmas morning, the families were amazed that the staff had gone to such lengths for them.

At mealtime, a son of one of the ICU patients volunteered to say grace.

"It was one of the most eloquent, moving prayers I've ever heard," Norma remembers. "He prayed for every family represented there and for all that they were going through. He prayed that God would give strength to the families whose loved ones weren't going to regain health. It was especially poignant because his father died just a few hours later."

That first ICU Christmas dinner has led to similar events in the years to follow. The Christmas 2006 dinner, with its abundance of food, involved families in all of the hospital's ICUs. Staff members now consider it a holiday tradition. Several

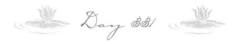

nurses with the day off have come in to help serve the meal, accompanied by their own family members.

"To me, it's like we're able to give these families a gift, and I think anybody who's helped with it can tell you how heartwarming it is and how it really is a gift to us as well," Norma says. "It's what Christmas is all about."

—Submitted by Cyndi Baxter, Central Baptist Hospital, Lexington, KY

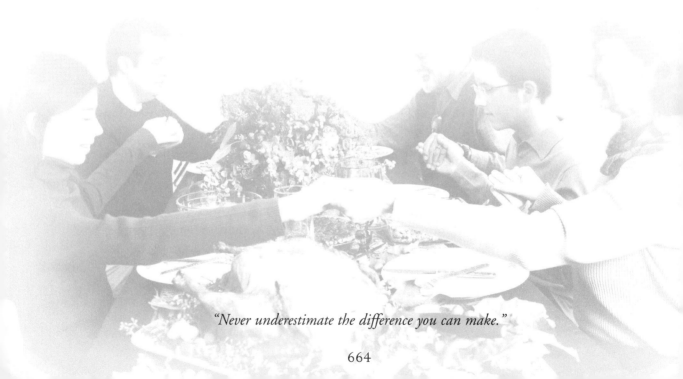

"Never underestimate the difference you can make."

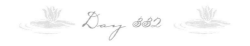

The Dance

What seemed to be an ordinary day in 4 Montvue turned into a moment that many of us will never forget. Paul, a new RN, is always up for a challenge and on this particular day, his attitude was no different. Admissions were arriving as usual, with Paul assigned to the less challenging cases on our busy Med-Surg/Stroke/Senior Friendly unit.

The shift leader that day, Leah, informed Paul he was getting an admission— an outpatient receiving two units of blood. Since Paul was already working with five patients, Leah reassured him it would not be too much for him to handle.

These admissions normally go smoothly and are in and out quickly, with minimal paperwork. Mrs. Smith arrived with her daughter and was offered a gown but wanted to stay in her own clothes. She was in her eighties, from an assisted living facility, and had a history of Alzheimer's and dementia. Although pleasant, Mrs. Smith seemed to be somewhat confused but the admission process went effortlessly for Paul. Mrs. Smith's daughter provided pertinent history, the IV site was successfully started on first attempt, and the blood was drawn for type and cross match.

As Paul waited for the blood to be ready for transfusion, Mrs. Smith started to become restless and agitated and pulled out her IV. Her daughter became tearful and stated that her mother typically acted this way when she got out of her normal environment. Mrs. Smith just wanted to go home. She needed to be pre-

medicated with Tylenol and Benadryl, but she informed Paul that she did not have a headache and did not need any Tylenol. He kept trying, explaining in his calm voice as to why she needed to be there. She stated she was just fine, did not need any blood, and just wanted to home.

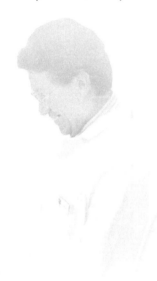

While Paul placed a call to her MD, different staff members took turns walking Mrs. Smith around the unit to keep her occupied. She grew tired of this and Paul took her back to her room. She was still persistent about going home. Paul again quietly explained that she could not go home, but he also asked if there were anything else she might like to do. Quickly she responded with a big smile on her face, "I would like to dance."

Paul, who is not a dancer, said, "You will have to lead." She agreed, and so—they danced.

What a wonderful sight, seeing this lovely lady calmed by the impromptu dance. It was at that moment we all knew Paul had a place at Parkwest Medical Center. The love and care that he showed Mrs. Smith was very touching to me as well as the others who were witnessing the moment.

On our journey to excellence, such moments capture how we touch lives and make a difference everyday. Thanks to Paul, Mrs. Smith received her blood transfusion later that night and was able to go home the next morning.

I often wonder what small acts we can perform to help other patients "dance."

—Submitted by Linda Minton, Parkwest Medical Center, Knoxville, TN

"Never underestimate the difference you can make."

THE MANY FACETS OF CARE

Eileen, in her forties, was a patient at St. Vincent's, diagnosed with lung cancer. Following surgery, she was referred to the Oncology Clinic and met with an oncologist, an oncology fellow, a clinical nurse specialist, and a social worker. As a single parent of a seven-year-old son and 15-year-old daughter and having minimal resources, Eileen felt the recommended daily radiation therapy would be impossible for her to complete.

We identified her specific areas of concern and, as a team, worked on creating practical solutions. We devised strategies for the management of symptoms such as fatigue and shortness of breath, we worked on financial assistance applications, found transportation for treatments, and located baby sitting services through a local church. We even worked with Eileen to reach out to a cousin living in New Jersey.

After completing radiation therapy, Eileen and her two children moved to New Jersey, not far from her cousin's home. We arranged for oncology and pulmonary consults at a nearby hospital, sent medical records as well as a case management summary, to facilitate the transition.

The move and persistent respiratory symptoms remained significant sources of stress for Eileen. With this in mind, we continued to provide emotional support, sending "thinking of you," holiday and birthday cards to her.

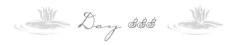

Later, Eileen wrote to us. "Thank you for the cards," she said. "I wrote to you many times mentally. I miss everybody at St. Vincent's. [The New Jersey] Hospital has a very good reputation. For me, it is like going to a new school, new teachers. I hate it. You spoiled me."

Getting that note confirmed to us that we'd made a difference. Several months later, we received another note from Eileen. It read, "Doc said he sees no mass in the lung…my breathing is still bad…But I'm still here. Thanks to [all of you] and St. Vincent's. With love, respect and hugs, Eileen."

We develop relationships with our patients and their families. So often, people assume caring for cancer patients is depressing. It's not. It can be very sad, but we learn to help patients in many ways—with physical symptoms, emotional issues, financial questions, and lending a sympathetic ear. Even in the worst-case scenario, where we could do little about the cancer, we found a way to help.

—Submitted by Marion Smith, Richmond University Medical Center,
(formerly St. Vincent's Hospital), Staten Island, NY

"Never underestimate the difference you can make."

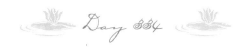

WHEN TRAGEDY STRIKES

It was a typical weekday morning in June. The Davis family's modest duplex on the grounds of Fort Detrick Military base in Frederick, Maryland, was alive with the hustle and bustle of family life—breakfast dishes in the sink, sorted laundry piled in the hallway, and tiny voices vying for TV channel control. But on this day, the street in front of the house was being paved, and cars needed to be moved from street parking into driveways to clear the road for the heavy equipment.

The car keys jingled in mom's hand as she told her four-year-old daughter to wait at the front door "where I can see you," while she moved the family car into the driveway. With a constant watchful eye on her daughter standing on the front porch, the car was pulled into the driveway, and put into park. Upon trying to exit the vehicle, mom noticed that she had perhaps parked a bit too close to her neighbor's car. A small parking adjustment to give her neighbor a few extra inches would be a courteous thing to do.

She put the car in reverse and moved only a few feet before the car suddenly bucked as if it had backed over the curb. She slammed both feet on the brake pedal as she heard her neighbors scream "pull up, pull up." She did. The car jolted again as if righting itself back over the curb. She looked at her front door. The porch was empty. Her daughter was nowhere in sight.

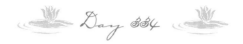

The paramedics arrived at the scene within minutes after receiving the 911 call. CPR was initiated and the critically injured, unresponsive child was loaded into the ambulance for the five-minute transport to Frederick Memorial Hospital (FMH).

The Emergency Department (ED) at FMH was ready when the ambulance pulled into the receiving bay. The ambulance doors flew open. Dr. Brian Rader, and emergency team members Patrick Keeling, RN; Lisa Jackson, RN; and Jackie Pettit, CN, rushed to the side of the gurney to take over the desperate fight to save the child's life. But just as the paramedics efforts were unable to elicit a response from the horribly injured child, the best efforts of the ED crew were likewise unsuccessful. The child was pronounced dead.

FMH Assistant Chaplain Mary Ann Braham recalls that within a matter of minutes the ED was filled with personnel from Fort Detrick. Clergy and commanding officers surrounded the mother as she was told of her child's death.

Despite the private quarters that were made available to the family, the nurses vividly remember the inconsolable cries of the child's mother as she tried to come to grips with the horror of what had happened. The nurses held her as she wailed in disbelief, doing their utmost to comfort the anguished parents.

Dr. Rader, the nurses, and Chaplain Mary Ann promised both of them that they would remain by their sides, and do all that they could to help them through the difficult hours ahead. They were true to their words.

The head trauma the child had sustained left her tiny body in a condition that required some time to make presentable. The nurses remember washing her body with loving care as they prepared her for her parents to see. They washed and brushed her hair, and removed what evidence they could of the injuries that had caused her death.

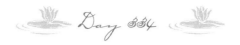

The parents were provided the privacy to hold their child in their arms, and the dignity to take as much time as they wished to say goodbye. Chaplain Mary Ann and Ft. Detrick Garrison Commander, Colonel Mary Deutsch, knelt with the mother at the side of the bed and cried.

As the ED filled with military personnel, friends, family, superior officers, and the Fort's commanding general, the FMH ED staff continued to support the family and see to their needs. Dr. Rader spoke with the medical examiner, who considered the facts of the case and determined no autopsy would be necessary.

The nurses made all of the arrangements with the funeral home so that the family could continue to receive colleagues and friends. Chaplain Mary Ann made phone calls to inform relatives and friends.

At the end of the day, just as there were no more tears to shed, there were no words to express what the family was feeling in their hearts for the compassionate care they had received at FMH. Words of thanks simply proved too difficult to find.

It was not until six months later that the hospital was to know what their care had meant not only to this family, but also to the entire military "family" FMH cares for every day of the year. At the December Leadership Roundtable, a contingent from Fort Detrick, including Base Commander, Major General Eric Shoomaker, MD, and the Garrison Commander, came to thank Frederick Memorial Hospital, and recognize specifically the outstanding care and consideration of the Emergency Room team on that terrible day.

In presenting the hospital with a beautiful plaque framed with commemorative medallions from every branch of the military, Dr. Shoomaker spoke eloquently of the extraordinary care FMH has given to Fort Detrick's military families over the years. He expressed his gratitude on behalf of the family

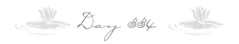

who suffered so terribly that day in June, and wanted all of us to know the difference we had made by treating an unspeakably horrific event with professionalism, dignity, and compassionate care.

General Shoomaker said that the tears that were shed that day by nurses Patrick, Lisa, and Jackie, and everyone else that was involved, had "anointed the day with the dignity that only tears can bestow." He spoke of the personalized care that the entire military base had come to expect from the hospital that they consider their own.

Speaking from personal experience as a trauma surgeon, he reminded us that in health care, the praise so richly deserved is not immediate, and oftentimes never conveyed at all. He said that we should pause everyday to remind ourselves of the extraordinary contributions we make to the health and well-being or our community, and that what we do matters in real and meaningful ways.

If we ever need a specific event to remind us of those valued contributions, we stop and remember that day in June, because it wasn't just another weekday morning.

—Submitted by Harry Grandinett, Frederick Memorial Hospital, Frederick, MD

"Never underestimate the difference you can make."

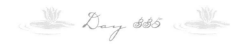

Not a Dry Eye

rs. C. had been ill with pneumonia and congestive heart failure and was admitted to 4ICU North in early May. Despite a series of stressful procedures, Mrs. C. kept a positive attitude because she trusted the staff caring for her. Trust, hope, and love of family kept Mrs. C moving forward.

Mrs. C.'s grandson was coming home from overseas military duty and planned to visit his grandmother. This particular grandson was, according to her family, "the apple of her eye." The grandson and his fiancée were to be married in July, and Mrs. C. was looking forward to the wedding. Her family feared she wouldn't live to see his special day.

Thanks to the work of the nursing staff and the family, Mrs. C.'s favorite grandson arrived at her hospital bedside May 12 with a bouquet of flowers and news that she would be participating in a wedding that very afternoon.

Family members of both the bride and groom, Mrs. C.'s pastor, several of 4ICU North's staff members, the housekeeper, dietitian, and physical therapist were all at Mrs. C.'s bedside to witness and share in this beautiful union of the grandson and his fiancée. There were no dry eyes in 4ICU North that warm and sunny afternoon.

Mrs. C. passed away three days later.

Health care workers not only touch patients, but they touch a whole network of family and friends. That is what nursing is all about—making a difference,

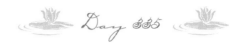

easing the journey, helping to start anew and reminding us all what really is important.

—Submitted by Cyndi Baxter, Central Baptist Hospital, Lexington, KY

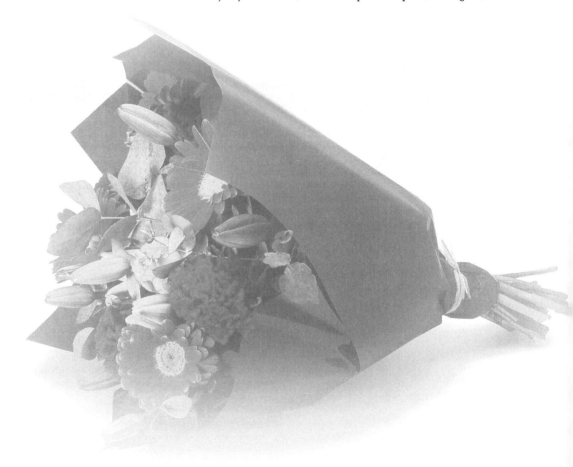

"Never underestimate the difference you can make."

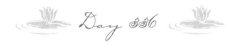

Volunteer Hero

While staffing the front desk of the Same-Day Surgery family waiting area, Lou Cot, a volunteer, noticed a patient looking weak and possibly close to passing out. He recognized her symptoms as possibly being those of a diabetic reaction, due to his diabetic wife's medical history.

Lou quickly alerted the nurses' station. As they prepared to move the patient to a room, Lou grabbed some cookies to give the patient to raise her blood sugar level.

Lou's keen observation and unhesitating action likely saved the patient's life, making this volunteer a hero!

—*Submitted by Darlene English, Lake Hospital System, Painesville, OH*

"Never underestimate the difference you can make."

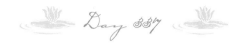

Butterscotch Pudding

I am the pharmacy director of a small in-patient pharmacy. We do not typically have daily interaction with patients, but my pharmacy technician still found a way to make a difference in the life of a special patient.

Our pharmacy is located directly across from patient rooms, and we notice when patients are out for walks with the physical therapist. One such patient was Ms. X., who was a wee bit of a thing and had been very sick. She had throat cancer and could not speak. She had a tracheostomy and subsequently, a feeding tube.

The pharmacy dispensed her tube feeding preparations every day. After many weeks of being with us, Ms. X. was improving. Her trach stoma was capped off and she started to speak in a raspy voice. She was quite a character and despite her health problems had a wonderful sense of humor.

Ms. X. had never married, and in the hospital, she had few visitors. In a casual chat with our pharmacy technician one day, it turned out they had acquaintances in common. After that, she greeted us in a low gravelly growl whenever she was out for her daily walks. Soon, she knew that the pharmacy dispensed her tube feedings, and with a twinkle in her eye, she started referring to the feedings as her "butterscotch pudding."

Margaret, our pharmacy technician, took a real interest in Ms. X. and began speaking to her every day. We followed her progress as the days passed. The day

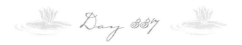

finally came that Ms. X. was going to be allowed to try one soft meal per day by mouth, rather than via the feeding tube.

As soon as Margaret saw that order, she had an idea. She checked with the patient's nurse and then with dietary. She suggested that Ms. X. be brought some REAL butterscotch pudding. Margaret pulled off the surprise and it was a big hit.

Ms. X. continued to improve and finally was discharged home. Margaret realized Ms. X. had few visitors during her long hospital stay, so on Valentine's Day, Margaret had flowers delivered to Ms. X.'s home. A fast friendship has been formed.

Now when Ms. X. comes in for a follow-up visit, she always pokes her head in the pharmacy. Margaret really made a difference in the life of this patient—all because of butterscotch pudding.

—*Submitted by Bonnie Orris, Greene County Medical Center, Jefferson, IA*

"Never underestimate the difference you can make."

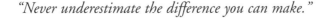

Special Care in Special Situations

*P*aul and Lauren, brother and sister, both had cystic fibrosis. They spent a lot of their time at St. Christopher's.

"With two kids in the family with CF, there is no way you cannot get close to the family," explains Claire Alminde, pediatric nurse, "so all of our hearts went out to this family. We knew what they were headed for."

It was February, and Lauren and Paul had both become ill, so they were admitted to the hospital. Lauren, who was the older sibling, took a turn for the worse.

At the time Lauren passed away, Paul was quite sick, so it was very difficult for Paul to be at the hospital. One of the things that Paul's mom was most concerned with was the impact Lauren's death would have on Paul.

"Paul's mom was especially worried about how Paul would feel being on the same unit where his sister had died," Claire recalls. "So I just tried to spend a little more time with Paul…knowing he was upset about how things had gone with Lauren. He was a great kid."

Claire realized it was important for Paul to have some normalcy while at the hospital, so she worked to make him smile and provide some activities that boys enjoy.

"I remember Paul's mom being so appreciative," Claire recalls, "when she would come in and see Paul laughing again."

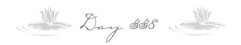
"Any family that has one child die," Claire says, "that's horrible enough for them to go through, but to have to go through it twice…and this is a family that knew they had another child who was going to soon meet the same fate."

Claire's attentive care helped ease the pain everyone was experiencing.

Paul's mother explains that, had Paul lived, he would have been 16.

"I know that if he was here," his mother says, "he probably would have had a big party, and he probably would have had a car out front. He always loved life and Claire made him happy. It's really important to have that kind of care."

—Submitted by St. Christopher's Hospital for Children, Philadelphia, PA

"Never underestimate the difference you can make."

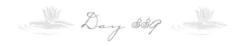

Out of the Ordinary

erek Chan, a physical therapist, is known for his engaging habit of whistling as he walks down the hallway, which is just one indication of the joy he brings to his work and to his patients. He doesn't consider what he does to be anything out of the ordinary. Derek says he is just doing what comes naturally, but his sincerity and warmth touch everyone he meets.

One day, Derek noticed that a patient's wife was not looking well, so he assisted her to the Emergency Department for treatment. Derek returned to work but was bothered by the notion of her being alone. Knowing she was still in the Emergency Department by herself, Derek returned after his shift and stayed with the woman until her family arrived.

On another occasion, Derek took the initiative to ensure his patient could participate in a very special life event. Derek's patient, an amputee, was concerned that he would not be able to walk his daughter down the aisle for her upcoming wedding.

Derek made a special trip to the church after work one day, surveyed the floor plan, and incorporated the proper treatments into the patient's physical therapy plan so that he was able to walk his daughter down the aisle.

Derek's special attention to the concerns and desires of his patients makes him a true Star of Excellence Employee.

—Submitted by Tonia Campbell, Henry Ford Wyandotte Hospital, Detroit, MI

"Never underestimate the difference you can make."

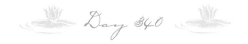

Volunteer Gives Back

Antoinette Marmar, 83, has always hated hospitals. So the St. Anne Mercy Hospital Intensive Care Unit waiting room is the last place you would expect to find her volunteering. She was inspired to overcome her fear of health care settings after she and her husband received outstanding care and service at St. Anne. Her husband passed away two years ago, but Antoinette says she knows he is smiling down on her from heaven while she works her volunteer shift at St. Anne every Thursday morning.

"I think Archie is probably really proud of me for doing this," Antoinette said. "I don't like hospitals at all, but they just treated us so wonderfully.

"This is a difficult time for me as the anniversary of Archie's death approaches. I miss him so much," Antoinette continued. "I think about him every day, and recently, as I was doing so, the thought just occurred to me, 'Why don't I volunteer at St. Anne?' So I hurried up and called right away before I had a chance to change my mind. Now I keep saying, 'Archie, I'm doing this for you—and for me!' "

Archie had been diagnosed with cancer of the bladder in 1987.

"He had to have cystoscopies every three months, and every once in a while, urine built up and he needed a catheter," Antoinette said. "When we went to St. Anne after having been to other hospitals, Archie couldn't believe how good they

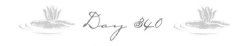

were. They were so gentle with him, so careful, and so concerned that he not suffer."

One night, Archie became so weak that Antoinette had to call an ambulance. After an Emergency Department visit at St. Anne, he became a patient in the ICU. He had been suffering from internal bleeding, and at St. Anne, he immediately received several pints of blood.

"He was in the ICU for seven days, and every day I sat in the waiting room, and 'wonderful' is the only word for the nurses and volunteers who came and talked to me," Antoinette said. "And the care and service Archie received was beyond compare."

"I also was an inpatient at St. Anne in September 2005, when I fractured my ankle. The moment I pressed my call button, they were right there. They checked on me all the time. That is the only hospital I can remember either of us being in where you never had to wait on the staff when you needed something," Antoinette explained.

When Archie was discharged from the hospital, Antoinette said his doctors warned her that he was likely to experience the internal bleeding and resulting weakness again.

"They said he had diverticulitis, and his intestines had been damaged beyond repair," Antoinette said. "The doctor said all we could do at that point was make him as comfortable as possible. A short time later, he began receiving Hospice care, and he passed away on Oct. 23, 2004, just two days before his 90th birthday."

Antoinette said she is grateful for the opportunity to volunteer at St. Anne as a way to honor her husband's memory.

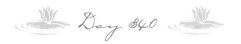

"We are fortunate to have a hospital like St. Anne in our neighborhood," she said. "The building is beautiful, parking is convenient and the staff and volunteers are just so pleasant and sincere. The care given to me and my husband really impressed me, and I hope I can give just a little bit back in return for all that we received."

—*Anonymous Contributor, St. Anne Mercy Hospital, Toledo, OH*

"Never underestimate the difference you can make."

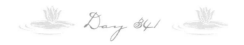

Selfless Acts of Compassion

A busy December day in the Operating Room turned out to be very special because of three compassionate nurses—Rebecca Baugh, RN; Judy Rhode, RNFA; and Gwendolyn Allen, RN.

The three nurses learned that one of their patients lived out of state and had been helping a friend move to Michigan. The patient's friend had promised her an airline ticket home, but due to a personal situation, couldn't honor that promise. For the four days prior to her surgery, the patient had been living in a car and was longing to return to her family. Rebecca, Judy, and Gwen quickly agreed to buy the patient a bus ticket home.

While the story could have ended there, it didn't. These nurses followed their hearts and acted as though the patient were a family member.

When Judy went to the patient's room to visit, she discovered the lady was being discharged the next day. Judy offered to take her to the bus station. The patient was overjoyed!

Rebecca brought in clean clothes for the patient to wear on her return trip. That evening, Judy and her teenage son drove the discharged patient to what they believed was the correct Greyhound terminal in Detroit, only to find it closed. They rushed to find the correct terminal and purchase a ticket. To Judy's dismay, the ticket agent told her the bus was full and there were no more tickets to be sold.

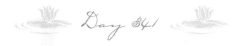

Unwilling to disappoint her patient, Judy approached a different agent and begged her for a Christmas miracle—which is just what she received! The agent sold her one last ticket!

Judy and her son stayed with the patient until the bus arrived. As the patient boarded the bus, Judy handed her a bag with enough food for her trip. As an extra special touch, Judy tucked a small Bible into the pocket of the lunch bag, wishing her a safe trip.

The next day, Judy called the patient to be sure she arrived home safely, just as she would have done for a member of her own family.

These three nurses say they feel blessed for being able to help this patient in a time of true need. Henry Ford Wyandotte Hospital and the patients we serve are truly blessed to have Judy, Rebecca, and Gwen on our staff.

—Submitted by Tonia Campbell, Henry Ford Wyandotte Hospital, Detroit, MI

"Never underestimate the difference you can make."

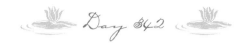

Aunt Marian

*I*n April of this year, my husband's 91-year-old Aunt Marian died. I met her when I was 22 and she was 60. She was a single woman who chose not to marry, but instead chose to take care of her aging parents, as well as her 100+ nieces, nephews, their spouses, and her grandnieces and nephews, not to mention the children she taught throughout her 42-year career as an educator.

In the early evening hours, just prior to her wake, approximately 10 of her loved ones were present at the funeral home. My sister-in-law, Jackie, and I were discussing our last few moments with Marian, marveling at what she was most concerned about. It was not her health condition, which was deteriorating, but rather for all the nieces and nephews to whom she had been unable to create and send her handmade birthday cards.

Since 1973, when she warmly welcomed me into her extended family, I had received a hand-drawn birthday card from her every year. No family member can recall a time when her cards were late or never received, since she was constant in her dedication to those she cared about and one of the ways she demonstrated her love was through her cards.

While Jackie and I marveled at Marian's dedication to all of us, a woman I did not know approached me. I stood up and extended my hand and said, "Hello." She inquired, "Is this the Marian K. who taught school at Jefferson Elementary in 1933?"

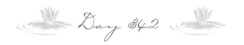

I didn't know where Marian taught school in 1933. At that point, I introduced myself, shared my relationship with Marian and while still holding her hand, walked over to Rose, one of my husband's cousins. I introduced the woman, Maria, to Rose. Yes, we found out, Marian had taught at the school at Jefferson Elementary.

Maria proceeded to share her story with us, crying as she did so. Her third grade teacher, now my dear aunt, learned quickly that Maria could speak English, but could not read and write. She spent many hours before, during, and after school with Maria until she learned how to read and write English. Maria said she learned quickly and by February 1934, her teacher asked her to help teach her peers. She came to tell us that Marian was the first person, outside her own family, who had made a difference in her life. By the time Maria finished her story, we were all crying.

Maria did not stay for the wake service. Before and after the service, Rose and I shared Maria's story to Marian's many extended family members who were present. Our family all knew how Marian enriched our lives. It was an awesome experience to hear someone else talk about the impact Marian had on her life.

I was not expecting to see Maria again, yet I noticed her at the funeral mass the next day. I stopped to introduce my husband and two children to her, thanking her for attending the funeral and telling her how much her presence and story comforted us. Again, we all cried.

I have learned how important it is to inform those people in our lives who have made a difference and let them know the impact they have had. In addition, I come to work knowing I must lead by example, set high standards, pursue excellence, and share successes. Our actions send out ripples, and we don't always know who we have influenced in a positive way.

—Submitted by Margaret (Peggy) Strawhecker

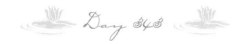

One by One...

Although she had been in the hospital since January 24th, I met Jane and her husband on February 9th. She had been admitted with chronic obstructive pulmonary disease (COPD) exacerbation and hypotension (low blood pressure).

At 65, Jane had a lengthy medical history including lung cancer, congestive heart failure, and depression, among other ailments. Now she was dealing with a long stay in the medical ICU and had expressly wished no ventilator support and no CPR.

Because of her condition, Jane was experiencing a great deal of pain, which was naturally a major concern for her. The nurses had been trying for two days to get her pain under better control, but to no avail. One evening a night nurse suggested starting her on Neurontin®, a medication for nerve pain, and left a note on the front of the patient's chart for the MD to address.

I had two patients other than Jane, but she was always my main priority. Even before I met her, I requested that the unit secretary and/or the charge nurse alert me when her two physicians came to the floor.

On going into her room, I was met with her husband, whose eyes were filled with tears as a result of watching his wife endure so much pain and suffering. Jane was saying her pain was a "12" on a 0 to 10 scale, but unfortunately it was too soon to give her any other pain meds. The medication that had been given

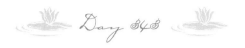

was obviously inadequate. She was extremely short of breath, could hardly swallow a drink of water (let alone eat a meal), and she too was in tears. Jane and her husband reported that the day and night before had been terrible. Neither of them had been able to get much sleep. I comforted them as much as I could, and I assured them I would be their advocate.

"Dr. X" (her primary physician) was rounding, and I introduced myself as Jane's nurse. I told him about her current condition and what was happening in her room. I told him our highest priority should be getting her pain under control. In her room, we discussed her current pain medications. I suggested increasing her oral morphine to a more frequent schedule as needed, adding a pain patch for more prolonged effect, and also adding the Neurontin, per the night nurse's suggestion, to help with nerve pathway pain. We also discussed increasing her anti-anxiety medication to a larger, more frequent dose as needed. We had a plan!

As Dr. X and I were walking toward the nursing station, the doctor said, "Watch for respiratory depression." I replied to him that she needed these meds and palliative care. He responded, "She is *not* dying!" I explained to him that palliative care means "to relieve" and we were, indeed, trying to relieve her suffering.

A while later, "Dr. Y" came to see her. When I saw him at the nurse's station, I immediately started updating him at the station about Jane. He said, "I know, I know. Dr. X has already called me. I guess it's okay. I'm not going to change anything." We went to see Jane together, and already she was feeling better and seemed less anxious. He too voiced his concerns about the possibility of respiratory depression with the medications and advised me to keep a close eye

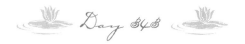

on Jane. That afternoon Jane slept the first real sleep she had enjoyed in a long time.

During my visits to her in the following days, I was glad to see she was eating more and was in less pain. One day she was actually knitting! Another day when she was alone, we sat and talked. During the conversation she asked me, "What is my condition?" I'm not sure if she really didn't understand or didn't know how to ask her doctors. I was honored she felt she could trust me and share her fears and hopes.

I saw Dr. X in those days after that first encounter, and I thanked him for helping Jane feel better and told him how well her medication plan was working.

A shining moment for me was Jane's day of discharge, February 14th, just five days after we first met. I was charting at the nursing station, and she was being wheeled by. She and her husband both had big smiles on their faces. I got up and gave them both a hug.

She went home on the same regimen of medications we had started her on. The only difference was that she needed less morphine and anti-anxiety medications as her condition improved.

Her husband sent a note in early March stating that Jane was back at home and doing well. One of the nurses on the unit asked me what it was that I did to make such a difference for this patient. I explained it to her, and added that it takes *Awareness, Knowledge, Practice, Patience, Compassion, and Success*…one by one.

—Submitted by Lois Leveque, St. Mary's Hospital, Madison, WI

"Never underestimate the difference you can make."

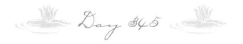

Clara

I don't remember a time when we did not worry about our daughter. She was born perfect, except for some blue, blood-filled masses on her back, growing along her spinal cord and compressing it into her lung fields and around her ribs and vital organs.

By the age of five, she was already an experienced patient with several major surgeries behind her. She had been dragged to the best medical centers in the nation with little to show for it. In spite of every blood draw, every procedure, and every MRI, her disposition remained decidedly sunny and tolerant. It was not uncommon for the anesthesiologist to hand her the mask, smile and say, "Put yourself to sleep, Clara."

At the age of seven, she was given, after much confusion and little headway in keeping her healthy, the diagnosis of a rare, fatal vascular disease. Health care gave up on her then. Wherever we took her, the answers began to sound strangely unified. "She has Cobb's Syndrome; there is not much that can be done," or "We have not seen it before," or finally, "Poor outcome."

Clara persisted in her determination that she was not her disease and never did we hear her complain about pain or being short of breath or being too tired to play softball, which she loved.

When she reached age 13, we were discouraged. Clara's hemoglobin was chronically low, and she developed significant scoliosis. She often needed IV therapy before school. The saddest day was when she stood in the kitchen and told us that none of the doctors cared about her or even really knew her. We were losing hope.

I am a nurse. Clara's grandmother, my mother, is also a nurse, and Clara talks often of going to nursing school. Every health care provider who did not care was our lesson. Every health care provider who took the time to care was our reassurance.

Then, Dr. Lisa entered into our lives. A new, young pediatrician, she cared enough to search the Internet to find information on Clara's disease, and to find a doctor who could help Clara maintain quality of life. We found Dr. Denise Adams at Cincinnati Children's. She asked for all of Clara's records, and we sent everything.

At a week short of "sweet 16," Clara met Dr. Adams, who asked her what she wanted from the visit. Clara said "Nothing." She had stopped believing that anyone cared. This doctor had, however, meticulously reviewed Clara's history and began to tell us slowly and carefully that Clara had been misdiagnosed. She was confident that with the right interventions, based on the correct diagnosis, Clara would be happily playing softball for the rest of her long life.

We all sat in stunned silence, not quite processing what we were hearing, except for Clara, who the doctor noticed was smiling for the first time since they had met.

What I did not tell you is that I am a Studer Group coach. Every time I coach an organization to be a better place for patients, I am coaching to impact better care for my daughter–or your daughter–or anyone you love.

Healthcare is not a building, nor a floor, nor a unit. Healthcare is the people who care about the people who need their caring.

Thank you, Dr. Lisa; thank you, Dr Adams!

—Submitted by Julie Kennedy, Studer Group, Eau Claire, WI

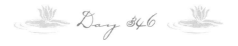

LUNCH ON US

*A*n 86-year-old couple recently visited our cafeteria well after the "rush hour." The wife had been at our facility to undergo a test for which she had to fast, so she was quite hungry and looking forward to having something to eat. After looking at the various choices, they started to leave and whispered to the cashier that they were sorry, they didn't have any cash with them, so they wouldn't be able to buy anything.

A staff member who overheard the conversation urged them to get whatever they wanted because the hospital would be happy to buy their lunch.

"No, no," the woman protested. "We can't ask you to do that." She looked at her husband.

"Well," he said, "to tell you the truth, I am kind of hungry."

They finally agreed to have lunch on us but, in parting, the woman commented to our happy employee, "Do you know why we always come back to Mercy? Everyone here is so nice—everyone. Do they train you to be that way?"

—Submitted by MaryEllen Combs, Provena Mercy Center, Aurora, IL

"Never underestimate the difference you can make."

695

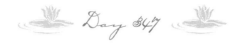

Finding Solutions

Rachel Gallaga-Roman and Sue Sekel, both patient representatives with the Hospital Eligibility Link Program (HELP) at our facility, will never forget a patient they worked with as he lived out his final days before succumbing to cancer.

"I received a referral from Radiation/Oncology, asking me to see a patient who was diagnosed with cancer," Rachel said. Michael was 49. He was thin and frail, and he had no family nearby. He lived in Bowling Green but was traveling to Toledo to receive treatment.

Michael was beside himself with worry over his health insurance ending. He explained that he had been so sick and weak, he had not been able to get to the phone to call in sick to work or to call for help. He lay on his floor, never realizing how much time was going by. Because he missed three days of work without calling in, he was fired, and he lost his insurance.

Rachel explained the Medicaid process to Michael, who was grateful to know that HELP would assist him with it. Working as a team, Rachel and Sue were able to get Michael approved for Medicaid, which covered all of his medical expenses. They also helped him get Social Security benefits for himself and his son.

"Michael had an 11-year-old son for whom he was supposed to be paying child support to his ex-wife, and he was so worried about not being able to since he had no income," Sue said. "When we expedited his Social Security claim, we

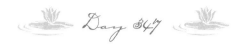

were able to get his son added as the dependent of a disabled person, so Michael's ex-wife started receiving funds for the son right away."

Sue noted that the doctors at St. V's helped a lot in getting both the Medicaid and Social Security benefits expedited by quickly completing the necessary forms to prove the seriousness of Michael's condition.

Meanwhile, Michael was so weak he didn't even have the strength to eat. A real estate company in Bowling Green had begun providing free transportation services, using their realtors to drive patients like Michael to their medical appointments.

"Every time Michael came to a doctor's appointment, I also had an appointment with him to gather further information or documents," Rachel said. "I spaced things out so as not to overwhelm him with the process."

Employees in Radiology/Oncology contacted Rachel because they were concerned about Michael's health. He had lost eight pounds over one weekend.

"Michael was too weak to fix meals and had a limited appetite," Rachel said. "I contacted Sue for help with getting Michael information about Meals on Wheels. Sue called me back and told me that Meals on Wheels would begin service to Michael as soon as they heard from him about the time and place to begin delivery. On Michael's fifth visit to me, he was embarrassed to ask me to help him, because he couldn't pay his rent, and, where he was renting, he was told that a late payment would mean eviction proceedings."

Rachel and Sue worked with the Marguerite d'Youville Program to try to help Michael with his housing situation.

"Initially, the program sent Michael's landlord a rent check, but because the check arrived late, eviction already was underway," Sue said. "Michael received the check back from his landlord, and the d'Youville program instead paid to

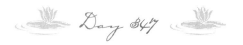

move Michael into a new apartment in Toledo, bringing him closer to St. Vincent. Rachel and I had been on standby, prepared to bring our own trucks to move him ourselves, but the d'Youville program came through and paid for movers."

Shortly after his move to Toledo, Michael underwent the amputation of his leg, but it only briefly extended his lifespan. He succumbed to his battle with cancer, but he left a lasting impression on many lives.

"I would see Michael in the halls, coming to and from treatment, and he would ask every time what color of flowers I wanted," Rachel said. "He asked when he could take Sue and me out to eat. He was elated to have all of his medical expenses covered through Medicaid and to be receiving Social Security benefits after struggling for so long without any type of income. Sue was such an integral part in fulfilling happiness for Michael. He is gone now, but I will always remember him."

—*Anonymous Contributor, St. Vincent Mercy Medical Center, Toledo, OH*

"Never underestimate the difference you can make."

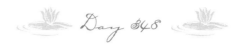

FULFILLING A NEED

Tammy Shather assists the Physicians of Downriver Surgeons in caring for patients during their office visits. Her care and compassion, however, extends far beyond the four walls of the office.

One Friday, a mastectomy patient came to the office. Her physician decided to continue her home care nursing visits, but it was too late in the afternoon to make the arrangements for weekend visits. The patient was very distraught over having to wait until Monday for her home care.

In a true demonstration of ownership and initiative, Tammy voluntarily went to the patient's home on Friday evening to change her bandages and help her shower. Tammy didn't stop there. She also went to the patient's home on Saturday and Sunday to change her dressings. And there's more! Tammy discovered that the patient was having out-of-town visitors on Monday. Without hesitation, Tammy told the patient that she would come over to help her shower and prepare for her guests.

Tammy treated this patient as she would one of her own loved ones, demonstrating true compassion. We are proud to recognize Tammy as a special Star of Excellence.

—Submitted by Tonia Campbell, Henry Ford Wyandotte Hospital, Detroit, MI

"Never underestimate the difference you can make."

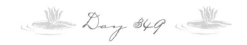

The Courage to Look

My father was dying from Alzheimer's disease. It had struck him at a young age—when he was in his mid-to-late 50s, my mother estimates—and for more than a decade my family had sorrowfully watched the slow, painful decline of a once strong and healthy man. My mother was able to keep him home for most of his illness, but eventually, he deteriorated to the point that he had to have professional care. He had become violent, and Mama could no longer control him. He entered the VA Hospital in Salisbury, North Carolina in 1997, and there he remained until his death 18 months later.

I was in my late 20s when my father was hospitalized. Every Sunday Mama and I would drive to Salisbury to visit him. The VA Hospital was the best place for Daddy—the staff was caring and competent and there was a spacious, plant-filled atrium where Alzheimer's patients could wander—but nonetheless, these were terrible days. We would make the long drive filled with a sense of dread, and we always left the hospital weeping. Earlier in his hospitalization while he was still somewhat cognizant, Daddy seemed unbearably sad and (understandably) angry. Sometimes, he didn't recognize Mama and me. Other times he did—and to me, those times were far worse.

Perhaps it was irrational, but I just felt so guilty. *Did he think we had betrayed him by leaving him in the care of strangers?* I wondered. *Was he still aware enough to know what was happening to him? Was he frightened and lonely? Did he know that he would die in this place—and when the time came, would I have the emotional strength to be present at his death?*

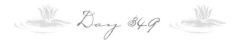

Eventually, Daddy collapsed and had to be put to bed. There he spent the last months of his life, unable to walk any longer, drifting in and out of lucidity. It was late in 1998, during one of our heart-wrenching Sunday visits, that Mama and I encountered "the nurse." I do not remember her name. I only recall her wisdom and quiet compassion—and the lesson she taught me about facing the harsh realities of life.

The nurse was discussing some aspects of Daddy's care with us when I broke down sobbing. "I just can't stand to see him like this!" I cried.

She comforted me as best she could, and said that even though Daddy may not truly be aware of our presence, spending as much time with him as possible was the right thing to do. "So many of these veterans never have visitors," she told Mama and me. "Their loved ones can't bear to see them suffer, so they just don't come. We do everything we can for them, of course, but a lot of these patients die with no family members by their side. It's a real shame. It may seem easier for family members to turn away from the suffering, but being present with people during the dark times is what love is all about," she explained.

"Life is not always pretty, and it takes courage to look full in the face at the parts which are not," she added. "Be with the people you love when they are sick and dying and you will never regret it."

A few months later, the nurse called us to say Daddy was dying. She had witnessed death many times and she felt sure it would happen in only a matter of hours. Mama and I rushed to the VA hospital. I was consumed with dreadful anxiety, mingled with an odd sense of anticipatory relief. The ordeal was almost over…but could I really be there when my Daddy left this world? Was I strong enough not to break down?

As it turned out, we didn't have long to wait. Daddy passed away within an hour after we arrived. Mama and I and the pastor from our church were present, talking softly to Daddy and praying over the dying shell that had once housed such a vibrant spirit. I held onto my Daddy's arm and looked into his face as his soul left his body. I do not know how to describe that moment, except to say it was nothing like I had imagined. It was one of the most powerful, spiritual and strangely beautiful moments of my life.

I often wonder if I would have been there at all, had it not been for that nurse. Perhaps I would have elected to hide out until it was over. I am so glad I found the courage to look. Life can be messy and painful and overwhelming, but in order to live (and love) fully, we must embrace the dark as fervently as we do the light. It's all a gift, even the not-so-pretty parts. And for me, the fact that a nurse cared enough to tell the unvarnished truth—and the fact that she has doubtless held countless similar conversations with grieving family members over the years—is what's right in health care.

—Submitted by *Anna E. Campbell, Granite Falls, NC*

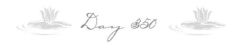

One Pebble

An older gentleman was upset with his bill and wanted to talk to a "higher up." I was available and talked to him for some time. By the end of our conversation, he seemed satisfied. Feeling pretty confident at this point, I boldly offered him my business card and wrote my home phone number on it.

Several months passed. Then, on a Saturday morning, I received a call from this gentle soul who was desperate for someone to talk to.

"LeeAnn," he said, "do you remember me? You helped me with my hospital bills several months ago."

Of course I remembered him—he had been pretty tough on me!

For a split second, I thought, "What was I thinking…writing my home phone number on my card?"

As I listened, he explained that his wife was very ill and was in a facility where he perceived that she was not receiving care that was of the "Hocking Valley standard." He was all alone and didn't know where to turn. He had carried my business card in his wallet for months, and he hoped I could help him.

I made some calls, got the right people involved, and after several hours, arrangements were made to move his wife back to HVCH the next day. I realized he had needed someone to listen to him and help him sort out his thoughts. He thanked me over and over and called me an angel.

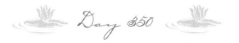
It was one of the best Saturdays of my life. Since then, I've never regretted offering my home number. "Never underestimate the difference one pebble can make." (Quint Studer, *Hardwiring Excellence*)

Quint planted the phone number idea at the first "Taking your organization to the next level" I attended. Practicing the skills gave me the courage to reach out—and the reward came back tenfold.

—Submitted by LeeAnn Lucas Helber, Hocking Valley Community Hospital

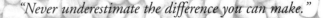

"Never underestimate the difference you can make."

Dedication to Profession

I am Linda Olive, the CEO of Creighton University Medical Center in Omaha. We're sometimes known as the heartland of this country and if there is one thing that Laura Peet-Erkes has, it's a big heart.

Laura is somewhat a modern day Renaissance woman. In just two and a half years with Creighton University Medical Center, she's amassed an incredible list of achievements and we are so proud of her.

What makes Laura different from her peers in her profession of Social Work is her dedication to her job. She has a true passion for what she does. She wants to help others. She comes in every day with a positive attitude, and she's willing to take that extra step for those she works with.

Our Emergency Department has been designated as a type of holding area for multiple psych patients and we needed a tool to help assess these patients. Laura worked with the ED manager to help develop a guide for the social workers to use when assessing individuals who might be suicidal.

"People that come into the hospital are usually in crisis," Laura says, "and they really need somebody who can be their advocate in a setting where a lot of people aren't very comfortable."

Using the system Laura developed has helped staff determine if patients could use step-down facilities and avoid an inpatient psychiatric stay–and it has worked very well.

Because of Laura's creative problem-solving, the whole psych issue in the Emergency Department has been effectively addressed and been turned around 100 percent.

—*Submitted by Linda Olive, Creighton University Medical Center, Omaha, NE*

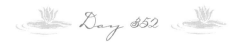

DINNER FOR TWO

I work in the Antepartum unit, where some of our moms stay for weeks or months at a time.

One particular mom was here for several weeks, expecting twins, and her husband and a family friend wanted to surprise her with dinner. With the help of maintenance, food, and nutrition services, as well as the nursing staff, we created a fabulous romantic dinner for two.

Maintenance moved a nice table and chairs into our healing garden area and placed a white linen table cloth and napkins on the table. With the help of the family friend, steaks were cooked and the husband was waiting in the garden area, wearing a tuxedo and holding a bouquet of flowers.

Because of a caring staff, husband and wife enjoyed a candlelit steak dinner for two before their twins arrived.

—Submitted by Lisa Barfield Price, Medical Center of Plano, Plano, TX

"Never underestimate the difference you can make."

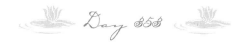

Ben's Story

Our second child, Benjamin, was born at approximately 2 a.m. on April 3rd, 1999. I held him for a brief moment before they took him away. Although he was only about three weeks premature, his breathing was very shallow and labored. Within hours, Ben was emergency transported to Arkansas Children's Hospital in Little Rock, Arkansas. Due to an en route intubation, Ben was reported in serious condition upon arrival.

As I made the two-hour drive to Arkansas Children's' Hospital, the images of the little boy I held for a moment were fresh in my mind. I remembered the fat little cheeks, the hoarse cry, the dark, soft hair and the beautiful blue eyes. I couldn't wait to see and hold him again.

Upon arrival, I hurriedly scrubbed in to the NICU with anxious anticipation of seeing Ben. My husband escorted me over to the place Ben would call home for the next month. I was overcome by what awaited me. The child I saw didn't appear to be the same one I had held just a few hours before. No longer was Ben free to wiggle and cry. He was now in the NICU, with wires and tubes, beeping monitors, and machines all around him. Each was a constant reminder of the danger hanging over my son.

As I stood there, the seriousness of the situation hit me. What was going on? Was he in pain? Why was he laying so still? Was he okay? What did all those numbers on the monitor mean?

It was then I met Ben's nurse, Carolyn. Carolyn knew instinctively what to do. She gently put her arm around me, brought me closer to Ben's bedside, and

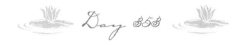

began to explain to me, in terms I could understand, all that was going on with Ben.

During the following days, I noticed many of Carolyn's special touches. None were flashy; none were enormous feats. All were simple, small acts of kindness and compassion that helped Ben survive and helped us better cope with an extremely difficult situation.

When I visited Ben's crib, his wires and tubes were always in perfect order and music was playing softly in the background. After a few days, Carolyn decided to speak with the physician to gain permission for me to hold Ben. She set up a screen to allow us privacy, and placed Ben in my arms for the second time. She stood close by to make sure the wires and tubes didn't interfere and that Ben was safe.

Even now, I can hear her voice commenting on how beautiful Ben was. I still recall how Ben's hair was neatly brushed for the special occasion.

Carolyn encouraged me to write in a journal to record the first days of his life. Although difficult to do at the time, it is now a treasured reminder of Ben's difficult start and what a miracle he is today.

Ben is now a healthy and vibrant eight-year-old boy who does well in school and loves to play soccer, baseball, and computer games. I thank the Lord each day for him. The memories of his first days are still close and precious to me.

There were a multitude of nurses, physicians, respiratory therapists, and clinicians we met during our time in the NICU. All of them were wonderful, and experts in their fields. But, as I remember back to those days, I remember Carolyn and think of the impact she made on us.

Never underestimate the difference your kindness, words and actions can make in someone's life.

—Submitted by Margaret Stanzell, Studer Group, Tupelo, MS

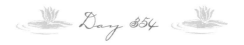
HANDLING THE LITTLE THINGS

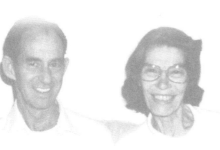

When both of my parents were suffering from emphysema, a very special hospice nurse—Sherry Wakefield of Burke Hospice and Palliative Care—showed me that you don't have to be a miracle maker to provide great care. She proved that by simply taking care of all the little things, one hospice nurse can make a huge difference.

Both of my parents suffered from emphysema for 12 years. During this time I lived 45 minutes away from them, and for the most part could see them only on the weekends. Even though my sister lived with them, she was working a full-time job during the daytime, which left my parents to take care of themselves during the day. My brother also came home frequently, but as he lived out of state he couldn't be with them as much as he would have liked. I knew my parents received great care from my sister, and I will be forever grateful for the sacrifice that she made for them. However, I still felt guilty when I couldn't be with them myself during the week.

Sherry instantly connected with my parents. She always did a great job. Her close attention to taking care of all the little things is what truly made her special—she always showed up on time, always voiced her concerns for them to

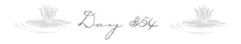

me, told us we could call with questions anytime day or night, and regularly coordinated with their doctors to ensure they received all the care they needed. Her reliability and attentiveness to my parents' needs gave me the peace of mind I needed to focus more of my attention on taking care of my own family and business during the week.

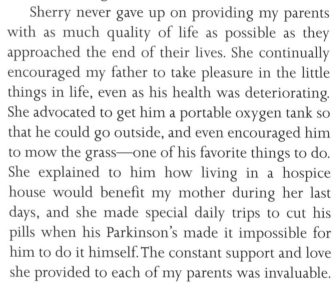

Sherry never gave up on providing my parents with as much quality of life as possible as they approached the end of their lives. She continually encouraged my father to take pleasure in the little things in life, even as his health was deteriorating. She advocated to get him a portable oxygen tank so that he could go outside, and even encouraged him to mow the grass—one of his favorite things to do. She explained to him how living in a hospice house would benefit my mother during her last days, and she made special daily trips to cut his pills when his Parkinson's made it impossible for him to do it himself. The constant support and love she provided to each of my parents was invaluable.

It was Sherry's close attention to taking care of all of these little things that made her such a special health care worker. She helped navigate my parents, my siblings, and myself through a very difficult time and for that I will always be grateful.

—Submitted by *Andra Keller, Hickory, NC*

"Never underestimate the difference you can make."

A FLOWERED GOWN

hen I was in my early twenties, I worked at Peninsula Hospital (where I now coach it as Mills-Peninsula Health Services) as a ward clerk. I liked my job and found it interesting and rewarding, but it was really just a job.

Then, my mother was diagnosed with cancer and suddenly my perception of hospitals and the work accomplished within those walls changed. Here are two of the situations that occurred during my mother's treatment.

After my mother's surgery, the pathologist came to talk to my mother and during the conversation, said, "Mrs. G., you have a 25 percent chance of survival."

Several hours later, her surgeon came to her room and said, "Mrs. G., you have a one-in-three chance of survival."

My mother turned to me and said, "Don't they talk to one another?" Before I could answer, she said, "Don't they know that when it's life or death, 8 percent is a big deal?"

My mother required radiation treatments, and the hospital was very kind about my schedule, so I was often able to make it to her appointments. This was so long ago that the flowered patient gowns were new, quite a novelty, and my mother really liked them. Unfortunately, her appointment times were in the afternoon, so the flowered gowns were always gone by the time she got there.

However, when one particular Radiation Technician was working, she would hide a gown and then present it to my mother with great ceremony! On those

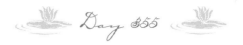

days when she received the flowered gowns, my mother did better. It often made the difference between her going home directly to bed, or staying up for a cup of tea and a chat with me.

After my mother died, my view of hospital work was forever changed. I loved it more, but frankly, saw that it was flawed. I decided that I would work in healthcare toward two goals—that communication between patient, physician and staff would have less "8 percent stories," and that hospital employees would see the value in flowered gowns for their patients.

—Submitted by Zani Weber, Studer Group, Eureka, CA

"Never underestimate the difference you can make."

712

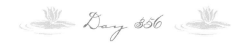

Laughter Through the Tears

"I met Kenniesha the day that she came into St. Chris," says Claire Alminde, pediatric nurse. "She was admitted here on my unit. That was before we knew she had any kind of cancer at all.

"She was terrified coming in here. She was five years old at the time and instead of getting her history and all of that, I played with her first. So instantly, we connected."

"It was hard when I had cancer," Kenniesha says. "I was scared when I had the surgery."

Kenniesha's surgery involved putting in a port. Then she had chemotherapy, which made her very sick. Eventually, she had extensive leg surgery.

"They actually amputated her upper leg, moved her lower leg up, and then rotated her foot backwards," Claire explains. "That was done so when they made a prosthesis for her later, it would fit better."

Claire was able to work with Kenniesha, who had a devastating diagnosis and who was going through the most horrible time in her life, and help her still enjoy the things that kids enjoy–and even to laugh in the course of a day.

"My stethoscope is my work tool, but in my opinion, it's not my most important tool," Claire says. "I have a whole bag of toys. Sponge Bob flashlight and flashing lights…"

Observers can attest—Claire has a complete menagerie of toys designed to make kids laugh.

Claire explains that her job has many rewards, but she knows she has made a difference for the whole family, when parents, as well as patients, thank her.

"When a mother comes up and hugs me and says, 'Thank you. You taught me to help my child with this disease,' or to have a kid run up and give me a big hug…That's a reward that everyone should get in their job everyday."

—Submitted by St. Christopher's Hospital for Children, Philadelphia, PA

"Never underestimate the difference you can make."

A NOSE IS A NOSE IS A NOSE...

The event described in this story took place at North Central Baptist Hospital in San Antonio:

Whitney, an 18-year-old facing sinus surgery, was pretty nervous. She brought her favorite childhood stuffed animal with her: a Pooh Bear that she had gotten at Disney World when she was seven.

Unfortunately, Whitney's dog had bitten off Pooh's nose, so Whitney joked that Pooh had a nose problem, just like hers. Whitney told her nurse, Michele Haley, RN, that she would like for Pooh to go with her to surgery, because his presence would calm her nerves. She also teased Michele by requesting that while she was in surgery, perhaps someone could fix Pooh's nose, too.

You guessed it! Michelle did just that: she used a black rubber stopper from a syringe and a little super glue to fix Pooh's nose. But she did not stop there. She put a dressing on Pooh's new nose that looked exactly like the dressing Whitney would have when she woke up. She then placed Pooh beside Whitney in the recovery room.

You cannot imagine the delight and surprise when Whitney woke up and found Pooh's nose fixed, and saw that he looked just like she did. It sure helped Whitney to not be so self-conscious about how she looked.

Whitney wrote a poem to Michele as a "thank you." Here is the poem:

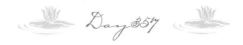
"Miracle Angel"

I couldn't believe
When the doctor told me
I needed surgery
Especially since needles make me uneasy
Luckily I had my Pooh bear
Whenever I'm scared, he's been there
I got him at Disney World when I was seven
But my dog got a hold of his nose when I was eleven
I was really sad
A nose he no longer had
But he seemed all right
And I still slept with him every night
My Mom said not to take him to into surgery
She said he didn't look sanitary
But I told Mom I was eighteen
And Pooh was going
After all, he had nose problems too
He knew what I was going through
I was just kidding when I asked if his nose could be worked on
After all, I had a nose but his was gone
Then when I regained consciousness
I couldn't believe Pooh was FIXED!!
I don't think you could ever know how much that meant to me
Pooh got to have plastic surgery

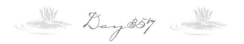

I've always heard amazing stories about what nurses do
Even though it was just sewing on a nose for Pooh
It meant a great deal
Faster it made me heal
Michelle, you didn't have to, but you did
It was a favor I'll never forget
People say that I'm silly because it's just a stuffed bear
But this is <u>my</u> Pooh bear
Every night I pray for you and wish you the best
As I snuggle Pooh to my chest
Thank you
For all that you do
I hope one day I can be a nurse just as special as you

My favorite part is the last line. I think we don't stop often enough to realize that the difference we make for our patients can be role modeling what nursing is—and inspiring them to pursue this profession of which it is a privilege to be a part. Whitney went in that day for surgery—and she came out with a successful surgical outcome and a passion/inspiration to become a nurse. Wow!

—Submitted by Lucy Crouch, Studer Group, Pensacola, FL

"Never underestimate the difference you can make."

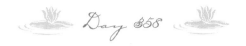

Last Goodbye

"It was late on the day before Thanksgiving when I was called into the ER," explains Laura Peet-Erkes, Social Worker. "A trauma patient had come in and they couldn't figure out who the girl was or where her parents were."

The girl had been in a motor vehicle accident and when she arrived, she went immediately into surgery.

The doctor explained to Laura that whatever she could do to get the girl's mom here, she should just do it, because "we don't know if she is going to make it until the morning."

The mother received a call explaining that her daughter was in a serious accident. Laura worked with the mother to help make arrangements to get her to the hospital.

"The hardest part was finding a way to get her on an airplane," Laura relays. "Everyone that I called was saying, 'Ma'am, it's the day before Thanksgiving, there is nothing we can do.' I begged and pleaded with them."

Because of her persistence, Laura finally worked out arrangements to get the mother to the hospital.

The staff rallied around the mother at her daughter's bedside, where the mother was able to say goodbye to her daughter. Laura made all of this happen.

—Submitted by Creighton University Medical Center, Omaha, NE

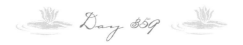

The Power of a Great Front Desk

Front desk staffers are the first people you see when you arrive, so this is where your experience with a medical practice really begins. They are also the last people you see when you leave, so that is the impression you take away.

I would like to give a "thumbs up" to Catawba Pediatrics, the largest pediatric practice in western NC, for understanding that a great front desk can make all the difference in the world. I've been taking my children there for nearly 10 years, so I've watched them go through a lot of changes. One of the most significant changes I've seen them make is really investing in their front desk. They hired a front desk team leader named Angela Wurth. She really "gets it." Not only does she greet you with a wonderful smile, she always seems genuinely glad to see you. She never gives the impression that she's bothered or interrupted by your presence, which is the feeling I get from some front desk staff.

Angela knows my children by name and knows how old they are (which is tough to do in a practice of this size). She's always approachable. If you have a complaint, she listens intently and never gets defensive. If you've waited a long time, she notices. If something goes amiss in the waiting room, she takes care of it before you have a chance to be annoyed.

What I love most about her is that she's not only wonderful to my children and me, she's wonderful to everyone! Working the front desk at a busy pediatric practice has to be an incredibly stressful job. She works quickly and efficiently, answering the phone with a jovial hello and greeting each patient as though he or she is a long lost friend. This is her attitude every day—no matter how busy she is!

One of the most touching things about her is her patience and kindness with underprivileged children and the non-English-speaking population. I've seen her patiently answer the same question five times without ever changing her original upbeat tone. One of the best things Angela has done since joining the team at Catawba Peds is to raise the level of professionalism for everyone at the front desk. I suspect she attracts good people because they enjoy working with her— and I likewise suspect she quickly gets rid of bad apples who are rude to patients. My theory is that people respect her and try harder because she's there.

In short, I'd like to offer a heartfelt thanks to Angela Wurth for making a real difference in healthcare…and congratulations to Catawba Pediatrics for realizing that she could.

—Submitted by Dottie DeHart, Conover, NC

"Never underestimate the difference you can make."

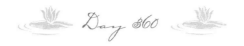

Long Trip Home

"I first came to know this patient when he was in the intensive care unit," Laura Peet-Erkes explains. "When he came in he was unresponsive, and he had an extended period of time when he was in a coma and they weren't even sure if he was going to live."

When the patient eventually came out of the coma, it was determined that he had months or less to live. In her role of Social Worker, Laura's primary goal was to allow him to return to El Salvador so he would be able to spend his final months with his family there.

"I had to work with the Salvadoran Consulate, the government in El Salvador, and the US State Department to make sure that they would allow him out of the country when he got to Customs," Laura relays.

Trying to coordinate this feat was daunting. Laura spent quite a bit of time and effort contacting the airlines, arranging his transportation and contacting the family in El Salvador.

"There were a couple of times he was scheduled to go that things kind of fell through and we had to postpone," Laura says.

When that occurred, Laura had to start all over again, making new arrangements.

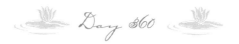

Once it was time for the patient to leave the hospital, he wasn't strong enough to go by himself. He needed someone to administer medicine en route, so a doctor was selected to go with him.

Laura gave the physician a packet with all of the needed information for the trip. The patient was ecstatic to be leaving but was also in a state of disbelief that the trip was truly going to take place.

Upon his arrival in San Salvador, the patient was met by his family. He had a 12-year-old daughter there and re-connecting with her was immensely important to him.

The physician who traveled with the patient reports that it was quite moving to see the patient reach his goal of returning home to his family before he died.

This extraordinary act was the direct result of Laura's persistence and dedication to providing assistance to a dying patient.

—Submitted by Creighton University Medical Center, Omaha, NE

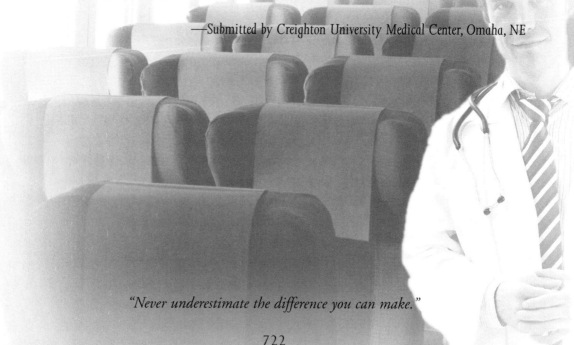

"Never underestimate the difference you can make."

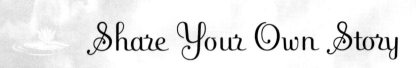

Share Your Own Story

Please share an experience that connected you back to purpose, worthwhile work, and making a difference. You are a big part of what's right in health care!

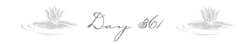

PUTTING THE "CARE" BACK IN HEALTH CARE

*A*t the age of 43, I was admitted to the hospital for a stress test after complaining of chest pains. I was totally aggravated by having to spend the night in the hospital when I truly believed nothing was wrong with me. While I was hospitalized, I suffered two heart attacks. (Imagine my surprise!)

I've heard complaints about how some doctors don't care and don't listen, but after my experience, I just don't think that's true. Dr. William Young, a physician at Hickory Family Practice, probably saved my life. No one would have ever believed it could have been my heart, especially not me. I am a young woman with no bad health habits, and I have always been amazingly healthy. I think back to that day and how easy it would have been for him to send me home. If he had, I might not be here to tell you how much I appreciate a doctor who really knows what it means to take "care" of a patient.

While I was hospitalized, I had another amazing experience that reiterated my newfound philosophy that the health care field attracts a special group of people. While I was in the Critical Care Unit at Frye Regional Medical Center in Hickory, NC, I had the good fortune of being cared for by a nurse whose name was Randy Madison.

Randy did an amazing job of nursing me back to health, but that's not where it ended. I had been transferred to a regular floor and was recovering nicely.

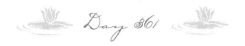

The door opened and in walked Randy. Of course, I was thrilled to see him, as we had really connected (which I bet he does with all his patients). We exchanged pleasantries and he began to go over all the new medicines I would be taking, what I could expect in terms of recovery, dos and don'ts, and so forth.

At the end of our visit, I happened to ask what his shift was that day, assuming he would just be going back up to CCU and this was standard procedure in patient care. He told me he had just finished his shift and was headed home, but wanted to make sure I was doing okay and understood everything. I can't tell you how much it meant to me to have someone show that kind of personal concern for my wellbeing. He actually came by to check on me several times during my stay, all "off the clock."

When I think about my experience of having a heart attack and being hospitalized, I don't ever think of it in a negative way. I actually smile to think of how fortunate I was to have such amazing people take such a personal interest in my wellbeing!

—Submitted by Bridgette Braswell, Hickory, NC

"Never underestimate the difference you can make."

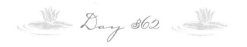

Moment of Recognition

A patient arrived from another hospital to LakeEast Hospital for rehab after suffering a stroke at age 50. The stroke left her paralyzed on the right side and unable to speak.

During the admission interview, her husband mentioned she had not had a bath in 18 days. When the patient's husband left to run errands, Stephanie Lawson, LPN, along with a coworker, treated the patient to a shower. They washed her hair and immediately noticed the joyful expression on her face.

Afterward, they dried and styled her hair, applied some lipstick they found in her bag, dressed her in clothes brought from home, and settled her into a wheelchair before her husband returned.

As her husband entered the doorway, he stopped abruptly, and began to cry. He said, "Now, that's my wife."

There wasn't a dry eye in the room. Obviously, it had been a while since this husband and caretaker had been able to enjoy seeing his wife as something other than a sick patient. Helping this couple deal with illness in such a basic way had reminded her husband who his wife really was. And it had given his wife some new hope when she looked in the mirror—and realized there was a spirit within her that was still very much alive.

—Submitted by Darlene English, Lake Hospital System, Painesville, OH

"Never underestimate the difference you can make."

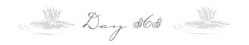

A Special Cross

As a Catholic nurse at a Catholic hospital, the cross is an important symbol for me. But over my many years of nursing, one cross in particular has become especially important.

I've come to rely on a very special cross necklace to help me through the challenging times of my job. I only wear this necklace at work and I've actually become quite superstitious about it, often relying on it to help me and those I work with, through the most trying of situations.

Here's how it works: If a bad situation arises, for example–difficulty placing a child's IV–I hold the cross and pray Hail Marys, often adding a personal prayer at the end. In this case, it is usually something like, "Help this IV find it's place."

It's a routine that has become very natural for me and one that has never failed me or the countless patients who have needed a prayer. It shows there truly is a higher power watching over us nurses!

—Submitted by Lisa McCann, St. Mary's Hospital, Madison, WI

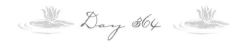

The Sacred Act of Healing

I work at a hospital in far northern Vermont, just a few miles from the Quebec border, serving the poorest (and proudest) two counties in Vermont.

For the past six years, I have had thyroid cancer, and during that time, I've undergone five surgeries. Recently, my doctors discovered metastasis to the lung. To the best of anyone's guess, I have three to five years to live. I am 59 years old, have raised six children, and have three more at home (one granddaughter and two nieces).

Friends have asked me what I am going to do. Quit my job? Travel? Be wild and crazy? You know the routine: how would you live if you were dying?

My answer is that I am going to continue doing exactly what I am doing now. Our jobs are sacred, and I know this first hand. We have a dream to deliver the very best health care possible to our community. And I am proud to say that we are on our way. As long as I am well enough to meet the need of our wonderful staff, I will be here.

I hope healthcare workers never forget, nor let their organizations forget, that we are not about marketing or selling or growing. We are fundamentally about the sacred act of healing. As I know all too well, we can't always cure, but we can and do heal every day.

—Submitted by Karen A. Weller, North Country Health System, Newport, VT

"Never underestimate the difference you can make."

Brian's Story

As I travel the country talking to Fire Starters in health care, I always carry a baseball cap from the University of Illinois, Chicago (UIC), with me in my briefcase. On the cap is a picture of a flame. Sometimes people see the cap on the table and ask if it is a Fire Starter cap. It is, but not in the way they think.

The cap belonged to my nephew, Brian Fitzpatrick, who played for the UIC Flames on a baseball scholarship. Brian was pretty excited about his baseball prospects because he was going to be a starter on the team.

That December he took a trip with the team to Australia. On his return, his dad, Mike Fitzpatrick Sr., and his older brother, Mike Jr., picked him up from the airport. Brian was enthusiastic about sharing all the stories from his trip with his mom Kathy, so they went back to the Fitzpatrick home. Then he hopped in the car to go visit his high school buddies. Afterwards, he stopped by Mike Jr.'s house to talk some more and fell asleep on Mike Jr.'s couch.

At 5:00 the next morning, on Christmas Eve 1995, Brian woke up, got in the car, and started to drive home. But he never made it. Brian was killed in a car accident that Christmas Eve morning.

We were devastated when we got the terrible news in an early morning phone call. You just don't expect to hear that your 19-year-old nephew, with his whole life ahead of him, has suddenly died.

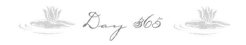

We quickly dressed and headed for the Fitzpatrick house, where many relatives, neighbors, and friends were already gathered. All one can really do in these situations is just be there and say, "I'm so sorry." The entire day saw people coming and going, sharing their pain and grief with Brian's family.

Since you can't have a wake on Christmas Day, we went back to the Fitzpatrick house and did it all over again, as more family and friends arrived from out of town.

December 26 was Brian's wake. As it began, the entire UIC baseball team walked in in their uniforms and lined up along the casket, just as a team lines up along the infield foul line on Opening Day. They stayed that way for five hours until the wake ended. Brian's Mount Carmel High School baseball cap and baseball from his first win as a Division 1 college pitcher shared the space in that casket with him.

Early the next morning, I got a phone call from Brian's dad. Mike said, "Kathy and I have been up all night talking about the funeral. We've decided we would really like you to do the eulogy."

When I am stunned, I have a bad habit of blurting something out without thinking so I just said, "Why me, Mike?"

And he said, "Brian really liked you."

Now, let me tell you what I did for Brian. All I ever did was role model what Mrs. James, Mr. King, and Mr. Fry did for me. I noticed the positive and helped him feel purpose. I rewarded and recognized his successes in small ways. It's the little things that make a big difference in a relationship. It's all about role modeling.

Well, I had never given a eulogy before. And I was to go last, after Brian's high school religious education teacher and his college baseball coach. When I stepped

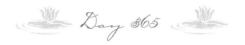

up on the altar, I noticed Brian's college baseball cap and the emblem of the flame on the front of it. Just 13 months earlier, I had been called a Fire Starter.

So I talked about being a Fire Starter. I said that Brian carried a flame, and I shared examples of the difference he had made. I said that Brian's flame had been extinguished on this earth much earlier than any one of us would have imagined. And I asked each person at the service to leave with a little of Brian's flame and to take it with them wherever they went. I suggested that it is up to each of us to determine how bright our flame burns.

Since then, I travel with Brian's cap to remind me of my own commitment to be a Fire Starter and carry Brian's flame with me wherever I go. It also reminds me of how quickly a flame can go out. All we have is each day, each moment to write that note or make that difference.

And that's how the story ended—until I was asked to speak at Christ Hospital in Oak Lawn (suburban Chicago) in January 1999. I thought that was the hospital Brian was taken to, but I wasn't sure, because there are a lot of hospitals in Chicago. So when I got to the hotel that night, I called up the Fitzpatrick home to tell them where I was speaking.

Mike Sr. said, "That's where Brian was taken." Then he held out the phone to his wife in the kitchen and said, "Kathy, Quint is speaking at Christ Hospital tomorrow."

I heard her say in the background, "Will you please tell Quint to say thank you to them? They were so kind to us."

Now let me put this into perspective. The Fitzpatricks were called Christmas Eve morning and told to hurry to the hospital where they were informed that their 19-year-old son was gone. They heard the worst news a parent can hear. But what Brian's mother chose to remember was the kindness of the hospital.

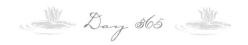

So when I spoke the next morning at Christ Hospital, I told them I wanted to thank them on behalf of the Fitzpatrick family for that kindness and shared some of the story. I spoke for 90 minutes and flew back home to Pensacola, Florida.

A few weeks later, I received a card from a nurse. It wasn't what I expected. It read:

> Dear Quint,
> I am an ER nurse at Christ Hospital. I heard you speak a couple of weeks ago and I want you to know that I was working that morning when Brian came in and was with Brian's parents that morning when they were told. I want you to know that there's not a Christmas that goes by that I don't think about that family.
> > Nurse
> > Christ Hospital, Oak Lawn

If I hadn't been asked to speak at Christ Hospital—or if I hadn't called the Fitzpatricks first before I spoke—I wouldn't have been able to say thank you and let the staff know the impact they had.

If you are like many who attend Studer Group Institutes, perhaps you've cried a little more than you were planning on as you read this book, and also laughed a little more too.

One of the special things about people who work in health care is that we've been given the unique ability to handle tremendous swings of emotions. Moments after delivering the worst news in the world to someone, we may experience a medical miracle that fills us with a burst of joy.

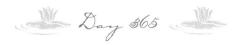

That's why God chose you and me to go into health care. We can handle that range of emotions. Not many people can. What a gift we've been given to have that strength to make a difference in the lives of others. In return for our willingness to serve, we receive a great gift: purpose, worthwhile work, and making a difference.

—Submitted by Quint Studer, Studer Group, Pensacola, FL

"Never underestimate the difference you can make."

StuderGroup.

Studer Group is an outcomes-based health care consulting firm devoted to teaching evidence-based tools and processes that organizations can immediately use to create and sustain service and operational excellence. Partner organizations see clear results in the areas of higher employee retention, greater patient and customer satisfaction, healthy financials, growing market share, and improvements in various other quality indicators. Studer Group has worked with hundreds of health care systems, hospitals, and medical groups since the firm's inception in 1999 and currently operates in the United States, Canada, Australia, and New Zealand.

<u>Mission and Vision</u>: Studer Group's mission is to make health care better— creating extraordinary places for employees to work, for physicians to practice medicine, and for patients and families to receive care. Our vision is to be the intellectual resource for health care professionals, combining passion with prescriptive actions and tools to drive outcomes and maximize the human potential within each organization and in health care as a whole.

<u>Harvesting Best Practices from a National Learning Lab:</u> CEO Quint Studer and Studer Group's coaches teach, train, and speak to thousands of leaders at health care organizations worldwide each week, through both on-site coaching sessions and frequent speaking engagements at industry events. This ongoing "in the trenches" dialogue provides ample opportunity to spot best practices in action from "first mover" innovators at many organizations. These best practices are then harvested and tested in other organizations, refined, and shared with the entire health care industry through peer-reviewed journal articles, Studer Group publications, and products to accelerate change.

Best-selling Books by Quint Studer

Results That Last: Hardwiring Behaviors That Will Take Your Company to the Top, by Quint Studer (Wiley, 2007, ISBN: 978-0-471-75729-0). This *Wall Street Journal* bestseller helps you build an organizational culture that develops great leaders *today*…and instills the mechanism and the mindset that will continue to foster great leadership *tomorrow*. The result is better strategy, better employee and customer relations, and bigger long-term profits. With the right practices in place, your organization's success won't depend on individuals. Excellence is hardwired into your culture, giving you a sustainable, tangible advantage over the competition.

Hardwiring Excellence: Purpose, Worthwhile Work, Making a Difference, by Quint Studer (Fire Starter Publishing, 2003, perfect-bound ISBN: 0-9749986-0-5, case-bound ISBN: 0-9749986-1-3). In this best-selling book, Studer helps individuals and organizations to rekindle the flame and offers a road map to creating and sustaining a Culture of Service and Operational Excellence that drives bottom-line results. His tools, tips, and techniques help readers hardwire key behaviors to increase employee, physician, and patient satisfaction; lower employee turnover; improve quality; grow market share; and increase revenue while reducing costs.

101 Answers to Questions Leaders Ask, by Quint Studer (Fire Starter Publishing, 2005, ISBN: 0-9749986-2-1). Informed by best practices in a national learning lab of health care organizations, Studer shares his insights on how to deliver excellent patient care, engage employees, and improve physician relations for access, growth, and strong financial performance. In short, his answers accelerate the leadership learning curve. Questions are organized by topic, making the book valuable as a reference point for specific issues or on-the-spot problem solving.

For more information on Studer and his books, please visit
www.quintsbooks.com.

How to Order Additional Copies of *What's Right in Health Care:*
365 Stories of Purpose, Worthwhile Work, and Making a Difference

Orders may be placed:

Online at: www.firestarterpublishing.com

By phone at: 866-354-3473

By mail at: Fire Starter Publishing
913 Gulf Breeze Parkway, Suite 6
Gulf Breeze, FL 32561

(Bulk discounts are available.)

What's Right in Health Care: 365 Stories of Purpose, Worthwhile Work, and Making a Difference is
also available online at www.amazon.com.

How to Use *What's Right in Health Care*
(Suggestions for industry professionals)

The stories in *What's Right in Health Care: 365 Stories of Purpose, Worthwhile Work, and Making a Difference* chronicle this journey we're all on—a journey to make health care better. The book provides a story a day that serves as a reminder about why we answered this calling and why we stay with it. We hope you will order additional copies to share with your employees, patients, and community.

A few ways you might use the book:

- Read it yourself whenever you need an emotional or spiritual boost (Yes, the stories are that uplifting!);
- Give a copy to each of your leaders;
- Use as a welcome gift for new employees and physicians;
- Place a copy in the employee breakroom;
- Leave one in each patient waiting area;
- Use for inspirational readings at shift changes;
- Use as part of your chaplaincy program;
- Let it inspire stories from your own employees—stories that can be published in newsletters, shared at meetings, posted on your website, and so forth.

This book can be a powerful tool for any health care organization. It's a moving reminder to anyone and everyone who works in this field that we serve a valuable purpose, that we perform worthwhile work, and that we really do make a difference.

Wanted:
Still More Great
Health Care Stories!

We hope you've enjoyed the stories in this book. If you're like us, they've inspired you to think, laugh, shed a tear or two, feel a greater connection to your calling, and perhaps open your heart just a little wider.

We also hope that reading them has sparked ideas for new stories drawn from your own work life. If you have a story you'd like to share, please submit it at www.studergroup.com/story. We may feature it on our website, in a future issue of *What's Right in Health Care*, or even both.

Thank you for reading, writing, and living the stories in this book and those that are yet to be written—and for continuing to be a shining example of what's right in health care.

www.studergroup.com/story